Henry Oakeley

AF873755

THE EVAN BEDFORD
LIBRARY OF CARDIOLOGY

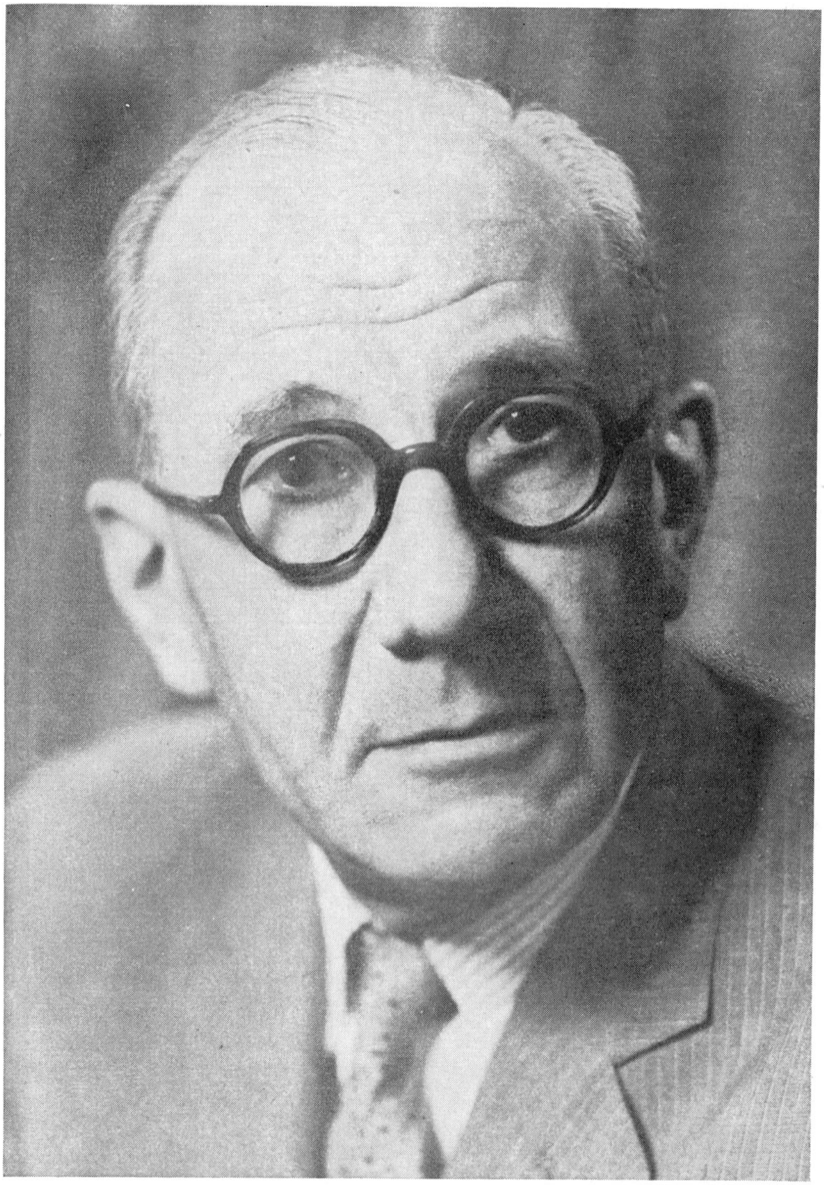

D. Evan Bedford, C.B.E., M.D., F.R.C.P.

THE EVAN BEDFORD LIBRARY OF CARDIOLOGY

Catalogue of books, pamphlets and journals

LONDON
ROYAL COLLEGE OF PHYSICIANS
1977

Royal College of Physicians of London

© 1977

ISBN 0 900596 40 6

Printed and bound in England by
STAPLES PRINTERS LIMITED
at The Stanhope Press, Rochester, Kent.

CONTENTS

INTRODUCTION

by

Charles Newman, CBE, MD, FRCP

Harveian Librarian

Dr. D. Evan Bedford was always most generous in giving to the College those books from his library that did not constitute part of his main interest, which was the collection of a complete library of all the important books bearing on the history of cardiology in all its branches. The ultimate fate of this great collection remained undecided: he hoped to preserve it permanently as a unity, and the United States, not unexpectedly, made most tempting offers. There were also institutions in this country which would have been glad to have it. Dr. Bedford finally decided to give it to the Royal College of Physicians, which had accommodation for it and was an obvious place where scholars would look for a medico-historical collection of this kind. The College set aside its general policy of putting all books into a single arrangement, so as to maintain the cardiological collection as a unit, accessible as such to scholars.

The gift is a landmark in the history of the College library. It is the greatest benefaction it has received in this century, which has already contributed the Lloyd-Roberts bequest and the Spencer and Dawson gifts. It is of the same order as the Matthew Baillie bequest and the Farre obstetric collection in the nineteenth century; the latter was, like Dr. Bedford's, a specialist collection. It is bigger than the Hale bequest in the eighteenth; not, of course, so big as the Dorchester Library, but more important than the Holsbosch collection of 680 books or any of the other seventeenth century accessions, although we do not know how valuable they would have become if they had not been lost in the Fire of London. The Evan Bedford Library of Cardiology is over a thousand volumes and pamphlets in extent; in range it covers most aspects of the subject, and includes all the important works, mostly in first editions and of very good quality. It took a lifetime—from 1926 to 1971—to get them together, and as a final labour of love Dr. Bedford prepared his own catalogue. This is made very readable by the notes he has written for many of the volumes indicating their significance. The collection is housed in the gallery of the main library, where it is visibly an independent unit, and is available, with maximum convenience, to all those who in the future wish to investigate, or write about, any aspect of cardiology up to about the middle of the twentieth century.

ON COLLECTING A CARDIOLOGICAL LIBRARY

by

Evan Bedford, CBE, MD, FRCP

Bodley cited leisure, knowledge, friends and pursability as the necessary qualifications for building up a library, to which might be added the collector's instinct, sometimes described as bibliomania. I have had little leisure, but have acquired some knowledge of cardiology and the history of medicine, and have had the help of many generous friends. Pursability is related to the value of money at any given time, and at today's prices the cost of the Osler and Harvey Cushing libraries would require a very deep purse indeed. From the start, the library has been restricted to the heart and its diseases, but much overlap into the history of medicine, anatomy, physiology and physical diagnosis was inevitable. My quest for books in this field covers about half a century of time.

The sources of books are bookshops, booksellers' catalogues, auction sales, and the generosity of friends. Before the last war, when I was a resident and registrar at the Middlesex, it was possible to pick up older books at reasonable prices in Charing Cross Road and elsewhere in London, and later I had opportunities of visiting many provincial bookshops. The late James Brown and I sometimes played truant for an afternoon from meetings of the Association of Physicians to visit the local bookshops, and he had an eagle eye for any item of interest among a pile of old books.

While working in Laubry's clinic in Paris in 1926, I acquired many French books from the second-hand bookshops round the Ecole de Médecine where books were displayed on trays outside the shops, and the selection was constantly changing. While in Lyon I bought a two-volume history of the Hôtel Dieu Hospital where I was working and where Rabelais had been physician in the past.

Even during my travels in the last war I managed to acquire a number of books at Aldershot, Salisbury, Liverpool, Leeds, Cairo, Jerusalem and Beirut. I recall particularly the last Latin edition of *De motu cordis* (Edinburgh 1824) purchased for a shilling in Liverpool, and Gowers's *Borderland of epilepsy* for ten piastres in Cairo. A quest for Testa's *Delle mallatie del cuore* (1810–11) in Rome in the company of the late Edward Cullinan was unsuccessful, as he was a stamp collector and stamp shops proved very numerous. It was not until fifteen years later that I succeeded in acquiring a copy from Dawson's in London.

One must be on good terms with the booksellers and be prepared to burn the midnight oil to peruse their catalogues promptly and to order items needed by telephone next day. The late Dr. Ernst Weil, the most learned of booksellers, was a very good friend who gave me much useful advice and sought and obtained many early books for me, including the Fludd (1631). Mr. R. D. Gurney has been another good friend who has supplied many books in the library including the Albertini (1648), described by Paul White as the earliest book on heart disease. Many of my earlier acquisitions came from David Low, Davis and Orioli, Feisenberger, Eisemann, and Sotheran's; in Paris from Thiébaud and Chamonal, and German works from Rothacker.

One tends to recall particular items acquired in the early days. The first Corvisart came from a visit to Davis and Orioli who many years later supplied the Alos (1694). Sotheran's supplied the Bulgetius *De affectionibus cordis* (1657), one of the earliest books on heart disease, and also Frank Nicholls' illustrated account of the necropsy on George II (1762) who died of a ruptured heart and a dissecting aneurysm. The Kreysig (1814–17) and the von Dusch, together with other German classics, came from Rothacker, and many later acquisitions came from Dawson's. David Low supplied the Primrose and the von Basch, the Allan Burns was found for me by H. K. Lewis, and Gilles de Corbeil's poem on the pulse (1514) came from Francis Edwards whose bid at Sotheby's exceeded the commission I had arranged. Many books were acquired at Sotheby's and Hodgson's book auctions but I have never had the courage to bid in person in the presence of the high priests of the book trade. A list of buyers and prices at each auction can be obtained so that one can still pursue a particular book by applying to the bookseller before it is entered in his catalogue.

The rising prices of old medical books since the last war has been remarkable and is probably due not only to inflation, but to the fact that more medical libraries and private collectors have joined the quest for old books, those on the heart being especially in demand. Yet before the war, many hospital libraries were disposing of nineteenth century books to make room for modern ones and often sold the lot for a song to local booksellers. For example, Hebb's translation of Corvisart (1813) which was among the castouts from the Middlesex Hospital library, eventually came into my possession at a price probably greater than the bookseller paid for the whole lot.

It is interesting to compare present booksellers' prices with those just after the war. Corvisart's translation of Auenbrugger's *Inventum novum* (1808) purchased from Thiébaud for less than £5 in 1947 is now catalogued in Paris at £125–£150. Piorry's *Percussion médiate* purchased in 1952 for £5–£10 is now listed at £80–£110. Many books purchased before the war for a matter of shillings would now cost more in pounds. At the start, I limited myself to £10 for any single book and although I have had to raise this limit progressively, only two books have cost £100 or more, namely *De circulatione sanguinis* (1649) and Gilles de Corbeil's poem on the pulse (1514).

To the collector, first editions are naturally prized, but to the cardiologist later editions may be far more important. For example, the third edition of Hope (1839) may be regarded as a masterpiece outclassing anything previously written and is mandatory reading for the cardiologist even today, but in the case of Laennec, the first edition is the one to read, for though he made serious errors in regard to the heart sounds, he fell into far worse errors in regard to murmurs in the second edition.

Many friends have kindly presented me with copies of their books, some of which have already become cardiac classics, such as Mahaim's *Diseases of the bundle of His* (1931) and his monograph on cardiac tumours (1945), Orias and Braun-Menendez's *Ruidos cardiacos* (1937) now translated into English, and Gallavardin's *Les Angines de poitrine* (1925). Dr. O'Donovan generously presented me with his copy of Williams's *Nervous and sympathetic palpitation of the heart* (2nd ed. 1852) which he acquired in Nottingham and which I had long sought in vain. An Irish RAMC officer presented me with Stokes's *Introduction to the use of the stethoscope* (Edinburgh, 1825) which he told me he had obtained for a few shillings from a barrow of books in a market in Dublin. Randolph Kaufmann's copy of Krehl's *Die Erkrankungen des Herzmuskels* was given to me by Hugo Roesler as a memento of my visit to the Herzstation in Vienna in 1929.

Many years ago, a friendly bookseller in Soho offered to seek a Withering on the foxglove of which he had never heard, but by ransacking the dusty basements of Charing Cross Road for botanical books he found a Withering in original boards which he purchased for five shillings and sold to me for £4, vastly below its market value even in those days. Many years later, I took the Withering to Claridges to show to my friend Mr. Arpad Plesch, whose famous botanical library in France I have visited, and curiously enough he had never seen a copy, but his librarian soon acquired one which was later exhibited at the Nice Flower Show. In return for this small service he generously presented me with first editions of Corvisart and Laennec which Quaritch obtained for him at Sotheby's

One tends to collect in sections and in each section there is generally a key book which serves as a guide to the literature. For example, on the pulse, Ozanam's *La Circulation et le pouls* (1886) is a veritable encyclopaedia of sphygmology; on Harvey and Harveiana, Bayon's papers in the *Annals of Science* and Sir Geoffrey Keynes's bibliography are important source books. I have managed to acquire the English, American, French, German, Spanish, Russian and Danish translations of the *De motu cordis*, but not the Dutch edition of 1650. The copy of Bykov's Russian translation, alleged to be out of print, was acquired by a Russian friend from an antiquarian bookshop in Moscow.

Bibliographies are essential for the collector, and Garrison and Morton, and Dezeimeris' *Dictionnaire historique de la médecine* in four volumes have been indispensable, together with the French translation of Sprengel's history of medicine, as a good guide to early literature.

An annotated catalogue was embarked upon, and evolved gradually over several years, with the unfailing help of my secretary, Mrs. Mervyn-Smith. There are various methods of cataloguing a library, alphabetical, chronological and so forth. Experience in using the library has indicated the most convenient arrangement of the books for personal reference. As long as the author index is complete, the grouping of books is not so important.

It has always been my ambition to preserve the collection intact as a reference library for those interested in the historical aspects of cardiology. In the course of discussions with Dr. Newman and Mr. Payne the plan to house it as a separate unit in the Harveian Library was approved by the President and other officers.

Harvey may be regarded as the founder of modern cardiology, which dates from the publication of *De motu cordis*, and it seems appropriate that the Harveian Library should contain a special section devoted to the heart and circulation, which I hope may long be of service to Harvey's disciples.

EDITORIAL NOTE

In preparing the catalogue of the Bedford Library for publication, the arrangement devised by Dr. Bedford and the text of his own catalogue have been generally followed with the following exceptions. Apart from the first section reference to the binding is infrequent; thereafter it can be assumed that in the majority of the items the binding is original. Additional bibliographical information has been incorporated and some entries have been amplified. This is the work of Gordon H. Smith, formerly senior assistant in the College Library, who also checked all the entries and supervised the typing. The whole has been edited and seen through the press by Leonard M. Payne, formerly College Librarian, who would like to acknowledge the advice and patience of the printer, in particular that of Mr. D. H. Tuckey.

The arrangement in each section is chronological by date of first publication or composition. Where the first edition is not held, that information usually appears in the annotation. Biographies are placed with an author's works, where possible. Histories of special aspects will generally be found at the end of the appropriate section instead of in the history of cardiology.

The use of abbreviations has been kept to a minimum; but it may be helpful to point out that Callisen refers to A. C. P. Callisen *Medicinisches Schriftsteller-Lexicon* (Copenhagen and Altona, 1830–45. 33 vols), Osler to *Bibliotheca Osleriana* (Oxford, 1929) and Wing to D. G. Wing *Short-title catalogue . . . 1641–1700.* (New York, 1945–51. 3 vols). No attempt has been made to include here the complete holdings of the Royal College of Physicians in this subject, but the addition of (RCP) to a title indicates that it is held in the College library.

Thanks are due to Dr. A. Stuart Mason for permission to reproduce in an adapted form the articles by Dr. Newman (College *Commentary*, 1970–71, **5**, 79–80) and Dr. Bedford *Journal of the Royal College of Physicians of London*, 1971–72, **6**, 227–234).

THE PULSE

The art of feeling the pulse dates back to a legendary antiquity. Knowledge of Chinese sphygmology was brought to Europe by Jesuit missionaries whose accounts were published by Cleyer in 1682 (translated in Floyer, no. 27). The best accounts are given by Capt. Dabry (no. 76), Ozanam (no. 61), Floyer (no. 27), Gruner (no. 43) and Menuret (no. 75).

Galen's voluminous works on the pulse (nos. 3–4) give details of Greek sphygmology before his time, and Struthius (no. 18) simplified and clarified Galen's pulse doctrines which dominated clinical practice up to the 19th century. Solano de Lucques (see no. 44) revived Galenic pulse lore in 1731 and knowledge of his work was published by Nihell (no. 29) in 1741, and Rucco's work of 1828 (no. 48) is the last of this revival.

Heberden (no. 42) renounced the Galenic pulse doctrines at the College of Physicians in 1768. The advent of the sphygmograph, much acclaimed as a new method of investigating the heart, merely replaced the classical pulses by a profusion of sphygmograms, one for every sort of disease. Mackenzie's *Study of the pulse*, 1902 (no. 67), finally terminated the ancient *ars sphygmica* and established graphic methods of recording the arterial and venous pulses as a scientific method of investigating the functioning of the heart.

The most comprehensive bibliography is that given by Amber and Babey-Brooke, 1966 (no. 78); but the catalogue of the exhibition, Ars Sphygmica (1966) (no. 79) in the library of the Royal College of Physicians gives details of many of the more important works.

KANĀDA, Maharishi, *fl.* 5th–6th cent. B.C., supposed author

1 Science of sphygmica; or, Sage Kanād on pulse, an English translation with Sanskrit passages by K. R. Lall Gupta. *Calcutta, S. C. Addy, 1891.* [i], [ii], [xi], 105 pp. 12mo, 12 cms.

According to RENOU (Louis) and FILLIOZAT (Jean), *L'Inde classique; manuel des études indiennes . . .* (Paris, 1953, vol. 2, p. 160), this work, the *Nadï vijñana*, dates from after the 10th century A.D. and is only attributed to Kanāda. Kanāda, author of the *Vaisesika Sutra*, lived probably in the 5th–6th century B.C. (S. PRAKASH. *Founders of sciences in ancient India*, New Delhi, 1965, c. 8). This kind of attribution is not uncommon in Indian texts. [Information from India Office Library].

RUFUS, of Ephesus, *fl. c.* 100

2 Oeuvres de Rufus d'Ephèse, texte collationné sur les manuscrits, traduit pour la première fois en français, avec une introduction. Publication commencé par le Dr Ch. Daremberg, continuée et terminé par Ch. Emile Ruelle. (*Greek and French.*) *Paris, J. B. Baillière, imprimé à . . . l'Imprimerie Nationale, 1879.* [iii], lvi, 678 pp. 8vo, 25 cms.

Traité abrégé sur le pouls, with notes, pp. 219–32 and 610.

This treatise is identical with the *Synopsis librorum de pulsibus* (Synopsis of the pulse) included in the Kühn edition of Galen (see no. 4). It was identified by Daremberg as pre-Galenic, and attributed by him to Rufus. The French translation was first published in 1845, and later included in this edition of the works of Rufus. Rufus described a number of the classical pulses which Galen detailed later.

GALEN, *c.* 130–*c.* 200

Some of Galen's books on the pulse have probably been lost, notably his commentaries on Archigenes, but 18 books preserved are regarded as authentic. For a bibliography of Latin editions see *An Investigation of the date and authorship of the Latin versions of the works of Galen* in Campbell (no. 1046, vol. 2, pp. 13–220). *De pulsuum usu*, the only one translated by Linacre, is listed as genuine by Choulant (no. 1061) and Horine (*Bulletin of the History of Medicine*, 1941, **10**, 217), but not included by Broadbent (no. 62) or Ozanam (no. 61). *Compendium pulsuum* included in the Kühn edition, is listed by Choulant as doubtful and is identical with the treatise translated by Daremberg and attributed by him to Rufus of Ephesus (no. 2, pp. 219–32). Those who are not latinists may consult the works of Paulus Aegineta (Adams's translation, no. 9), Daremberg's notes appended to the treatise of Rufus (no. 2), Le Clerc's *Histoire de la médecine* (no. 1022), Wetsch (no. 41), Gruner (no. 43), Menuret (no. 75) and Ozanam.

3 Claudii Galeni Pergameni Commentariolus de pulsibus ad medicinae candidatos. Joanne Guinterio Andernaco interprete. *Parisiis, Ex officina Simonis Colinaei, 1531.* 18 ff. Illus. 4to, 23 cms.

[*and*] Claudii Galeni De alimentorum facultatibus libri tres. Joachino Martinio interprete. *Parisiis, apud Simonem Colinaeum, 1530.* [4], 110 ff. Illus. 4to, 23 cms.

Contemporary MS notes. Original blind stamped calf, vellum spine.

The commentator Joannes Guinterius (1505–1574)—his date of birth is disputed, as is the form of his name—wrote many interpretations of Galen. While professor of anatomy in Paris he taught Vesalius and Servetus.

4 Opera omnia; editionem curavit C. G. Kühn. (*Greek and Latin*). *Hildesheim, Olms, 1965.* Tom. 8–9. 8vo, 22 cms.

Facsimile reprint of edition published at Leipzig, 1821–33.

Tom. 8 ([vi], 961 pp.) contains *De pulsibus libellus ad tirones* pp. 453–92; *De differentia pulsuum* (4 books) pp. 493–765; *De dignoscendis pulsibus* (4 books) pp. 766–961. Tom. 9 ([i], viii, 941 pp.) contains *De causis pulsuum* (4 books) pp. 1–204; *De praesagitione ex pulsibus* (4 books) pp. 205–430; *Synopsis librorum de pulsibus* pp. 431–549.

SARTON (GEORGE ALFRED LÉON) 1884–1956

5 Galen of Pergamon. (Logan Clendening Lectures on the History and Philosophy of Medicine. 3rd series, 1952). *Lawrence, Kansas University Press, 1954.* [xii], 112 pp. Map, plan, bibliog. 8vo, 22 cms.

TYLDEN (HENRY JOHN) 1857–1892

6 Galen: an essay. *London, Pardon & Sons, printers, 1894.* 59 pp. 8vo, 22 cms.

Autograph: Charles Singer (Charles Joseph Singer, 1876–1960, medical historian).

Published posthumously by Tylden's mother from a manuscript among his papers (see *Preface*).

MARKELLINOS, *fl.* 2nd cent.?

7 Markellinos' Pulslehre. Ein griechisches Anekdoton von Hermann Schöne.

Extract from *Festschrift zur 49. Versammlung deutscher Philologen und Schulmanner*, Basel, 1907, pp. 448–71. Bibliog. (ftn. refs).

The Greek text of Markellinos' treatise on the pulse, written probably in the 2nd century A.D., was first made available by Schöne in this edition, to which he has added an introduction and notes.

Markellinos cites Herophilos (*fl.* late 4th century B.C.), Erasistratos (*fl.* early 3rd century B.C.) and Archigenes of Apamea, Syria (*fl.* late 1st, early 2nd century A.D.), but neither Galen (*c.* 130–*c.* 200) nor Celsus (*fl.* early 1st century A.D.). Since Markellinos does not cite Galen, he may have lived before him, although linguistic evidence suggests a later date.

THEOPHILUS PROTOSPATHARIUS, *fl.* early 7th cent.

8 Liber de pulsibus.

Pp. 2–77 in Ermerins (Franz Zacharias) 1808–1871. *Anecdota medica graeca e codicibus MSS expromsit.* (*Greek and Latin*). Lugduni Batavorum, apud S. et J. Luchtmans, 1840. 327 pp. 8vo, 23 cms.

Other works: Leo, Archbishop of Thessalonica, the Iatrosophist or the Philosopher, *fl.* 9th cent. *Conspectus medicinae*, pp. 79–221; Incerti auctoris *Tractatus de cibis, e libro de medicina ad Constantium Pogonatium*, pp. 228–75; Hippocrates, *c.* 460–*c.* 377 B.C. (supposed author). *Epistola ad regem Ptolemaeum de hominis fabrica*, pp. 277–97.

Theophilus, also known as Philaretus, was a Byzantine physician who lived at the Court of Constantinople under the Emperor Heraclius, 610–641 A.D. He is best known for his treatise on the urine. He was a contemporary of Paulus Aegineta and his pulse treatise is largely a compilation of Galen's doctrines. This text, in Latin and Greek, by Ermerins, is cited by Adams in his edition of Paulus Aeginata.

PAULUS, Aegineta, *fl.* late 7th cent.

9 The Seven books of Paulus Aegineta; trans. from the Greek with a commentary embracing a complete view of the knowledge possessed by the Greeks, Romans and Arabians on all subjects connected with medicine and surgery, by Francis Adams. (Sydenham Society). *London, Sydenham Society, 1844–1847.* 3 vols. Bibliog. 8vo, 23 cms.

Vol. 1, pp. 202–22. On the pulse, from the works of Galen. Francis Adams (1796–1861) was a Scottish country doctor and classical scholar; his commentary (p. 213 onwards) begins with a bibliography of "ancient authorities on the pulse". Throughout the work most sections have a bibliographical commentary.

KAO YANG-SHENG, *fl.* early 10th cent.

10 Secret du pouls, traduit du chinois [par le père Hervieu].

Pp. 384–410 in Du Halde (Jean Baptiste) 1674–1743. *Description géographique, historique, chronologique, politique et physique de l'Empire de la Chine et de la Tartarie chinoise. . . .* Paris, P. G. le Mercier, 1735. Tom. 3 ([2] ff., iv, 564 pp., [2] ff.). Illus, maps, plans, diagrs. Folio, 44 cms.

Original calf. Bookplate with crest and coronet of Fox, baron Holland (created 1762, extinct 1859) from Holland House (*cf.* British Museum. Franks Collection nos. 11130–11132). Similar crest and coronet stamped in gilt on front cover.

Wang-Shu-Ho or Wang-Cho-Ho (*fl.* 3rd cent.) was a court physician of the Western Chin dynasty and author of the *Mo Ching* (*Mei Ching* or *Meh Ching*) (Pulse classic) in ten volumes and one of the standard works on medicine. Father Hervieu's *Secret du pouls* was not the genuine treatise, but a spurious work called *Mo Chueh*, dated 907–960 A.D., often mistaken for the book of Wang-Shu-Ho, but probably written by Kao-Yang-Sheng. (*cf.* Amber and Babey-Brooke, no. 78, p. 41).

MERCURIUS, Monachus, 10th cent.?

11 Pernecessaria de pulsibus doctrina. Ex ms. Cod. Regiae Neapolitanae Bibliothecae edidit, atque illustravit Salvator Cyrillus. (*Latin and Greek*). *Neapoli, typis Vincentii Orsini, 1812.* 63 pp. Bibliog. (ftn. refs). 8vo, 22 cms.

Greek and Latin texts pp. 50–63.

Mercurius was a Greek-speaking Byzantine monk living in southern Italy, possibly in the 10th century, whose brief treatise, based on Galenic sphygmology, was edited and translated into Latin from a manuscript in the Royal Library (Biblioteca Reale, now Biblioteca Nazionale), Naples, by Salvadore Cirillo.

ALPHANUS I, Archbishop of Salerno, *d.* 1085

12 Il "Tractatus de Pulsibus" di Alfano I°, arcivescovo di Salerno (Sec. XI); [trascrizione di] Pietro Capparoni. *Roma, Istituto Nazionale Medico Farmacologico "Serono", 1936.* 51 pp. Illus. (original MS reproduced on six plates), bibliog. 8vo, 25 cms.

Transcribed from MS 1024 in the Bibliothèque de l'Arsenal, Paris. (*cf.* no. 79, item 13). This important treatise was discovered in 1930 by Dr Wickersheimer. Its authenticity has been verified by the bibliographical researches of Capparoni in the Vatican, British Museum, and Naples libraries.

Alphanus belonged to the early period of Salerno, about 1050 A.D., and is mentioned in Gilles de Corbeil's poem on the pulse.

AEGIDIUS (PETRUS), Corboliensis, known as Gilles de Corbeil, *c.* 1140–1224?

13 Tractatus de iudiciis urine metrice compositus cum ipsius commento. Una cum eiusdem... tractatu de pulsibus cum commentariis Gentilis de Fulgineo. Addito insuper Petri Leonis Spoletani... tractatu de urinis: nunc primum in lucem edito [ab Avenantio de Camerino].... *Venetiis, impensis heredum... Octaviani Scoti... per Georgium Arrivabenum, 1414 [i.e. 1514].* 50 ff. Folio, 32 cms.

Gothic letter, double columns, printer's device on last page. De urinis ff. 2–18; De pulsibus ff. 19–32; PETRUS LEO. De urinis ff. 33–49r.

Provenance: Sotheby's sale, 20 December 1965; purchased by Francis Edwards and from him by D.E.B.

VIEILLARD (CAMILLE)

14 L'Urologie et les médecins urologues dans la médecine ancienne. Gilles de Corbeil—sa vie—ses ouvres—son poème des urines. *Paris, Rudeval, 1903.* x, 390 pp. Illus, ports, bibliog. 8vo, 25 cms.

Includes La Doctrine urologique, pp. 17–205; Gilles de Corbeil..., pp. 207–313; Le Traité de l'urine de Jean de Cuba, pp. 315–77.

Aegidius Corboliensis (Gilles de Corbeil), born about 1140, studied at Salerno and later came to Montpellier and Paris. His poems on the urine and the pulse were a standard reference work for three centuries. The edition of 1494, published in Venice, was included in the R.C.P. Ars Sphygmica Exhibition 1966 (*cf.* no. 79, item 14). Flint (no. 1002, p. 21) gives a table of headings of the poem from MS Digby, in the Bodleian Library, Oxford.

The treatise of Joannes Cuba (Johann Dronnecke or Wonnecke von Caub or von Cube, *fl.* 15th century, second half) shows very little advance in urology since Gilles.

15 Essai sur la société médicale et religieuse au XIIe siècle: Gilles de Corbeil, médecin de Philippe-Auguste et chanoine de Notre Dame, 1140–1224?: avec un facsimile du manuscrit de la Hierapigra. *Paris, Honore Champion, 1909.* xix, 456 pp. Facsim., bibliog. 8vo, 23 cms.

Comprehensive bibliography at end, footnote references.

ROGANUS (LEO), Caietanus, *d.* 1558

16 In Galeni Libellum de pulsibus ad tyrones, commentarius... Eiusdem De urinis libri tres ex Hippocrate et Galeno collecti. *Venetiis, ad instantiam Iacobi Anelli de Maria, 1575.* [4], 254, [2] ff. 8vo, 16 cms.

De urinis libri tres has own title page. Last leaf (blank?) wanting. Leaves *A ii* and *A v* occur twice and are in different impressions. Device on title-pages and at end. Marbled boards, paper label. Rare.

LAVELLIUS (JACOBUS) *fl.* 1602

17 De pulsibus ad tyrones, liber et commentarii in primum librum prognosticorum Hippocratis. *Venetiis, apud Io. Baptistam Ciottum Senensem, 1602.* [4], 87, [1], [4], 75, [1] ff. 4to, 20 cms.

Part 2, *Commentarii,* has its own title-page. Colophon reads: Venetiis, apud Marcum Antonium Zalterium, 1601. Limp vellum.

A rare early commentary on Galenic pulse doctrines, not cited by historians of the pulse. (*cf.* no. 79, item 17). Salvatore de Renzi (*Storia della medicina italiana.* Bologna, Forni, 1845–48, tom. 3, p. 288) simply mentions the author's Italian name, Giacomo Lavellio. Haller (*Bibliotheca anatomica.* Tiguri, 1774, tom. 1, p. 292) records editions in 1601 (as in the colophon above) and 1602 (perhaps a reprint). Lavellius also wrote a *Compendium medicinae* (Venetiis, 1609) which includes both parts of the above.

STRUTHIUS (JOSEPHUS) 1510–1568

18 Ars sphygmica, seu pulsuum doctrina, supra MCC annos perdita & desiderata omnibus tamen medicinam cum nominis celebritate, maximaque utilitate facere volentibus summè necessaria . . . libris V conscripta, & iam primum aucta. Accessit Hieronymi Capivaccei De pulsibus elegans tractatus: & Caspari Bauhini Introductio pulsuum synopsin continens. *Basileae, impensis Ludovici Koenigs, 1602.* [10] ff., 23 pp., [2] ff., 460 pp., [10] ff. Diagrs. 8vo, 14 cms.

Contents: BAUHIN (Caspar), 1560–1624. *Introductio in doctrinam pulsuum ad tyrones,* pp. 1–23; *Ad Casp. Bauhinum . . . Io. Hendricus Krug* [poem] [3 pp.]; STRUTHIUS (J.), *Ars sphygmica,* pp. 1–356; CAPIVACCIO (Girolamo) *d.* 1589. *De pulsibus tractatus,* pp. 357–460. Last leaf blank. Folding table at end.

Half bound in calf (rebacked), marbled boards. Bookplate of Edward Waple, M.A., B.D. (1647–1712, vicar of St. Sepulchres, London, and canon of Winchester), book-stamp of Sion College Library, sold 1938, and bookplate of Dr David Assur Henry Moses.

The *Ars sphygmica* is the most important treatise on the pulse between Galen and Harvey. The first graphic representation of the pulse in the form of a sphygmogram was based on the movement of a leaf placed on the artery. Struthius was a Pole who became professor at Padua at the age of 25. He simplified Galen's pulses and gave a useful mnemonic of the five simple pulses in the form of a hand.

BUGIEL (V——) *b.* 1872

19 Un Célèbre médecin au XVIe siècle, Joseph Struthius (1510–1568): contribution à l'histoire de la médecine à l'époque de la Renaissance. *Paris, G. Steinheil, 1901.* 94 pp. Bibliog. 8vo, 24 cms.

An important work on Struthius with a bibliography of early sphygmology.

SASSONIA (ERCOLE) 1551–1607

20 De pulsibus libri tres nunc primum in lucem editi. *Patavii, apud Franciscum Bolzettam, 1603.* [26], 286, [2] ff. Diagrs. 4to, 21 cms.

Last of preliminary leaves blank. f. 286^v approbation; [287]^r errata; [287]^v colophon; [288]^v printer's device.

Old limp vellum; fine copy from the Liechtenstein Library (bookplate with coat of arms of the house of the Ruling Prince).

Sassonia (Saxonia) emphasised the importance of the pulse compared with the urine in diagnosis. He made a crude attempt at graphic representation of the pulse by using dashes of unequal length.

FLUDD (ROBERT), known as Robertus de Fluctibus, 1574–1637

21 Pulsus, seu nova et arcana pulsuum historia e sacro fonte radicaliter extracta, nec non medicorum ethnicorum dictis & authoritate comprobata. Hoc est, portionis tertiae pars tertia, de pulsuum scientia. [*Francofurti, in officina G. Fitzeri, 1630?*]. 94 pp., [1] f. Fol., 32 cms.

This is the last item in a volume made up of his *Integrum morborum mysterium: sive Medicinae catholicae tomi primi tractatus secundus, in sectiones distributas duas*... (Francofurti, typis excusus Wolfgangi Hofmanni, prostat in officina Guilelmi Fitzeri, 1631. [14] ff., 503 pp. Illus, port. (of Fludd)) [*and his*] *Καθολικον medicorum κατοπτρον*; ... *sive tomi primi, tractatus secundi, sectio secunda, de morborum signis.* ([Francofurti], 1631. [2] ff., 413 pp. Illus).

Vellum. Ex Biblioth. Gymnasii Regii Joachimici (library stamp). [?Joachimsthalsches Gymnasium, Berlin, later at Templin].

The whole volume, which is a continuation of his *Medicina catholica* (Francofurti, 1629) and is now very rare, contains Fludd's chief medical writings. The *Καθολικον* is divided into several parts; one is the *Ουρομαντια*, a comprehensive treatise on uroscopy with many engravings, including one of a uroscopist receiving a flask of urine from a messenger; another is the *Pulsus*; on p. 93 is the legend "Completum est istud opus 1629. Octob. 19"; and on p. [94]; Epilogus; the catchword "Medi-" refers to the folding table "Medicamentosum Apollonis oraculum", with the imprint: "Typis excudebatur Wolfgangi Hofmanni, Anno M.DC.XXX"; it also refers to "Tomus secundus" which never seems to have been published (see Weil, no. 139). As is usual the folding table is wanting in this copy.

WAITE (ARTHUR EDWARD) *d.* 1942

22 The Real history of the Rosicrucians founded on their own manifestoes, and on facts and documents collected from the writings of initiated brethren. *London, G. Redway, 1887.* viii, 446, 40 pp. Illus, bibliog. (ftn. refs). 8vo, 20 cms.

Chapter 11 (pp. 283–307) gives a full biography of Fludd and a list and analysis of his philosophical works. (See also MUNK (William) *Roll of the Royal College of Physicians of London* (London, 1878, vol. 1, p. 150); and CRAVEN (J. B.) *Dr. Robert Fludd: ... life and writings* (Kirkwall, 1902) (RCP).)

Fludd was a fellow student with Harvey at Padua, and must have been a close friend as he is mentioned in Harvey's lectures on anatomy (translation no. 107, p. 104). He is credited with the first published support of Harvey's discovery of the circulation (*cf. Pulsus*, p. 11, which was written in 1629). Fludd was a Rosicrucian who employed a mystical language. The circular motion of the blood agreed symbolically with Fludd's microcosm of man.

HAFENREFFER (SAMUEL) 1587–1660

23 Monochordon symbolico-biomanticum. Abstrusissimam pulsuum doctrinam, ex harmoniis musicis dilucidè, figurisq; oculariter demonstrans, de causis & prognosticis inde promulgandis fideliter instruens, & jucundè per medicam praxin resonans. *Ulmae, typis & impensis Balthasari Kühnen, 1641.* [7] ff., 146 pp. Illus (folding plates). 8vo, 16 cms.

Original vellum. An early work on musical notation of the pulse.

BELLINI (LORENZO) 1643–1704

24 De urinis et pulsibus, de missione sanguinis, de febribus, de morbis capitis, et pectoris ... dicatum Francisco Redi. Cum praefatione Hermanni Boerhaave.... Ed. 5. *Lugduni Batavorum, apud Joannem à Kerckhem, 1730.* [12] ff., 679 pp., [13] ff. Illus. 8vo, 20 cms.

Original calf. Bookplate of T. Armitage.

First edition 1683. Bellini belonged to the iatro-mathematical school and explained the circulation in terms of mechanical and hydraulic laws. He is best known for his work on the kidney.

ABERCROMBY (DAVID) *fl.* 1701

25 De variatione, ac varietate pulsus observationes. Accessit ejusdem authoris Nova medicinae tum speculativae, tum practicae clavis. Sive ars explorandi medicas plantarum, ac corporum quorumcumque facultates ex solo sapore. *Londini, impensis Samuelis Smith, 1685.* [6] ff., 54 pp., [1] f. (blank), [6] ff., 36 pp., [2] ff. 8vo, 16 cms.

Nova medicinae . . . clavis has separate title-page. Final two leaves: Books printed for Samuel Smith . . . (publisher's catalogue). Wing A60. Vellum. Bound with FRANCKE (Johann), 1648–1728. *Castorologia, explicans castoris animalis naturam & usum medico-chemicum.* (Augustae Vindel., impensis vidua Theophili Goebelii, 1685. [8] ff., 224 pp. Illus). Provenance: Bibliothèque Saint Victor (?), Muséum d'Histoire Naturelle (library stamps).

A Scottish physician practising in London, the author deals with the Chinese pulse lore, and regards the origin of the pulse as "more obscure than the source of the Nile".

HARVEY (JAMES) *fl.* 1706

26 Praesagium medicum, or, the Prognostick signs of acute diseases, established by antient observation, and explained by the best modern discoveries. *London, G. Strahan, 1706.* xxix, 216 pp. 8vo, 19 cms.

Original calf rebacked. Provenance: Ja[mes] Smith, W[illia]m Young 1830, to Dr. J. B. Codman[?] 1852, from Salhield[?] 1943, Dr. Hubert J. Norman. From Dr. Norman's library.

Ch. 5: Of prognosticks taken from the pulses. Some account of physiology of pulse and its state in various fevers, etc. A very early account in English on prognosis from the pulse, a year prior to Floyer's book. He mentions as a cause of the weak intermitting pulse, pressure on the aorta by tumours and too much water in the pericardium.

FLOYER (Sir JOHN) 1649–1734

27 The Physician's pulse-watch; or, an Essay to explain the old art of feeling the pulse, and to improve it by the help of a pulse-watch. In three parts. . . . To which is added, An Extract out of Andrew Cleyer, concerning the Chinese art of feeling the pulse. *London, Sam. Smith and Benj. Walford, 1707.* [12] ff., 440 pp. 8vo, 19 cms.

Pp. 49–64 wanting, supplied in photostat. Original calf. Bookplate of Sir D'Arcy Power.

The pulse-watch ran for one minute. Floyer made many observations on the pulse rate related to age, sex, emotions, diet, climate, drugs and disease (*cf.* no. 79, item 20). The appendix contains an extract on Chinese pulse lore from Andreas Cleyer's *Specimen medicinae Sinicae* (Frankfurt, 1682) (RCP).

GIBBS (DENIS DUNBAR) *b.* 1927

28 The Physician's pulse watch.

Reprinted from *Medical history*, 1971, **15**, 187–90. Illus, bibliog.

[*and*] Sir John Floyer, M.D. (1649–1734). *London, British Medical Association, 1969.* 10 pp. Port., bibliog. 8vo, 21 cms.

Reprinted from the *British medical Journal*, 1969, **1**, 242–5. Presentation copy with a letter from the author.

NIHELL (JAMES) *fl.* 18th cent.

29 New and extraordinary observations concerning the prediction of various crises by the pulse, independent of the critical signs delivered by the ancients; made first by Dr. Don Francisco Solano de Luque, late of the city of Antequera in Spain; and subsequently by

several other physicians. Illustrated with many new cases and remarks, to which are added, some general hints on the ancient observance, and modern neglect of crises. *London, the Society of Booksellers for Promoting Knowledge, 1741.* xxviii pp., [6] ff., 153 pp., [7] ff. Bibliog. 8vo, 22 cms.

Half-calf rebound. Signature of Ja[mes] Ferguson.

30 *The same.* Novae raraeque observationes circa variorum crisium praedictionem ex pulsu nullo habito respectu ad signa critica antiquorum: primum a Francisco Solano de Luque . . . ex Anglico Latine reddidit Wilhelmus Noortwyk, M.D. *Amstelaedami, apud Gerardum Tielenburgh, 1746.* [8] ff., 152 pp. Bibliog. (ftn. refs). 8vo, 23 cms.

First Latin edition (2nd ed. Utrecht 1753). [*and*] NOORTWYK (Wilhelmus) *fl.* 18th cent. *Dissertatio de natura humana.* [Amsterdam?, Tielenburgh?, 1746]. 48 pp. Original boards.

31 *The same.* Observations nouvelles et extraordinaires sur la prediction des crises par le pouls, faites premièrement par le Docteur D. Francisco Solano de Luques, Espagnol; & ensuite par différens autres médecins. Enrichies de plusieurs cas nouveaux, & de remarques. Traduites de l'anglois, par M. Lavirotte. *Paris, De Bure l'ainé, 1748.* xlvi pp., [1] f., 258 pp. Bibliog. (ftn. refs). 12mo, 17 cms.

Pp. 251–8 publisher's catalogue. Original calf.
James Nihell was an Irish physician practising at Cadiz. He spent two months with Solano de Luque in Antequera and published an account of his discoveries in London. As Solano's book (see no. 44) was inaccessible, Nihell's became the standard work on Solano's pulse doctrines, and two English, four Latin and one French edition were published.

MARQUET (FRANÇOIS NICOLAS) 1687–1759

32 Nouvelle méthode facile et curieuse, pour connôitre le pouls par les notes de la musique. 2ᵉ éd. Augmentée de plusieurs observations et reflexions critiques & d'une dissertation en forme de thèse sur cette méthode; d'un mémoire sur la manière de guérir la melancholie par la musique, et de l'éloge historique de M. Marquet par P. J. Buchoz. *Amsterdam, Didot, 1769.* [2] ff., vi, 216 pp. Diagrs (5 folding plates on different pulse beats). 12mo, 17 cms.

Éloge pp. 203–11. Original calf. Bookplate of Edouard de Laplane.
The first edition of his book was published in Nancy, 1747. This posthumous edition was published by his son-in-law, Pierre Joseph Buchoz of Metz (1731–1807), physician to King Stanislas of Poland, and later a renowned botanist who, like Marquet, devised a musical notation of the pulse, portraying the classical pulses in musical format.

BORDEU (THÉOPHILE DE) 1722–1776

33 Recherches sur le pouls par rapport aux crises. 2ᵉ éd. *Paris, Didot, 1768–1772.* 3 tom. en 4. Bibliog. (ftn. refs). 8vo, 18 cms.

Tom. 1 (1768): [2] ff., 3, xxx, 356 pp: sub-title reads: "Augmentée des *Recherches sur les crises* du même auteur, & des jugements portés sur la doctrine du pouls, depuis la publication des Recherches en 1756." (*Recherches sur les crises* was published in the *Encyclopédie* of Diderot.) Tom. 2 (1768): [2] ff., 3, 388 pp., [2] ff. (Approbation; Catalogue des ouvrages de M. Théophile de Bordeu): same sub-title. Tom. 3 (1772), 1ᵉʳᵉ partie: i–xxx, 31–323 pp. 2ᵉ partie: [1] f., 323–660 pp., [1] f. (Approbation; Errata) sub-title reads: "Contenant les decisions de plusieurs savans médecins sur la doctrine du pouls; avec des réflexions & quelques dissertations qui n'ont point encore vu le jour; on y a joint une dissertation nouvelle sur les sueurs critiques & leurs pouls." (Ce troisième volume . . . se vend séparément pour la commodité de ceux qui ont acheté les deux premiers. . . . On n'a fait aucun changement pour le fonds dans l'édition de 1756, non plus que dans celle qui fut faite en 1768.—Avis du libraire). Original calf. First edition 1756.

De Bordeu revived the organic pulses and classified the pulse into superior and inferior varieties—pectoral, guttural, nasal, gastric, intestinal, renal, uterine, etc.

LE CAMUS (ANTOINE) 1722–1772

34 Mémoire où l'on fait l'histoire des observations sur le pouls & quelques remarques sur le pouls de regles et des hémorroides.

Pp. 243–84 in his *Mémoires sur divers sujets de médecine.* Paris, Ganeau, 1760. [ii], xxvi, 338 pp., 7 ff. 8vo, 17 cms.

Last leaf blank. An historical account of the pulse. Very rare.

COX (DANIEL) *d.* 1750

35 Nouvelles observations sur le pouls intermittent, qui indique l'usage des purgatifs, & qui, suivant Solano & Nihell, annonce une diarhée critique. . . . *Amsterdam, Vincent, 1761.* lx, 246, 6 pp. Bibliog. (ftn. refs). 8vo, 17 cms.

Sub-title reads: Ouvrage traduit & augmenté de quelques remarques par M. D***, médecin de la faculté de Toulouse, & dans lequel on trouve de nouvelles preuves du plan proposé dans les *Recherches sur le pouls, par rapport aux crises* . . . par M. Théophile de Bordeu . . . (*cf.* no. 33). First French edition. Last 6 pp. publisher's catalogue. Original calf.

Daniel Cox, physician to the Middlesex Hospital (1746–49), following the ideas of Solano (no. 44) and Nihell (no. 29) related the intermittent pulse to diarrhoea.

36 *The same.* Nouvelle éd. *Amsterdam, Vincent, 1766.* lx, 246, 6pp. Bibliog. (ftn. refs). 8vo, 17 cms.

Straight reprint of the first edition (identical errata p. lx). Original calf. First English edition, 1758.

FOUQUET (HENRI) 1727–1806

37 Essai sur le pouls, par rapport aux affections des principaux organes, avec des figures qui représentent les caracteres du pouls dans ces affections. Ouvrage augmenté d'un abregé de la doctrine et de la pratique de Solano, d'apres les livres originaux et ouvrages espagnols et d'une dissertation sur la théorie du pouls, traduite du latin de M. Fleming [i.e. Malcolm Flemyng], Membre du College des Médecins de Londres. *Montpellier, la veuve de Jean Martel, 1767.* [6] ff., lxiv, 399 pp. Illus (figures and folding plate), bibliog. (ftn. refs). 8vo, 17 cms.

[*and*] FLEMYNG (MALCOLM) *d.* 1764

Dissertation sur les découvertes de Solano, concernant les modifications du pouls, & les prognostics qu'on peut en tirer; dans laquelle on explique ces phénoménes d'après les loix ordinaires de l'économie animale. *Londres, S. Bladon, 1753.* viii, 38 pp., [3] ff. Bibliog. (ftn. refs).

Last three leaves Fautes à corriger. Original calf.

38 *The same.* . . . Nouvelle édition, augmentée de l'article Sensibilité, inséré dans *L'Encyclopédie*, par le même . . . précedée d'une notice biographique sur l'auteur, par M.T-t. *Montpellier, Auguste Seguin, 1818.* 392, [6] pp. 8vo, 22 cms.

Half sheep, vellum tips, marbled boards. Fouquet's essay was first published in 1767, and contrives to combine the organic pulses of his teacher Théophile de Bordeu (no. 33) and critical pulses of

Solano (no. 44) and his disciple Nihell (no. 29). The book is notable for its remarkable graphic representations of the various pulses. He is described by Ewart as the father of modern tactile sphygmology (see Part VI of no. 64). (*cf.* no. 79, item 30). Solano's doctrine was brought to England by Nihell and the physiological comment on it by Malcolm Flemyng, a Scots physiologist (*d.* 1764) first issued in 1753.

GANDINI (Carlo) *fl.* 18th cent.

39 Gli Elementi dell'arte sfygmica, ossia la dottrina del polso ricavata dall'antica e moderna storia della medicina chinese, ed europea, indi combinata, e ridotta a regole non meno sicure, che facile. *Genova, Adamo Scionico, 1769.* vii, 296 pp. 8vo, 20 cms.

Half sheep, vellum tips, marbled boards. Book stamp: Prof. Rag Giovanni Appiani, Torino.

Deals with the history of the pulse in China, Asia, and Europe. Cited by Sprengel (no. 1026), and Amber and Babey-Brooke (no. 78).

STEDMAN (John) *d.* 1791

40 Physiological essays and observations. *Edinburgh, Kincaird and Bell; London, T. Cadell, 1769.* [2] ff., 140 pp. Diagrs (4 plates at end). 8vo, 21 cms.

Half calf, marbled boards, rebacked, new corners. Bookplate of Thomas Renwick, M.D. (graduated Edinburgh 1787. British Museum. Franks Collection no. 24827.)

In the first essay *Of the divisions of pulses* (pp. 1–30) he attempts to simplify classification and to define the various pulses. He notes that the pulses are rarely expressed in English so he uses the Latin names. He gives a graphic representation of the various pulses.

WETSCH (Ignaz Joseph) 1737–1779

41 Medicina ex pulsu, sive systema doctrinae sphygmicae. *Vindobonae, apud Rudolph Graeffer, 1770.* xxxvi, [iv], 268 pp., [11] ff. Illus (folding plate), bibliog. (ftn. refs). 8vo, 17 cms.

Half vellum, marbled boards. Wetsch was an Austrian physician who became professor at Moscow. His book gives a valuable historical review of Galen's pulse doctrines and those of Solano (see no. 44), Fouquet (see no. 37), Bordeu (see no. 33) and others, and was widely quoted.

HEBERDEN (William), the elder, 1710–1801

42 Remarks on the pulse.

Pp. 18–33 in Royal College of Physicians of London. *Medical transactions*, published by the College of Physicians in London. London, S. Baker and J. Dodsley, 1772. Vol. 2. (xv, 533 pp., [1] f.). 8vo, 23 cms.

This volume also contains (pp. 59–67) Heberden's paper on angina pectoris, described on p. 126, below.

Of the set of six volumes (1768–1820) Library has also vol. 1 (2nd ed. 1772. xv, 474 pp., [1] f.). This latter includes various papers by Heberden, including one on night blindness (pp. 60–63), and queries (pp. 469–74). Original boards. Both vols. have armorial bookplate of Sir Gervase Clifton (baronetcy, seat at Clifton Hall co. Nottingham: title dormant since 1869).

Heberden was the first to renounce the Galenic pulse doctrines at the College in 1768 as follows: "There can be no pretence before this audience for wasting time in shewing that such minute distractions of the several pulses exist chiefly in the imagination of the makers, or at least that they have little place in the knowledge and cure of diseases."

GRUNER (CHRISTIAN GOTTFRIED) 1744–1815

43 Semiotice physiologicam et pathologicam generalem complexa. *Halae Magdeburgicae, impensis viduae Gebaveri et filii, 1775.* xvi, 688 pp. Illus (2 folding plates), bibliog. (ftn. refs). 8vo, 20 cms.

Half calf, marbled boards. Book-stamp: Dr. Köster, Pract. Arzt.

Gruner, professor at Jena, was an authority on the history of medicine and an early historian of the pulse. He gives a detailed account of Chinese, Galenic and later sphygmology, citing all the important works (pp. 41–173). He recommends Struthius (nos. 18–19) to those studying Galen's books on the pulse.

SOLANO DE LUCQUES (FRANCISCO) 1685–1738

44 Observationes sobre el pulso; obra postuma. *Madrid, Imprenta Real, 1787.* [24] ff., 357 pp. Port. 4to, 21 cms.

Portrait of Solano as frontispiece. Original calf.

Solano de Lucques (or Luque) practised at Antequera in southern Spain. He devoted himself for many years to the study of the pulse and published a large folio volume entitled *Lapis lydius Apollinis* (Madrid, 1731), in which he described his method of predicting crises from the pulse. Solano revised his manuscripts with the help of James Nihell and they were republished in Spanish posthumously as above. Solano's work started a revival of the Galenic pulse doctrines in Europe.

FALCONER (WILLIAM) 1744–1824

45 Observations respecting the pulse; intended to point out with greater certainty, the indications which it signifies; especially in feverish complaints. *London, T. Cadell junior and W. Davies, 1796.* [2] ff., 158 pp. Tables, bibliog (ftn. refs). 8vo, 19 cms.

Original calf, new spine and fore-edges. Provenance: Sion College library, sold 1938.

Falconer devised tables to determine the degree of fever from the pulse rate.

CIRILLO (DOMENICI) 1734–1799

46 Tractatus de pulsibus. *Neapoli, expensis Lucae Marotta, 1802.* 139 pp., 1 f. 8vo, 21 cms.

Index on reverse of p. 139. Final leaf approbation. Typis Dominici Sangiacomo. Original boards.

A Neapolitan physician who became involved in political troubles and was executed in spite of intervention by Nelson and Sir W. Hamilton. He describes Galenic pulses, critical pulses of Solano, and deals with signs of aneurysm of the aorta. (*cf.* no. 79, item 34). He was not a Fellow of the Royal Society as is usually stated; this distinction belongs to Nicola Cyrillo (1671–1735), who was made F.R.S. March 9, 1727.

DANGLADE (MATHIEU) 1770–1848

47 Essai sur la connoissance de l'art sphygmique . . . [M.D. thesis]. *Montpellier, Auguste Ricard, 1804.* 28 pp. Bibliog. (ftn. refs). 8vo, 24 cms.

Mathieu Danglade was born at Mézin, Lot-et-Garonne, on 4 November 1770, the son of François Danglade and his wife Marie (*née* Rivière). He graduated M.D. at Montpellier on 8 November 1804. Danglade figures as resident at Mézin in the lists of physicians, pharmacists and public health officers compiled by the Prefecture of Lot-et-Garonne in 1818 and 1829. He was mayor of the commune of Andiran, Lot-et-Garonne. He married his niece Antoinette Virginie Bosseront, herself aged 50, by special dispensation 16 December 1847. He was then 77 and died the following year, on 24 September according to a declaration of succession but the following day according to his death certificate. (Research by J. Monteil, conservateur, Bibliothèque Universitaire (Section de Médecine), Montpellier).

RUCCO (JULIUS) *d.* 1874?

48 Introduction to the science of the pulse as applied to the practice of medicine. *London, for the author, 1827.* 2 vols. Bibliog. (ftn. refs). 4to, 27 cms.

Vol. 1, xii, xcviii, 353 pp.; vol. 2, viii, 452 pp. and errata slip. Signature on title-page (vol. 1): John Davenport, Doctors' Commons.

Rucco was an Italian practising in London, and his book is dedicated to Sir Henry Halford (1766–1844), President of the Royal College of Physicians. His lengthy work comprises a fantastic mixture of the pulse doctrines of Galen, China, Solano, and de Bordeu. It is the last treatise based on the *ars sphygmica* of ancient writers.

WEBER (ERNST HEINRICH) 1795–1878

49 De pulsu, resorptione, auditu et tactu. Annotationes anatomicae et physiologicae. *Lipsiae, prostat apud C. F. Koehler, 1834.* viii, 176 pp. Tables. 4to, 26 cms.

Quarter calf, marbled boards (rebound). A rare and important book by the great physiologist.

HÉRISSON (JULES) *b.* 1789

50 The Sphygmometer, an instrument which renders the action of the arteries apparent to the eye. . . . A memoir presented to the Institute of France . . . with an improvement of the instrument and prefatory remarks by the translator, E. S. Blundell. *London, Longman, 1835.* xvi, 46, [1], 6 pp. Illus, tables. 8vo, 22 cms.

The very rare translation of his *Le Sphygmomètre; instrument qui traduit a l'oeil toute l'action des artères.* (Paris, Crochard, 1834). (Garrison and Morton 2748.1). This instrument is mentioned by Marey, Landois, Ozanam and others.

FOSTER (BALTHAZAR WALTER) 1st baron Ilkeston, 1840–1913

51 On the use of the sphygmograph in the investigation of disease. *London, T. Richards 1866.* 32 pp. Illus, diagrs (tracings). 8vo, 19 cms.

Reprinted from *British medical Journal*, 1866, 1, 275–8, 330–3. Author's presentation copy to Dr. George Johnson (later Sir George Johnson, 1818–1896).

SANDERSON (Sir JOHN SCOTT BURDON) 1828–1905

52 Handbook of the sphygmograph; being a guide to its use in clinical research, to which is appended a lecture delivered at the Royal College of Physicians on the 29th of March 1867 on the mode and duration of the contraction of the heart in health and disease. *London, Robert Hardwicke, 1867.* vii, 83 pp. Illus, diagrs (sphygmograph tracings), bibliog. (ftn. refs). 8vo, 20 cms.

Lecture begins p. 49.

The advent of the sphygmograph substituted a profusion of sphygmograms often owing more to the instrument than to the pulse, for the classical pulses of Galen, and Galenic terminology were preserved.

LORAIN (PAUL JOSEPH) 1827–1875

53 Étude de médecine clinique faites avec l'aide de la méthode graphique et des appareils enregistreurs: le pouls, ses variations et ses formes diverses dans les maladies. *Paris J. B. Baillière et fils, 1870.* xii, 372 pp. Illus, diagrs (sphygmograph tracings), bibliog. (ftn. refs). 8vo, 24 cms.

Lorain, using Marey's sphygmograph (no. 59), investigated the pulse tracing in relation to exercise, food, sleep, etc. in acute and chronic diseases and in heart disease. (*cf.* no. 79, item 42).

GARROD (Alfred Henry) 1846–1879

54 On the law which regulates the frequency of the pulse. *London, H. K. Lewis, 1872.* 29 pp. Bibliog. (ftn. refs). 8vo, 23 cms.

Subsequently published in the *Journal of Anatomy and Physiology*, 1872–3, **7**, 219–32; 1873–4, **8**, 54–61.

LANDOIS (Leonard) 1837–1902

55 Die Lehre vom Arterienpuls nach eigenen Versuchen und Beobachtungen. *Berlin, Hirschwald, 1872.* xiv, 360 pp. Illus, tables, diagrs (sphygmograph tracings), bibliog. (ftn. refs). 8vo, 23 cms.

Landois was an early worker with the sphygmograph and invented his own instrument, the angiograph. He gives a historical review of sphygmology and early sphygmographs.

MOSSO (Angelo) 1846–1910

56 Die Diagnostik des Pulses in Bezug auf die localen Veränderungen desselben. *Leipzig, Veit, 1879.* viii, 65, [3] pp. Illus, diagrs (hydrosphygmograph tracings, including 8 folding plates), bibliog. (ftn. refs). 8vo, 24 cms.

Last [3] pp. publisher's catalogue.
Pulse recording by hydrosphygmograph by an Italian physiologist, who was professor of pharmacology at Turin University.

BRAMWELL (Sir Byrom) 1847–1931

57 The Examination of the pulse; including a description of the sphygmograph. *Edinburgh, Maclachlan and Stewart, 1881.* 15 pp. Illus, diagrs. (sphygmograph tracings). 8vo, 23 cms.

Reprinted from the *Edinburgh medical Journal*, 1880, **26**, 520–32. A lecture delivered in the Extra-Academical School of Medicine, Edinburgh.

58 *The same.* 2nd ed. Student's guide to the examination of the pulse and use of the sphygmograph. *Edinburgh, Maclachlan & Stewart, 1883.* 66 pp. Illus, diagrs (sphygmograph tracings), bibliog. (ftn. refs). 8vo, 22 cms.

Gives a rational account of the rate, rhythm, tension and volume of the pulse instead of the old pulse jargon. Recognises the high tension pulse of chronic Bright's disease and the completely irregular rhythm of mitral disease.

MAREY (Étienne Jules) 1830–1904

59 La Circulation du sang à l'état physiologique et dans les maladies. *Paris, G. Masson, 1881.* [iii], iii, 745 pp. Illus, diagrs (sphygmograph tracings), bibliog. (ftn. refs). 4to, 26 cms.

Half calf rebound with original paper covers. Marey was a pioneer in the application of graphic methods to the study of the pulse and circulation, and introduced the first clinical sphygmograph. In 1861, with Jean Baptiste Auguste Chauveau (1827–1917), he recorded intracardiac pressure curves in living horses with his cardiac sound.

DUDGEON (Robert Ellis) 1820–1904

60 The Sphygmograph: its history and use as an aid to diagnosis in ordinary practice. *London, Baillière, Tindall & Cox, 1882.* vi, 72 pp. Illus, diagrs (sphygmograph tracings), bibliog. (ftn. refs). 12mo, 17 cms.

Dudgeon's pocket sphygmograph, introduced in 1880, became the most popular instrument for clinical use, the tracing being recorded on strips of smoked paper. Sir James Mackenzie's original polygraph consisted of Dudgeon's instrument with an added recorder for venous pulse.

OZANAM (Charles) *fl.* 1846–1886

61 La Circulation et le pouls: histoire, physiologie, séméiotique, indications thérapeutiques. *Paris, J. B. Baillière et fils, 1886.* xiv, 1060 pp. Illus, tables, diagrs (sphygmograph tracings), bibliog. (ftn. refs). 8vo, 25 cms.

Première partie: *Histoire de la circulation du sang*, pp. 1–163.

Ozanam had been librarian of the Academy of Medicine at Paris and so was qualified to write a history of the circulation and pulse. Like most sphygmologists of this period, he had invented a sphygmograph and used it to record the pulse in every form of disease. The book is an encyclopaedia of the pulse and a valuable reference work in regard to Chinese and Greek sphygmology. (*cf.* no. 79, item 47).

BROADBENT (Sir William Henry) 1835–1907

62 The Pulse. *London, Cassell, 1890.* vii, 312 pp. Diagrs (sphygmograph tracings). 12mo, 17 cms.

Largely a reproduction of the Croonian Lectures 1887 (*Preface*).

Broadbent's classic record of what the unaided finger could appreciate, includes a translation of part of Galen's treatise on the pulse for beginners (*Libellus de pulsibus ad tirones*, *cf.* no. 4).

EWART (William) 1848–1929

63 How to feel the pulse and what to feel in it: practical hints for beginners. *London, Baillière, Tindall and Cox, 1892.* xv, 112 pp. Illus, tables, bibliog. (ftn. refs). 8vo, 19 cms.

Provenance (autograph): George Todd, Jan. 1893.

64 Heart studies, chiefly clinical. 1. The Pulse-sensations: a study in tactile sphygmology. *London, Baillière, Tindall & Cox, 1894.* xxiv, 486 pp. Illus, port., facsims, diagrs (sphygmograph tracings), bibliog. 8vo, 23 cms.

No more published. Provenance (autograph): George Hoy, August 1894.

Ewart is best known for his signs of pericardial effusion. His work on the pulse is a revolt against the sphygmograph and a last attempt to preserve the tactus eruditus of the old-time physician. Like Galen, he wrote a book for beginners, and a larger treatise. Part VI of *Heart studies* (pp. 417–46) is devoted to the observations and theories of Henri Fouquet (1727–1806), (*cf.* no. 37).

FREY (Max von) 1852–1932

65 Die Untersuchung des Pulses und ihre Ergebnisse in gesunden und kranken Zuständen. *Berlin, Julius Springer, 1892.* viii, 260 pp. Illus, tables, diagrs (incl. tracings), bibliog. 8vo, 21 cms.

Von Frey worked under Vierordt (no. 800) who first devised the sphygmograph. He was an early exponent of haemodynamics after Marey (nos. 59, 260), and investigated the pulse, the apex cardiogram, and intracardiac pressure curves. It was the standard scientific work on the pulse in its day.

MACKENZIE (Sir James) 1853–1925

66 The Venous and liver pulses, and the arhythmic contraction of the cardiac cavities. [*Edinburgh, Oliver & Boyd, 1894*]. 145 pp. Illus, diagrs (sphygmograph tracings), bibliog. (ftn. refs). 8vo, 24 cms.

Reprinted from the *Journal of Pathology and Bacteriology*, 1894, **2**, 84–154, 273–345.

Mackenzie's classic work on the pulse marked the end of the *ars sphygmica* of ancient sphygmology.

67 The Study of the pulse, arterial, venous and hepatic, and the movement of the heart. *Edinburgh and London, Young J. Pentland, 1902.* xx, 325 pp. Illus, table, diagrs (tracings), bibliog. 8vo, 23 cms.

68 *The same.* Die Lehre vom Puls. Arterienpuls, Venenpuls, Leberpuls, sichtbare Herzbewegungen. Aus dem Englischen . . . von Adolf Deutsch. *Frankfurt, Johannes Alt, 1904.* xvi, 306 pp. Illus, table, diagrs (tracings), bibliog. 8vo, 23 cms.

Provenance: interesting bookplate of Dr. L. Wauer of Eigen.

OLIVER (George) 1841–1915

69 Pulse-gauging: a clinical study of radial measurement and pulse pressure. *London, H. K. Lewis, 1895.* xv, 174, 16 pp. Illus, tables, diagrs, bibliog. (ftn. refs). 8vo, 17 cms.

Last 16 pp. publisher's catalogue. Stamp: Mr E. Cluneglas Davies, surgeon.

GRAVIER (Laurent) *b.* 1886

70 L'Alternance du cœur: étude critique et clinique. *Paris, Baillière et fils, 1914.* xii, 429 pp. Diagrs (sphygmograph tracings), bibliog. 8vo, 24 cms.

Historical introduction and full account of pulsus alternans based on Gallavardin's graphic records.

CHALLAMEL (Augustin)

71 De l'influence de l'horloge sur le rythme du cœur. *Paris, [priv. print.], 1919.* 9 pp. 8vo, 21 cms.

Half morocco by Blanchetière, with original covers and extra title-page, together with his *Discours de présidence [de la] Société Médicale de l'Observatoire.* Paris, [priv. print.], 1934. 7 pp. 8vo, 21 cms. Reprinted from *Journal des Praticiens*, no. 34, 31 mars 1934. Autograph presentation copy "a mon Ami Brissemoret, temoignage de mon affection".

Introduces a pulse lore worthy of Galenic times that the pulse rate can be synchronised with the clock.

WIGGERS (Carl John) 1883–1963

72 The Pressure pulses in the cardio-vascular system. *London, New York and Toronto, Longmans Green, 1928.* xi, 200 pp. Illus, diagrs (sphygmograph tracings), bibliog. 8vo, 23 cms.

Extensive bibliography alphabetically arranged (320 references).

POUMAILLOUX (Marcel) *b.* 1897

73 Le Pouls alternant: étude clinique et essai de pathogénie. Préface du Dr. [Charles] Laubry. *Paris, Masson, 1930.* 239 pp. Diagrs (sphygmograph tracings), bibliog. 8vo, 23 cms.

Extensive bibliography, 401 references.

BRAMWELL (JOHN CRIGHTON) 1889–1976

74 The Lumleian Lectures on the arterial pulse in health and disease, delivered at the Royal College of Physicians . . . 1937. *London, Lancet, 1937.* 56 pp. Illus, tables, diagrs (sphygmograph tracings), bibliog. 8vo, 22 cms.

Reprinted from *Lancet*, 1937, **2**, 239–47, 301–5, 366–71. Presentation copy.
Son of Byrom Bramwell, Crighton Bramwell brought knowledge of the pulse up to date.

History and Bibliography

MENURET DE CHAMBAUD (JEAN JACQUES) 1733–1815

75 Nouveau traité de pouls. *Amsterdam, Vincent, 1768.* xlviii, 280, [6] pp. 12mo, 17 cms.

First leaf of preliminaries blank except for signature, last leaf of preliminaries blank except for catchword. Last 6 pp. publisher's catalogue. Original calf.
An historical review of works on the pulse.

DABRY DE THIERSANT (PIERRE) *b.* 1826

76 La Médecine chez les Chinois. Ouvrage corrigé et précédé d'une préface par J. Léon Soubeiran. *Paris, H. Plon, 1863.* xii, 580 pp. Illus. 8vo, 24 cms.

Rebound in cloth with original paper covers. Gives a full account of the Chinese pulse lore.

BEDFORD (DAVIS EVAN) *b.* 1898

77 The Ancient art of feeling the pulse.

Reprinted from *British Heart Journal*, 1951, **13**, 423–37. Illus, ports, bibliog. 8vo, 25 cms.

AMBER (B—— B——) and BABEY-BROOKE (A—— M——)

78 The Pulse in Occident and Orient: its philosophy and practice in India, China, Iran and the West. *New York, Santa Barbara Press; London, Dawsons, 1966.* [vi], vii, 210 pp. Bibliog. 8vo, 23 cms.

The extensive bibliography contains many mis-spellings in the names and titles.

ROYAL COLLEGE OF PHYSICIANS OF LONDON. Library

79 Ars sphygmica: [catalogue of an exhibition]. *London, Royal College of Physicians, 1966.* 191–210 pp. 4to, 27 cms.

The exhibition included many items in this section of the catalogue.

THE WORKS OF WILLIAM HARVEY

De Motu Cordis

Exercitatio anatomica de motu cordis et sanguinis in animalibus, usually known by its short title *De motu cordis*, was first printed in Frankfort-on-Main in 1628 by William Fitzer. Fitzer, whose life and career have been traced by Weil (see no. 139), was also publisher for Harvey's friend Fludd (see no. 21). Soon after the publication of *De circulatione sanguinis* the two works were often published together; a list of editions of *De circulatione* published in this way is included in the introduction to that section (p. 22).

The Keynes numbers in each entry refer to his *Bibliography of William Harvey* (see nos. 143, 144) where fuller descriptions may be found. The majority of the items in this bibliography are in the library of the Royal College of Physicians.

Latin Texts

80 Guilielmi Harve[i] Doct: & Profess: Regii Exercitatio anatomica de motu cordis & sanguinis. Cum praefatione Zachariae Sylvii medici Roterodamensis. Accessit Dissertatio de corde Doct. Jacobi de Back, urbis Roterdami medici ordinarii. *Roterodami, ex officinâ Arnoldi Leers, 1648.* [20] ff., 215 pp., [2] ff., 219 pp., [4] ff. Illus. (2 plates). 12mo, 12 cms.

Keynes 7. Additional engraved title-page. "i" in "Harvei" of title missing (freak, type dropped out during printing?) Final errata leaf (numbered p. 216, verso blank) transposed with separate title-page of Back's *Dissertatio de corde.* "Sectionum & capitum elenchus" starts on reverse of p. 219.

Autograph: Sam[ue]l Hingeston 1765 (Samuel Hingeston, 1730–1807, Rector of Boyton, and later of Holton St. Peter, Suffolk).

81 Guilielmi Harveji Doct: & Profess: Regii Exercitationes anatomicae, de motu cordis & sanguinis circulatione. Cum duplici indice capitum & rerum. Accessit Dissertatio de corde Doct. Jacobi de Back, urbis Roterodami medici ordinarii. *Roterodami, ex officinâ Arnoldi Leers, 1660.* [16] ff., 285 pp., [9] ff., 252 pp., [12] ff. Illus (2 plates). 12mo, 13 cms.

Keynes 9. Additional (engraved) title-page dated 1661 (as Keynes). *Exercitationes duae de circulatione sanguinis* pp. 173–209, 210–85 with running titles as no 82. Index begins on reverse of p. 285. MS notes on fly-leaves at front.

Provenance: W [?] Boydang [?]. "Nunc B. J. Castellanus jure emptionis, me possidet". Jules Chatelassat 1828.

This volume also contains: Eyssonius (Henricus) 1620–1670. *Tractatus anatomicus & medicus, de ossibus infantis cognoscendis, conservandis, & curandis. Accessit Volcheri Coiteri eorundem ossium historia.* Groningae, typis Johannis Colleni, 1659. [12] ff., 216 pp.

82 Guilielmi Harveii Doct. & Profess. Regii Exercitationes anatomicae, de motu cordis & sanguinis circulatione. Cum duplici indice, capitum & rerum. Quibus accesserunt Jo. Walaei, De motu chyli & sanguinis, epistolae duae. Itemque Dissertatio de corde Doct. Jac. de Back, medici Roterodamensis. *Londini, ex officina R. Danielis, 1660.* [21] ff., 464 pp., [12] ff. Illus. 12mo, 13 cms.

Keynes 10, Wing H1089, the first English edition of the Latin text. As in all copies the additional (engraved) title-page is dated 1661, pp. 88–9 are blank, pp. 134–5 and 142–3 are transposed. This copy also lacks plates.

De circulatione sanguinis pp. 121–99: *Exercitatio I* (running title Exercitatio II, *De motu cordis* being Exercitatio I) pp. 121–46, *Exercitatio altera* (III) pp. 147–99.

Johannis Walaei Epistolae duae de motu chyli et sanguinis, pp. 201–82; for another edition see no. 169.

Bookplate of Frederick Cripps; book-stamp on title-page: M.B.

83 Guilielmi Harveii Doct. et Profess. Regii Exercitationes anatomicae de motu cordis et sanguinis circulatione. *Glasguae, in aedibus R. Urie, sumptibus D. Baxter Bibliopolae, 1751.* x, [ii], 299 pp. Illus. (2 plates). 12mo, 15 cms.

Keynes 15. *De circulatione sanguinis* pp. 169–278.

Book-stamp: Fort Pitt Medical Library.

This Glasgow edition was described by Laubry as easy to read, easy to handle, a veritable pocket breviary which he carried in his pocket when making his translation of Harvey (see no. 97) during the war.

84 Guilielmi Harveii Exercitationes de motu cordis et sanguinis; quas notis pauculis instruendas curavit Thomas Hingston, M.D., Societatis Regiae Medicae Edinburgensis Socius, nunc ex Collegio Reginae Cantabrigiensi. *Edinburgi, ven. apud Joannem Carfrae et Filium; atque Longman et Socios, Londini, 1824.* xviii, 250 pp. Illus. (2 plates), bibliog. (occasional ftn. refs). 8vo, 22 cms.

Keynes 16. *De circulatione sanguinis* pp. 159–250.

a1, half-title, wanting. Acquired 1942. Autograph: J [?] Wickham.

Excluding facsimiles, this is the last time that the *De motu* was published with only the Latin text.

85 Exercitatio anatomica de motu cordis et sanguinis in animalibus . . . *Florence, R. Lier, 1928.* 73 pp. 4to, 22 cms.

Keynes 17. Facsimile reprint of first edition, *Francofurti, sumptibus Guilielmi Fitzeri, 1628.* One of 250 copies printed for the Royal College of Physicians of London, Harvey Tercentenary. Has RCP bookplate, with legend "pro indicio amicitiae et in memoriam sempiternam Gulielmi Harveii."

English Translations

The first English translation of *De motu cordis* in 1653 was anonymous; it was reprinted in 1673 (*cf.* no. 86) and in 1928 in the Nonesuch edition edited by Keynes (no. 90). The second translation by Michael Ryan was published in the *London medical and surgical Journal*, 1832–33. The third translation was made by Robert Willis in 1847 and it became for long the standard version. It was reprinted in revised form by Bowie in 1889 (nos. 87, 1040), and in the Everyman edition of 1907 (no. 89). The fourth translation by Chauncey Leake in 1928 (nos. 91–2) was based on the Longhine edition of 1697, Moreton's facsimile of the 1628 edition (no. 88), and on Willis's translation. The fifth translation, made by K. J. Franklin in 1957 (no. 93), is probably the best.

86 The Anatomical exercises of Dr. William Harvey, Professor of Physick, and Physician to King Charles the First; concerning the motion of the heart and blood. With the preface of Zachariah Wood, physician of Roterdam. To which is added, Dr. James de Back, his Discourse of the heart, Physician in ordinary to the town of Roterdam]. [*London, printed for Richard Lowndes . . . and Math. Gilliflower . . . 1673*]. [12] ff.. 107 pp., [10] ff., 172 pp. 8vo, 18 cms.

Keynes 20. This is a reprint of the 1653 edition with some textual errors and omissions.

This copy has a made-up title-page (a later addition) which bears no resemblance verbally or typographically to the original, and reads: "Anatomical exercitations concerning the motions of the heart, and the circulation of the blood. By William Harvey, an Englishman, Professor of Anatomie and Chirurgery in the Colledge of Physicians at London, and Doctor of Physick to the King's most excellent Majesty. *London, printed 1673.*" Note the very close resemblance to the title page of *Two anatomical exercitations* . . . (see below), from which it was probably taken.

This copy also lacks the dedications to King Charles I (a2) and Dr Argent (a3–4) together with the preface of Zachary Wood (A1–7). The index of the chapters (A8) therefore follows directly after the made up title-page, followed by *The Proeme* pp. 1–13, *Anatomical exercises* . . . pp. 15–107; *The Discourse of James de Back*, pp. 1–91. *An Addition, in defence of Harvey's circulation*, pp. 92–104. *Two anatomical exercitations concerning the circulation of the blood* . . . pp. 105–72. Signature U3 does not have the misprint T3 as stated in Keynes, but T4 instead of U4 remains.

Bookplate: Dr Albert Grünbaum 1903 (Albert Sidney Frankau Grünbaum, later Leyton, 1869–1921, M.D., F.R.C.P.).

87 On the motion of the heart and blood in animals, by William Harvey, M.D.: Willis's translation, revised and edited by Alex. Bowie. (Bohn's Select Library). *London, G. Bell, 1889.* [i], xx, 147 pp. 8vo, 19 cms.

Keynes 22. Biographical introduction pp. v–xviii. Additional last 24 pp. Catalogue of Bohn's libraries (publisher's catalogue). Another edition in no. 1040.

Bookplate of Sir D'Arcy Power (1855–1941).

88 An Anatomical dissertation upon the movement of the heart and blood in animals, being a statement of the discovery of the circulation of the blood . . . privately reproduced in facsimile from the original edition printed at Franckfort-on-the-Maine in the year 1628, with a translation and memoir, for G. Moreton [pseudonym, i.e. George Blacker Morgan], 42, Burgate Street, Canterbury. (*Latin and English*). *Canterbury,* [*privately printed*], *1894.* x, 72, [4], i–viii, 9–91 pp. Illus, port. 8vo, 23 cms.

Keynes 23. Frontispiece National Portrait Gallery portrait of Harvey. Introductory memoir. Facsimile of 1628 text; English translation altered from that of Willis without acknowledgement (Keynes).

Autograph: Wm. Stirling (1851–1932, author of *Some apostles of physiology*).

89 The Circulation of the blood and other writings [translated by Robert Willis]. (Everyman's Library no. 262). *London, J. M. Dent; New York, E. P. Dutton, 1907* (*reprinted 1952*). xxvi, 230 pp. Bibliog. (occasional ftn. refs). 12mo, 18 cms.

Reprint of Keynes 24. Contents: An Anatomical disquisition on the motion of the heart and blood in animals, pp. 1–108; An Anatomical disquisition on the circulation of the blood to John Riolan, jun., of Paris, pp. 109–30; A Second disquisition to John Riolan, jun., pp. 131–72; Letters [to physicians], pp. 173–201; The Anatomical examination of the body of Thomas Parr . . ., pp. 205–11; The Last will and testament of William Harvey, pp. 212–19.

90 The Anatomical exercises of Dr. William Harvey: De motu cordis, 1628: De circulatione sanguinis, 1649: The first English text of 1653 now newly edited by Geoffrey Keynes. Issued on the occasion of the tercentenary celebration of the first publication of the text of De motu cordis. *London, Nonesuch Press, 1928.* xvi, 202, [6] pp. Illus (1 plate, 4 figs). 8vo, 21 cms.

Keynes 25. *De motu cordis*, pp. 16–118, *De circulatione sanguinis*, pp. 119–93. Editor's postscript to the present edition and textual notes pp. 195–202, a note on printing on the following (unnumbered) page. Copy no. 365 of 1450 copies printed for sale.

91 Exercitatio anatomica de motu cordis et sanguinis in animalibus by William Harvey, M.D.: with an English translation and annotations by Chauncey D. Leake. Tercentennial edition. (*Latin and English*). *London, Baillière, Tindall & Cox, 1928.* [xi], 72, [2] pp., 154 pp. Illus, ports, facsim., bibliog. 8vo, 25 cms.

Keynes 25a with British imprint. Facsimile reprint of 1628 edition.

92 Exercitatio anatomica de motu cordis et sanguinis in animalibus, by William Harvey, M.D. An English translation with annotations by Chauncey D. Leake. 3rd ed., 2nd printing. *Springfield, Illinois, Charles C. Thomas, 1949.* xvii, 150 pp. Illus, port., facsims, bibliog. 8vo, 23 cms.

Contains only the modern English translation. The third edition (1941) is treated as a re-issue of the second edition by Keynes (see note with Keynes 25b).

Dr. Leake used the Longhine Latin edition (Bonomiae, typis Longhi, 1697. Keynes 13, not in the library.), Willis's translation (no. 89) and Moreton's facsimile of the 1628 edition (no. 88) as a basis for his text.

93 The Movement of the heart and blood in animals: an anatomical essay by William Harvey: translated from the original Latin by Kenneth J. Franklin and now published for the Royal College of Physicians of London. (*Latin and English*). *Oxford, Blackwell Scientific Publications, 1957.* xii, 209 pp. Illus, port., bibliog. (occasional ftn. refs). 8vo, 22 cms.

R.C.P. portrait as frontispiece. Reprint of Latin text, pp. 113–209.

German Translation

94 William Harvey, der Entdecker des Blutkreislaufs und dessen anatomisch-experimentelle Studie über die Herz- und Blutbewegung bei den Thieren. Cultur historisch-medicinische Abhandlung zur Feier des dreihundertjährigen Gedenktags der Geburt Harvey's (1 April 1578) von Dr. Joh[ann] Hermann Baas. *Stuttgart, Ferdinand Enke, 1878.* [vi], 114 pp. Illus. 8vo, 25 cms.

Keynes 26. Numbering of pp. 114, 116 interchanged. Plate bound in at end. Contents include Einleitung pp. 1–6, Culturhistorische Skizze der Denkrichtung und Forschungsmethode der Medicin des 17. und des 19. Jahrhunderts pp. 7–20, Harvey's Leben und Schriften pp. 21–37, translation of *De motu cordis* pp. 38–116 [i.e. 114], Literatur pp. 115–114 [i.e. 116]. MS notes in German.

Autograph and book-stamp: J. K. Proksch.

French Translations

95 La Circulation du sang. Des movements du cœur chez l'homme et chez les animaux. Deux reponses à Riolan. Traduction française avec une introduction historique et des notes par Charles Richet. *Paris, G. Masson, 1879.* [iv], iii, 287 pp. Illus, diagrs, bibliog. 8vo, 24 cms.

Keynes 28, the first French edition of *De motu cordis* and *De circulatione sanguinis*.

Presentation copy signed by Richet to Mr. [or M?] G. Raynaud (possibly A. G. Maurice Raynaud, 1834–1910, of Raynaud's disease; there was also a Gaston Raynaud, 1850–1911, a medievalist at the Bibliothèque Nationale).

The historical introduction and notes by the great French physiologist make this edition especially valuable.

96 Harvey. Traité anatomique sur les mouvements du cœur et du sang chez les animaux. [Traduit par Charles Robert Richet]. (Les Maîtres de la Science). *Paris, G. Masson, 1892.* 128 pp. Illus. 12mo, 19 cms.

Keynes 29. The series, Les Maîtres de la Science, Bibliothèque Retrospective, was published under the direction of Charles Richet.

97 Guillaume Harvey. Étude anatomique du mouvement du cœur et du sang chez les animaux. Aperçu historique et traduction française par Charles Laubry. *Paris, G. Doin, 1950.* 224 pp. Port., bibliog. (ftn. refs). 8vo, 22 cms.

Keynes 29a. Contains preface, historical review of the discovery of the circulation, facsimile of *De motu cordis*, 1628, and French translation. Inserted are two autograph letters and a signed article, La postérité est à Harvey, from *Le Progrès medical* no. 22, 24 novembre 1948, pp. 570–3, by Laubry.

Charles Laubry, professor of cardiology in Paris, was trained in the classics before starting his medical studies and made this original translation from the Latin texts during the German occupation of Paris when he liked to carry the Glasgow edition of 1751 in his pocket while travelling on the Metro. For Laubry's presumed death in 1941 see the note and autograph letters at no. 409.

Russian Translation

98 [Exercitatio anatomica de motu cordis et sanguinis in animalibus. *Russian*]. Вильям Гарвей Анатомическое исследование о движении сердца и крови у животных: перевод, редакция и комментарии академика К. М. Быкова. (Классики Науки). Ленинград, Академия Наук СССР [*Leningrad, Soviet Academy of Science*], *1948.* 234, [1] pp. Illus, ports, facsims. 8vo, 23 cms.

Keynes 29c. Russian translation by K. M. Bykov with Pavlov's preface of 1924, two prefaces by Bykov and an oration on Harvey by A. F. Samoilov; *De circulatione sanguinis* pp. 101–67. 5,000 copies were printed for the Academy of Science.

The Russian translation of the *De motu cordis* was first published in 1927.

Purchased for DEB at an antiquarian bookseller in Moscow, by Dr. Herzberg.

Danish Translation

99 William Harvey's bog om opdagelsen af blodets kredslob. Oversat og udgivet af V[aldemar] Meisen. *København, [print.] "Hafnia" (Carl Kretzschmer), 1929.* xxvi, [iii], xxvii–xxviii, 103 pp. Illus, port., facsim. 8vo, 23 cms.

Keynes 29d.

Spanish Translation

100 Harvey, iniciador del metodo experimental. Estudio critico de su obra De motu cordis y de los factores que la mantuvieron ignorada en los paises de habla española, con una reproduccion facsimilar de la edicion original y su primera version castellana, por Jose Joaquin Izquierdo. (*Spanish and Latin*). *Mexico, Ediciones Ciencia, 1936.* xviii, 399 pp. Illus, ports, facisms, bibliog. 8vo, 24 cms.

Keynes 29e. First Spanish translation of the *De motu* with facsimile of original Latin text. Half-title (pp. i–ii) ? wanting. Facsimiles from the works of Galen and other pre-Harveian writers. Contains an important historical review of the circulation with particular reference to Servetus and to the Spanish reception of Harvey with a full bibliography of early Spanish literature on the circulation (pp. 1–124).

De Circulatione Sanguinis

The publication of *De motu cordis* led to Harvey being subjected to considerable misrepresentation and abuse. In 1649 he chose to reply to an opponent he thought specially worthy of a reply, Riolan the younger, one of the most famous anatomists of his day. The small book, usually known as *De circulatione sanguinis*, contains two essays addressed to Riolan. It was first published jointly by Roger Daniel at Cambridge (the title beginning *Exercitatio anatomica*) and by Arnold Leers at Rotterdam (the title beginning more descriptively *Exercitationes duae anatomicae*).

De circulatione soon became regarded as an appendix to *De motu cordis* and these joint copies have been placed in this catalogue, as in Keynes's bibliography, under the major work. Apart from those in the *Opera omnia* therefore, copies of *De circulatione* will be found with nos 81–84, 86, 89–90 and 95.

101 Exercitationes duae anatomicae de circulatione sanguinis. Ad Joannem Riolanum filium; Parisiensem medicum peritissimum, anatomicorum corypheum: in Academia Parisiensi Anatomes & Herbariae Professorem Regium egregium atque Decanum, Reginae matris Lodovici XIII. medicum primarium. Authore, Gulielmo Harveo anglo, in Collegio Medicorum Londinensium Anatomes & Chirurgiae Professore; serenissimaeque Majestatis Regiae archiatro. *Roterodami, ex officinâ Arnoldi Leers, 1649.* [1], 140, [1] pp. 12mo, 12 cms.

Keynes 32. This first edition of *De circulatione sanguinis* was published simultaneously with the Cambridge edition.

Bound with *De motu cordis* (Roterodami, Leers, 1648). Keynes 7, lacks errata (p. 216); see no. 80 for description of another copy).

Paste-downs (no fly-leaves) formed from blank verso of title-page of *The Vanity of self-boasters . . .* by E[dward] H[inton]. (London, R. Bishop for S. Gellibrand, 1643) (Wing H2066).

Autographs: J. G. Leath, M.D. (John Gogill Leath, 1776–1859). J. Jeffn. Hogg (probably Thomas Jefferson Hogg, 1792–1862, who greatly assisted his brother, John Hogg, 1800–1869, classical scholar and naturalist, in his studies).

102 The Circulation of the blood. Two anatomical essays by William Harvey, together with nine letters written by him. The whole translated from the Latin and slightly annotated by Kenneth J. Franklin. (*Latin and English*). *Oxford, Blackwell Scientific Publications, 1958.* xxiii, 184 pp. Illus, port., bibliog. 8vo, 22 cms.

Opera Omnia

103 Exercitatio anatomica de motu cordis et sanguinis in animalibus. Cui accedunt Exercitationes duae anatomicae de circulatione sanguinis ad Joannem Riolanum Filium; In Academia Parisiensi Anatomes & Herbariae Professorem Regium, Reginae Matris Ludovici XIII Medicum Primarium. Auctore Gulielmo Harveo Anglo, Anatomiae & Chirurgiae in Collegio Medic. Lond. Professore, Serenissimaeque Majestatis Regiae Archiatro. Hujusque operum pars prima. Editio novissima. Indice ornata. *Lugduni*

Batavorum, apud Johannem van Kerckhem, 1737. [8] ff., 170 pp. Illus (2 plates). 4to, 20 cms.

Keynes 46, first part, already published separately in 1736 (Keynes 14). *Exercitationes duae anatomicae de circulatione sanguinis*, pp. 105–67 (*Exercitatio . . . prima*, pp. 107–26, *Exercitatio altera . . .*, pp. 127–67), publisher's catalogue (*Libri aliquot medici et juridici quos excudit & in officina sua debinet J. a Kerckhem*) pp. 169–70; second part: *De generatione*, wanting.

Bookplate: William Johnston Esqr (BM. Franks Collection, no. 16619) of Holly Park, Co. Down; Autograph: E[dward] Cresswell Baber 1872 (1851–1910, M.B.).

104 Guilielmi Harveii Opera omnia: A Collegio Medicorum Londinensi edita. [Edita a M. Akenside cum Harveii vita a T. Lawrence]. [*Londini, excudebat Guilielmus Bowyer*], 1776. [viii], xxxix, 673 pp. Illus, port., bibliog. (occasional ftn. refs). 4to, 30 cms.

Keynes 47. Lacks frontispiece portrait of Harvey. Harveii vita, pp. i–xxxviii, *De motu cordis*, pp. 1–87, *De circulatione sanguinis*, pp. 89–141, *De generatione animalium*, pp. 159–603, *Anatomia Thomae Parri*, pp. 605–10, *Epistolae*, pp. 611–36, *Diploma*, pp. 637–42.

Autographs: Donum Collegii Medicorum Londin. Edvardo Fryer, Anno 1790. (Edward Fryer, 1761–1826, M.D., L.R.C.P. 1790). E libris Carolus A. Harries 1843 (Charles Alexander Harries, 1808–1871, M.R.C.S., L.S.A., of Bath).

105 The Works of William Harvey, . . . translated from the Latin with a life of the author by Robert Willis [1799–1878]. (Sydenham Society). *London, Sydenham Society, 1847.* xcvi, 624 pp. Illus, bibliog. (ftn. refs). 8vo, 23 cms.

Keynes 48. Life of William Harvey, pp. xvii–lxxxvii, Last will and testament, pp. lxxxix–xcvi *De motu cordis*, pp. 1–86, *De circulatione sanguinis*, pp. 87–141, *De generatione animalium*, pp. 143–586, *Anatomy of Thomas Parr*, pp. 587–92, *Letters* pp. 593–617.

Autograph: G. N. Pitt, Oct. 1879 (George Newton Pitt, 1853–1929, M.D., F.R.C.P.).

For many years this book was the standard English translation of all Harvey's works.

Prelectiones

106 Prelectiones anatomiae universalis by William Harvey. Edited with an autotype reproduction of the original by a committee of the Royal College of Physicians of London. *London, J. & A. Churchill, 1886.* viii, 98 ff. Facsims. 4to, 26 cms.

Keynes 52. Reproduction of Harvey's notes for his lectures from a MS in the British Library (Sloane 230) containing the first account of his observations on the circulation. Inserted between each pair of leaves are plates with the autotype reproductions of pages of manuscript on both sides. Thus each page of MS. faces its transciption made by Edward Scott of the Manuscript Department of the British Museum (now British Library).

107 Lectures on the whole of anatomy. An annotated translation of Prelectiones anatomiae universalis by C. D. O'Malley, F. N. L. Poynter, K. F. Russell. *Berkeley and Los Angeles, University of California Press, 1961.* [x], 239 pp. Illus, port., facsims, bibliog. (ftn. refs). 8vo, 24 cms.

Rolls Park portrait of Harvey as frontispiece. See no. 108 for another translation.

De Motu Animalium

108 William Harvey. De Motu locali animalium, 1627; ed., translated and introduced by Gweneth Whitteridge, Archivist of St. Bartholomew's Hospital, London. *Cambridge, published for the Royal College of Physicians [of London], at the University Press, 1959.* xii, 163 pp. Facsim., bibliog. 8vo, 25 cms.

Facsimile of manuscript page as frontispiece. Transcription and translation on facing pages. Copious footnote references, and bibliography of works cited in notes.

This work comprises notes made by Harvey for a treatise which is contained in the British Library, Sloane MS. 486, ff. 69–118v. These notes are of great interest as examples of Harvey's handwriting and Latin which Dr. Whitteridge has deciphered with much labour and skill. Dr. Whitteridge has published a transcription and translation of the rest of this manuscript and included it in a new annotated translation of the *Prelectiones,—The Anatomical lectures of William Harvey* (Edinburgh and London, 1964) (RCP).

Letters

Two small groups of Harvey's letters have been published—nine to contemporary physicians and eleven to Lord Feilding. The nine include a letter to Caspar Hoffman of Nuremberg (1572–1648) in 1636 and eight others in the period 1651–1657 (to Paul Marquard Schlegel of Hamburg, 1605–1653, in 1651; three letters to Giovanni Nardi of Florence, *c.* 1580–1655?, in 1651, 1653 and 1655; to Robert Morison then of Paris, 1620–1683, in 1652; two letters to Johann Daniel Horst, Chief Physician of Hesse-Darmstadt, 1616–1685, both in 1655; to Jan Vlackveld of Haarlem in 1657, the year of Harvey's death). These nine letters (text in nos. 89, 102 and 104–105) have never been published separately, but those to Lord Feilding have.

109 Some recently discovered letters of William Harvey, with other miscellanea by S. Weir Mitchell . . . With a bibliography of Harvey's works by Charles Perry Fisher. *Philadelphia, College of Physicians of Philadelphia, 1912.* 59, [3] pp. Illus (2 plates), bibliog. 8vo, 23 cms.

Keynes 53.

Weir Mitchell identified the signature of Harvey's will as that of Heneage Finch, his nephew, and also identified Harvey's writing in Goulston's edition of Galen in the British Library. On pp. 42–50 is a prose translation of Robert Grove's *Carmen de sanguinis circuitu* (1685; see no. 118) by Dr Astley Paston Cooper Ashurst. The list of Harvey's works was the only bibliography available prior to Keynes's of 1928. The principal item, however, is the text of Harvey's letters to Lord Feilding.

110 Eleven letters of William Harvey to Lord Feilding June 9th–Nov. 15th, 1636. Purchased from the Earl of Denbigh and presented to the Royal College of Physicians by Sir Thomas Barlow, Bt., President, Oct. 18, 1912. [*London, privately printed, 1912*]. [28 pp.]. 8vo, 23 cms.

Keynes 54.

The letters were also published in a paper by Sir D'Arcy Power in *Proceedings of the Royal Society of Medicine* (*Section of the History of Medicine*), 1916–1917, **10**, 33–59; and in his *Selected writings* (Oxford, 1931, pp. 141–71) (no. 136).

Anatomy of Thomas Parr

111 Other copies will be found in nos. 89, and 104–105.

The Anatomy of Thomas Parr; [trans. by Arnold Muirhead, introduction by Sir Geoffrey Keynes].

Reprinted from *St. Bartholomew's Hospital Reports*, 1939, **72**, 17–22.

Dr. Norman's (Hubert James Norman, *d.* 1948) copy, a gift from the translator, with a covering autograph letter. Also letter from Sir Richard Leighton to DEB.

Harvey performed a post-mortem on Thomas Parr, alleged age 152, by order of the King, on 16th Nov. 1635. The manuscript of Harvey's Latin report was given to Betts by Harvey's nephew, and was originally published by John Betts in *De ortu et natura sanguinis* (London, 1669). The report was first translated by Robert Willis, 1847, and Dr. Muirhead's new translation was made at Keynes's request.

Sir Richard Leighton of Loton Park, Shrewsbury, lord of the Manor, has investigated the trial records and it is recorded that Parr was in court for indecent assault on girl when advanced in age. He has a portrait of Parr (painting).

LEGRAND (MAXIMILIEN ALBERT HENRI ANDRÉ) 1857–?

112 La Longevité à travers les âges. *Paris, Ernest Flammarion, 1911.* [iii], 307 pp. Tables, bibliog. (ftn. refs). 8vo, 19 cms.

Autograph: A. D. Hutchison.

Deals with every aspect of longevity, and mentions Thomas Parr and Harvey's post-mortem, p. 239.

Biography and Criticism

AUBREY (JOHN) 1626–1697

113 Aubrey's brief lives. Ed. from the original manuscripts and with an introduction by Oliver Lawson Dick. 3rd ed. *London, Secker & Warburg, 1960.* cx, 342 pp. Ports, facsims. 8vo, 24 cms.

Aubrey's account of Harvey is on pp. 128–33. (See also Keynes' Harveian Oration for 1958, no. 188). Also includes short notes on Sir John Berkenhead (or Birkenhead, 1616–1679), whose commendatory poem on William Cartwright's verse in the latter's *Comedies, tragi-comedies and other poems*, London, 1651, contains a reference to Harvey (pp. 23–4; see no. 124), Descartes (pp. 94–5; see nos 163–4) and Walter Warner (*d.* 1640) (pp. 315–6) who claimed he told Harvey of the discovery of the circulation of the blood, and whose claims are discussed by George Rolleston (1829–1881) in *The Harveian Oration 1873* (London, Macmillan, 1873, pp. 50–65). (RCP).

CHAUVOIS (LOUIS) 1881–1972

114 William Harvey: his life and times: his discoveries: his methods. *London, Hutchinson, 1957.* 271 pp. Illus, ports, facsims, maps, bibliog. 8vo, 24 cms.

Translated from the French and published simultaneously with the French edition on the tercentenary of Harvey's death.

COHEN OF BIRKENHEAD (HENRY COHEN) baron, *b.* 1900

115 Harvey and the scientific method. *London, British Medical Association, 1950.* 17 pp. Bibliog. 8vo, 22 cms.

Reprinted from *British medical Journal*, 1950, **2**, 1406–10. The Harveian Lecture delivered before the Harveian Society of London, 22 March 1950.

CURTIS (JOHN GREEN) 1844–1913

116 Harvey's views on the use of the circulation of the blood. *New York, Columbia University Press, 1915.* xi, 194 pp. Illus, port., facsims, bibliog. 8vo, 20 cms.

Autograph: D. Fraser Harris, May 1916.

Based on a lecture delivered in 1907 to the Johns Hopkins Hospital Historical Club at Baltimore. Contains a scholarly analysis of Harvey's lines of thought and of the historical background to his work on the circulation with a bibliography.

FRANKLIN (KENNETH JAMES) 1897–1966

117 William Harvey, Englishman 1578–1657. *London, MacGibbon & Kee, 1961.* 151 pp. Illus, ports, bibliog. 8vo, 23 cms.

Enclosed with this book are the author's 'King Charles I and William Harvey'. (Extract from *Proceedings of the Royal Society of Medicine*, 1961, **54**, 85–91 (*Section of the History of Medicine*, 1–7). Illus, ports, bibliog.), and an obituary of the author (Extract from the *Lancet*, 1966, **2**, 1108–9. Port.).

GROVE (ROBERT) 1634–1696

118 Carmen de sanguinis circuitu, a Gulielmo Harveo anglo, primum invento. Adjecta sunt, miscellanea quaedam. *Londini, impensis Gualteri Kettilby, 1685.* [2] ff., 40 pp. 4to, 21 cms.

Wing G2148.

This volume also contains: *Responsio ad nuperum libellum qui inscribitur Celeusma seu Clamor ad theologos hierarchiae Anglicanae, &c.* Londini, pro Gualt. Kettilby, 1680. [2] f., 95 pp. Wing G2157. *Defensio suae responsionis ad nuperum libellum, qui inscribitur Celeusma, adversus refutationem, ab authore Celeusmatis editam.* London, impensis G. Kettilby, 1682. [2] f., 110 pp., [1] p. Wing G2150.

Manuscript dedication (by author?): Reverendo Viro Joanni Cory Cleri Dioceseos Eliensi In Sacra Synodo Provincia Cantuariensis Procuratori Dignissimo haec opuscula paterna observantiae ergo D.D., R.G.R.C.F. (John Cory M.A., B.D., 1651–1727, was rector of Landbeach, Cambridgeshire 1688–1727).

Provenance: E libris W. Whitehead Coll. Eman. (William Whitehead, M.A., B.D. was admitted sizar at Emmanuel 1711; rector of Stanground, Huntingdonshire, died 1754).

Robert Grove, Bishop of Chichester, had a large medical library but never practised medicine. A prose translation of parts of the *Carmen* by Dr Astley Paston Cooper Ashurst is given by Weir Mitchell in *Some recently discovered letters of William Harvey* (see no. 109, pp. 42–50). Keynes (no. 128, p. 314) describes the *Carmen* as "pure fiction, expressed in elegant scholarship, but not to be taken seriously as a contribution to the story of Harvey's life".

AGNEW (LESLIE ROBERT CORBET) *b.* 1918

119 Robert Grove, bishop of Chichester, and his *Carmen de sanguinis circuitu*, &c. (The Chichester papers no. 21). *Chichester, Chichester City Council, 1961.* 11 pp. Illus, facsims, bibliog. (ftn. refs). 8vo, 25 cms.

First published as "*De sanguine episcopoque:* a discussion of Bishop Robert Grove (1634–1696) and his *Carmen de sanguinis circuitu, &c.* (1685)" in *Bulletin of the History of Medicine*, 1960, **34**, 318–30, and reprinted with very minor alterations.

GUTHRIE (Douglas James) 1885–1975

120 Harvey in space and time. (Harveian Oration to Harveian Society of Edinburgh, 1956). *London, British Medical Association, 1957.* 14 pp. Bibliog. (ftn. refs). 8vo, 22 cms.

Reprinted from *British medical Journal*, 1957, **1**, 575–9.

HERRINGHAM (Sir Wilmot Parker) 1855–1936

121 William Harvey at St. Bartholomew's: a speech delivered at . . . the Harvey Tercentenary. *London, Adlard, 1928.* 9 pp. Bibliog. (ftn. refs). 8vo, 22 cms.

Reprinted from *St. Bartholomews's Hospital Journal*, 1927–28, **35**, 133–6.

122 The Life and times of Dr. William Harvey. *New York, Paul B. Hoeber, 1933.* [87 pp.]. Illus, ports, bibliog. 4to, 28 cms.

Reprinted from *Annals of medical History*, 1932, n.s. **4**, 109–25, 249–72, 347–63, 491–502, 575–89. Presentation copy. A fascinating account of Harvey and his family tree, medical education at Oxford and Cambridge in Harvey's day, and of important incidents in Harvey's life.

HILLS (Rowland) *d.* 1909?

123 The Life of William Harvey and his discovery of the circulation of the blood. *London, Henry Renshaw, 1893.* 40 pp. 8vo, 19 cms.

Autograph: Amy Smith, 1903.

HUNTER (Richard Alfred) *b.* 1923 and MACALPINE (Ida) 1899–1974

124 [Miscellaneous Harveiana].

William Harvey: his neurological and psychiatric observations.

Reprinted from *Journal of the History of Medicine and allied Sciences*, 1957, **12**, 126–39. Facsims, bibliog. (ftn. refs).

Dr. May's monster: a chapter in the history of the circulation of blood. [*London, St. Bartholomew's Hospital*], *1957.* [12] pp. Illus, facsims, bibliog. 8vo, 25 cms.

Reprinted from *St. Bartholomew's Hospital Journal*, 1957, **61**, 184–93. Inserted: a letter from Dr. Macalpine. Authors' presentation copy to DEB.

Harvey's "Boy abowt Holborn Bridg".

Reprinted from *Journal of the History of Medicine and allied Sciences*, 1960, **15**, 295–6. Illus., bibliog. (ftn. refs).

Sir John Berkenhead's lines on William Harvey.

Reprinted from *Journal of the History of Medicine and allied Sciences*, 1962, **17**, 403–5. Illus., facsim.

Daniel Oxenbridge, John Twysden, and William Harvey.

Reprinted from *Journal of the Royal College of Physicians of London*, 1970, **4**, 169–76. Facsim., bibliog.

(Macalpine is placed first as author). Authors' presentation copy to DEB.

125 KEELE (Kenneth David) *b.* 1909

William Harvey, the man, the physician, and the scientist. *London & Edinburgh, Nelson, 1965.* xi, 244 pp. Illus, port., facsims, map, bibliog. 8vo, 21 cms.

Regarded by Keynes as the best study of Harvey.

KEYNES (Sir GEOFFREY LANGDON) *b.* 1887

126 The Personality of William Harvey. The Linacre Lecture, delivered at St. John's College, Cambridge on 6th May 1949. *Cambridge, University Press, 1949.* 48 pp. Ports, bibliog. 8vo, 20 cms.

127 The Portraiture of William Harvey, with a catalogue and reproductions of the pictures. (The Thomas Vicary Lecture, 1948). *London, The Royal College of Surgeons of England, 1949.* vi, 42 pp., 32 pp. of plates. 8vo, 25 cms.

Insertion: A Christmas and New Year card from the President (1968) of the Harveian Society, Dr N. H. Moynihan, showing the Rolls Park portrait.

128 The Life of William Harvey. *Oxford, Clarendon Press, 1966.* xviii, 483 pp. Illus, ports, facsims, maps, plan, bibliog. 4to, 26 cms.

Inserted: a review of this book by Anthony Powell; cutting from the *Daily Telegraph*, July 28, 1966.

The most complete and authoritative work on Harvey so far published.

MALLOCH (THOMAS ARCHIBALD) 1887–1953

129 Finch and Baines, a seventeenth century friendship. *Cambridge, University Press, 1917.* x, 89 pp. Illus, ports, facsim., bibliog. (ftn. refs). 4to, 30 cms.

Malloch was persuaded to write this history by Osler, and it contains notes of interest about Harvey whose niece, Elizabeth, married John Finch's brother, Heneage. Both John Finch (1626–1682) and Thomas Baines (1624?–1681) studied medicine at Padua around 1652 and later Finch became professor of anatomy at Pisa. Harvey attended Anne Conway, Finch's sister. An account of the "Tabulae Harveianae" is given in the appendix in which Malloch, with Sir Thomas Barlow, first doubted whether they were actually used by Harvey and suggested they had belonged to Finch (see also *British medical Journal*, 1966, **2,** 38–9).

130 William Harvey. *New York, Paul B. Hoeber, 1929.* xi, 103 pp. Illus, ports, facsims, bibliog. 8vo, 20 cms.

Inserted slip gives publisher as Humphrey Milford of Oxford University Press.

MITCHELL (SILAS WEIR) 1829–1914

131 Some memoranda in regard to William Harvey, M.D. *New York, (privately printed), 1907.* 45 pp. Bibliog. (ftn. refs). 8vo, 23 cms.

Pp. 25–45 A List of portraits of Dr. William Harvey, with remarks by W[illia]m Roberts.

OWEN (Sir RICHARD) 1804–1892

132 Experimental physiology: its benefits to mankind with an address on unveiling the statue of William Harvey at Folkestone, 6th August, 1881. *London, Longmans, Green, 1882.* vii, 216 pp. Bibliog. (ftn. refs). 8vo, 19 cms.

Book-stamp: Liverpool Library 20 Jul. 1882.

Contains an account of the erection of the statue of Harvey on the Leas at Folkestone; sculptor, Bruce Foy. The ceremony took place during the International Medical Congress in London of 1881, members of which went by special train to Folkestone. Owing to the keen sea breeze blowing, the address including a defence of vivisection had to be condensed, but was published in full.

PADUA UNIVERSITY

133 [A Facsimile reproduction of the diploma of Doctor of Medicine granted by the University of Padua to William Harvey, 1602]. [*London, privately printed at the Chiswick Press, 1908*]. [7] ff. 8vo, 24 cms.
[*and*] Notes to accompany a facsimile reproduction of the diploma . . . , with a translation by J. F. Payne. *London, privately printed at the Chiswick Press, 1908.* 18 pp. 8vo, 24 cms.

J. F. Payne was Harveian Librarian at the Royal College of Physicians from 1899 to 1910. According to the inscription in Harvey's Diploma it was presented to the College in 1764 by Rev. Osmund Beauvoir, head master of King's School, Canterbury; this is an error in the roman numerals for 1766 (see R.C.P. *Annals* 30 Sept. 1766). The gift may have been in exchange for a copy of Harvey's works published by the College in that same year.

PAGET (Sir JAMES) 1814–1899

134 Records of Harvey: in extracts from the journals of the Royal Hospital of St. Bartholomew; with notes by James Paget. *London, J. Churchill, 1846.* viii, 43 pp. Bibliog. (ftn. refs). 8vo, 22 cms.

Inscribed Dawson Turner Esq. with the author's compliments.
Literal copies of all that is recorded concerning Harvey in the Journals of St. Bartholomew's Hospital, with explanatory notes.

POWER (Sir D'ARCY) 1855–1941

135 William Harvey. (Masters of Medicine). *London, T. Fisher Unwin, 1897.* xi, 283, [4] pp. Port., facsim. 8vo, 20 cms.

Last [4] pp. publisher's catalogue. A classic life of Harvey.

136 Selected writings, 1877–1930. *Oxford, Clarendon Press, 1931.* x, 368 pp. Illus, ports, facsims, map, bibliog. 8vo, 23 cms.

Autograph: A.L.C. ii/31.
Includes chapter 7 (pp. 127–40) Dr. William Harvey and St. Bartholomew's Hospital, and chapter 8 (pp. 141–71) Revised chapter in the life of Dr. William Harvey, 1636. (This describes Harvey's travels, with a map).

137 Sir Thomas Bodley's London house.

Pp. 203–05 in *The Bodleian quarterly Record.* Oxford, Bodleian Library, 1936. Vol. 8 (203–26 pp.). Plan. 8vo, 25 cms.
Bodley's house was near St. Bartholomew's Hospital. Lord Montagu lived opposite, and his daughter, Elizabeth, married Sir Daniel Harvey, William Harvey's nephew. Bodley was treated by Harvey.

ROYAL SOCIETY OF MEDICINE. Historical Section.

138 Portraits of Dr. William Harvey. *London, Humphrey Milford* [*at the*] *Oxford University Press, 1913.* v, 50 pp. Illus, ports. Folio, 35 cms.

Plates 1–19, portraits; plate 20, Harvey's coffin. Preface and notes by Sir D'Arcy Power.
Inserted is a criticism by Keynes from *British medical Journal,* 1944, **2**, 669–70. Sir Geoffrey Keynes regards some of these portraits as recent forgeries or of others yet unidentified, and only considers nine as possibly genuine portraits or early copies.

WEIL (Ernst) 1891–1965

139 William Fitzer, the publisher of Harvey's *De motu cordis*, 1628. *London, the Bibliographical Society, 1944.* [26 pp.]. Bibliog. 8vo, 22 cms.

Reprinted from *The Library*, 1943–44, 4th ser. (*Transactions of the Bibliographical Society*, 2nd ser.), **24**, 142–64.

Presentation copy. Fitzer, an Englishman, born about 1600, married a daughter of de Bry, the Frankfurt publisher, and started as a publisher there. He also published Fludd's works. Weil gives an erudite study of Fitzer and the publishers of Frankfurt. (See no. 21). Also gives a list of 46 extant copies of the first edition of *De motu cordis* (1628), with their location.

WILLIS (Robert) 1799–1878

140 William Harvey: a history of the discovery of the circulation of the blood. *London, Kegan Paul, 1878.* xvi, 350 pp. Port. 8vo, 23 cms.

Publisher's catalogue (32 pp.) bound in. Although the preface is dated October 1878, this possibly refers to the publication date, for Willis died on September 21st. The text probably only needed a short general conclusion anyway.

Two copies. One copy has the pencilled autograph "Matheson Cullen" on the title-page (George Matheson Cullen, M.D., F.R.C.P. Ed., 1867–1935, medical officer at the Scottish Department of Health), and marginal notes in the same hand. This copy lacks portrait, but line engraving is inserted.

WYATT (Raymond Benedict Hervey)

141 William Harvey (1578–1657). (Roadmaker Series). *London, Leonard Parsons; Boston, Small, Maynard, 1924.* 214 pp. Port, bibliog. 8vo, 19 cms.

Harvey's life with historical notes of his precursors, and some of his contemporaries.

Bibliography

BETT (William Reginald) 1903–1968

142 A Guide to the literature on William Harvey. *London, Smith, Kline & French, 1957.* [40] pp. 8vo, 25 cms.

Published for the Harvey Tercentenary Congress 1957. Contains a list of Harveian Societies, Harveian Orations and a select list of writings on William Harvey.

KEYNES (Sir Geoffrey Langdon) *b.* 1887

143 A Bibliography of the writings of William Harvey, M.D., discoverer of the circulation of the blood, 1628–1928. *Cambridge, Cambridge University Press, 1928.* xii, 67 pp. Ports, facsims. 4to, 27 cms.

First edition, limited to 300 copies.

144 *The same.* A Bibliography of the writings of Dr. William Harvey 1578–1657. 2nd ed. *Cambridge, Cambridge University Press, 1953.* xiii, 79 pp. Ports, facsims. 4to, 26 cms.

Second edition limited to 750 copies. Inserted are facsimiles of title-pages extracted from sale catalogues.

An authoritative and exhaustive bibliography of Harvey's works (1928 and 1953). Keynes states that the Latin text of *De motu cordis* (see nos 80–85) has been printed twenty-three times, the English translation (see nos 86–93) eleven times, the French (see nos 95–7) thrice, the German (see no. 94) thrice, the Russian (see no. 98) twice, the Spanish (see no. 100) twice, the Dutch and Danish (see no. 99) once.

De circulatione sanguinis was first published separately at Cambridge and Rotterdam (no. 101) in the same year (1649), and there is no proof as to which was printed first; both are very rare. It was published separately in Paris (1650) but since 1654, it has been included as an appendix to *De motu cordis*, until again published separately with Franklin's translation in 1958 (no. 102).

ROYAL COLLEGE OF PHYSICIANS OF LONDON. Library

145 William Harvey, (1578–1657): an exhibition of books and manuscripts illustrating his life and work [by L. M. Payne]. *London, Royal College of Physicians, 1957.* 25 pp. Port., bibliog. 8vo, 25 cms.

Rolls Park portrait as frontispiece. Thirty-nine exhibits are catalogued and annotated; with a brief note on portraiture and genealogy.

THE DISCOVERY OF THE CIRCULATION OF THE BLOOD

Before Harvey

This section comprises works attributing knowledge of the circulation to King Solomon and Hippocrates, and works dealing especially with the forerunners of Harvey arranged chronologically.

SOLOMON, King of Israel, 10th cent. B.C.

SMITH (JOHN) 1630–1679

146 *Γηροκομία βασιλικη*: King Solomons portraiture of old age. Wherein is contained a secret anatomy both of soul and body. And a perfect account of the infirmities of age incident to them both. And all those mystical and ænigmatical symptomes, expressed in the six former verses of the 12th chapter of Ecclesiastes, and here paraphrased upon, and made plain and easie to a mean capacity. *London, printed by J. Hayes for S. Thomson, 1666.* [8] ff., 266 pp., [3] ff. (index). Tables (one on folding plate). 8vo, 17 cms.

Wing S4114. Leaf A1 (Ecclesiastical approbation on verso) wanting. Autograph: Z. R. pr[ice] 2s:6d. This copy, from the library of Dr A. F. Voelcker (Arthur Francis Voelcker, 1861–1946, M.D., M.R.C.S., F.R.C.P.), was sold at Sotheby's in 1948.

This first edition is of great rarity possibly because most copies perished in the Great Fire of London. A second edition, *The Pourtract of old age*, was printed in London by J. Macock for Walter Kettilby 1666 (Wing S4115) another "second edition" was also issued in 1676 (Wing S4116). A third edition (London, E. Withers, 1752) is recorded in the *Index-Catalogue of the Library of the Surgeon-General's Office* [1st series], vol. 13, p. 214.

John Smith graduated M.D. at Oxford in 1659 and was elected F.R.C.P. in 1672. From an ingenious paraphrase of part of the Old Testament book Ecclesiastes (ascribed to King Solomon), he concluded that Solomon perfectly knew and described the circular motion of the blood, but this knowledge lay buried for 2500 years until Harvey retrieved it, so that the Harveian doctrine was at first Solomonian. Nevertheless, he was a whole-hearted admirer of Harvey.

HIPPOCRATES *c.* 460–*c.* 377 B.C.

MEYSSONNIER (LAZARE) 1602–1672

147 Les Aphorismes d'Hippocrate, traduits nouvellement en françois suivant la vérité du texte grec; avec un meslange de paraphrases, d'éclaircissement és lieux plus obscurs, et la clef de cette doctrine par le moyen de la circulation du sang, & d'autres nouvelles découvertes de ce siecle en anatomie & chymie. [*anon.*] *Lyon, Pierre Compagnon, 1668.* [18] ff., 290 [i.e. 288] pp. 12mo, 15 cms.

Final pages misnumbered. Les Aphorismes (pp. 1–99); la lef de cette doctrine . . . (pp. 100–234).

New method of understanding the aphorisms of Hippocrates according to the doctrine of the circulation. A very rare book: no copy in the British Library, Bibliothèque Nationale nor National Library of Medicine.

[*and*] Le Médecin charitable abbregé. Pour guérir toutes sortes de maladies avec peu de remèdes. Et l'almanach perpetuel ou régime universel . . . 2e éd. *Lyon, de l'imprimerie de Marcelin Gautherin, 1668.* 59 pp. Port. 12mo, 15 cms.

Title page has initials D.D.R.C.F. (an abbreviated motto?). Woodcut portrait of Meyssonier.

IBN an-NAFIS, *c.* 1308–1388

CHÉHADÉ (ABDUL KARIM) *b.* 1922

148 Ibn an-Nafis et la découverte de la circulation pulmonaire. *Paris, Faculté de Médecine, 1951.* [*Printed in Beyrouth, 1955*]. viii, 55 pp. Facsims, bibliog. 8vo, 25 cms.

Paris Thesis, No. 1143, 1951. The MS in Arabic in the Bibliothèque Nationale, Paris, (Fonds Arabes no. 2939) is reproduced in 19 plates.

A valuable account of the history of Ibn an-Nafis by a physician of Damascus who studied the Arab MS while in Paris. Ibn an-Nafis, who was physician at Damascus and later at Cairo, described the pulmonary circulation in his commentary on anatomy in the Canon of Avicenna (Šarh tašrih al-Qanūn). His actual description is so similar to Servetus that it has been suggested that Servetus may have been influenced by the Arabic account to which he might have had access in Spain. A good account of Ibn an-Nafis is given in the Harveian Oration for 1939 by R. A. Young (see no. 186).

LEONARDO DA VINCI, 1452–1519

KEELE (KENNETH DAVID) *b.* 1909

149 Leonardo da Vinci on movement of the heart and blood . . . with a foreword by Charles Singer. *London, Harvey and Blythe, 1952.* xviii, 142 pp. Port., facsims. 8vo, 25 cms.

No. 76 of edition limited to 1000 copies.

Leonardo's MS remained unpublished after his death in the hands of Francesco Melzi (1493–*c.* 1570) until 1570. William Hunter (1718–1783) first called attention to Leonardo's drawings in his posthumous *Two introductory lectures* . . . (London, J. Johnson, 1784). Leonardo had made 30 autopsies and studied not only the anatomy of the heart but also the hydraulics of the blood current, and he depicted the coronary arteries and veins.

PAZZINI (ADALBERTO) *b.* 1898

150 Leonardo nella storia della cardiologia. *Firenze, Edizioni Mediche Italiane, 1960.* 47, [2] pp. Port. 12mo, 14 cms.

In a case with medallion of Leonardo da Vinci struck for the third European Congress of Cardiology, Rome, 18–24 September 1960.

SERVETUS (MICHAEL) 1511–1553

BARÓN FERNÁNDEZ (JOSÉ) *b.* 1904

151 Miguel Servet (Miguel Serveto): su vida y su obra. *Madrid, Espasa-Calfe, 1970.* 337 pp. Illus., ports, facsims, bibliog. 8vo, 23 cms.

A coloured photograph of the Servetus Monument in Geneva with Lukl, D.E.B., Harley Williams and Vega Diaz (an expert on Servetus) inserted.

Presented by Dr. Vega-Diaz and described by him as the best biography of Servetus. This monumental historical study has a bibliography of 299 books and 15 manuscripts. See also part 4 of Bayon (no. 200).

DRUMMOND (WILLIAM HAMILTON) 1778–1865

152 The Life of Michael Servetus, the Spanish physician who, for the alleged crime of heresy, was entrapped, imprisoned, and burned by John Calvin the reformer, in the city of Geneva, October 27, 1553. *London, John Chapman, 1848.* xvi, 198, [2] pp. Bibliog. (ftn. refs). 12mo, 19 cms.

Final 2 pp. "Works by the same author". A theological work on Servetus with many bibliographical references, and details of Calvin's defence and judgements of contemporaries.

HODGES (Sir BENJAMIN) supposed author

153 An Impartial history of Michael Servetus, burnt alive at Geneva for heresie. *London, Aaron Ward, 1724.* [1] ff., 216 pp. 8vo, 18 cms.

Osler 853. A coloured photograph of the Servetus Monument in Geneva inserted. Autograph: Samuel Sandison, Adelaide Road, Surbiton; bookplate: T.D.S.

The first English account of Servetus's life and trial. His passages on the pulmonary circulation are given in Latin and English; also his speech delivered before he was burnt at the stake. The authorship of this book was wrongly attributed by Linde to George Benson. It seems almost certain that the author of this work was Sir Benjamin Hodges; the *Dictionary of National Bibliography* notes that John Lewis (1675–1747) wrote a manuscript life of Servetus in answer to Hodges's book.

TOLLIN (HENRI) 1833–1902

154 Die Entdeckung der Blutkreislaufs durch Michael Servet (1511–1553). *Jena, Hermann Dufft, 1876.* [viii], 81 pp. Bibliog. (ftn. refs). 8vo, 24 cms.

Tollin spent twenty years in seeking information on Servetus in many parts of Europe and is said to have written 75 papers on the subject. He also wrote on Caesalpinus. He gives a German translation of the passages on the pulmonary circulation from *Christianismi restitutio.* Tollin's views are reviewed at length by Bayon (see no. 200), Doby (see no. 204) and Arcieri (see no. 159).

WILLIS (ROBERT) 1799–1878

155 Servetus and Calvin: a study of an important epoch in the early history of the Reformation. *London, Henry S. King, 1877.* xvi, 541 pp. Ports, bibliog. (ftn. refs). 8vo, 22 cms.

Publishers' catalogues, H. S. King (2 pp.) and C. Kegan Paul (32 pp.) (the latter took over the business of Henry Samuel King (1817–1878) in 1877) bound in at end. Autograph and bookplate: William Stirling (1851–1932, author of *Some apostles of physiology*, no. 195).

For early bibliography of Servetus see "Servetus Notes" by L. L. Mackall, in no. 1045, vol. 2. pp. 767–77.

WOTTON (WILLIAM) 1666–1726

156 Reflections upon ancient and modern learning. To which is now added a defense thereof, in answer to the objections of Sir W. Temple, and others. With observations upon the *Tale of a Tub*. Also A Dissertation upon the epistles of Themistocles, Socrates, Euripides, &c. and the fables of Aesop, by R. Bentley D.D. 3rd ed. *London, Tim. Goodwin, 1705.* [3] ff., xxxiv, 542 pp. 8vo, 20 cms.

Osler 5602. Wotton first drew attention to Servetus's account of the pulmonary circulation in the first edition of 1694 (2nd ed., 1697). The account in the third edition is the most complete (pp. 215–16) and is supplemented by a section in the postscript (pp. xxiii–xxix) taken from a manuscript copy of Servetus's theological work, *Christianismi restitutio.* When Servetus was burned at the stake in Geneva, 1000 copies of his book, printed in 1553 at Vienne, near Lyon, were burned with him. Only three copies are known to have been preserved: one in Edinburgh (incomplete), one in Paris, and one in Vienna.

The controversy of Wotton and Richard Bentley (1662–1742) with Sir William Temple (1628–1699) and Charles Boyle, 4th earl of Orrery (1674–1731), led to the *Battle of the Books* by Jonathan Swift (1667–1745), published with his *Tale of a Tub* in 1704.

COLOMBO (REALDO) 1515?–1559

157 De re anatomica libri xv. *Bruxelles, Culture et Civilisation, 1969.* [1], [4] ff., 269, [3] pp. Folio, 32 cms.

Facsimile reprint of the original edition, *Venetiis, ex typographia Nicolai Bevilacquae, 1559.*

Colombo studied anatomy under Vesalius whom he succeeded in 1543 as professor of anatomy at Padua, and described the pulmonary circulation in this work. The correct date of Colombo's death as against 1577 and 1564 is established by Edward D. Coppola in "The discovery of the pulmonary circulation" in the *Bulletin of the History of Medicine*, 1957, **31**, 44–77. The date 1577 refers to the death of Colombo's daughter-in-law, her epitaph being misleadingly indexed as Colombo's in F. Arisi's *Cremona literata (Parma, 1702–41).* The date 1564 is based on an epitaph bearing a dedication to Colombo's son Epiphanio by the *parentes maestissimi* of the deceased, but here *parentes* means kinsmen instead of the associated meaning of parents. The dedication by Colombo's sons to Pope Pius IV in *De re anatomica* (*2r) implores the protection of the pope for the book so that their dead father's memory might live again ("Ut igitur Beatissime Pater Realdi demortui memoria Pontifice reuiuiscat . . .").

CAESALPINUS (ANDREAS) 1519–1603

158 Questions péripatéticiennes: traduction de Maurice Dorolle. *Paris, Félix Alcan, 1929.* viii, 241 pp. 8vo, 20 cms.

Autograph: Charles Singer (1876–1960, M.D., D.Litt., D.Sc., F.R.C.P.).

This is the only translation of *Quaestionum peripateticarum libri V . . . Ed. 2* (Venetiis, apud Juntas, 1593), and has a historical introduction by Dorolle.

ARCIERI (GIOVANNI P.) *b.* 1897

159 The Circulation of the blood and Andrea Cesalpino of Arezzo. *New York, S. F. Vanni, 1945.* 193 pp. Illus, ports, facsims, bibliog. 8vo, 21 cms.

This anti-Harveian work with useful citations from Caesalpinus (Cesalpino) was critically reviewed by Charles Singer in the *Bulletin of the History of Medicine*, 1946, **19**, 122–4, and *British medical Journal*, 1946, **1**, 436. Earlier claims for Caesalpinus are dealt with by Johnson in his Harveian Oration of 1882 (see no. 179) and his *Defence* (no. 193), Willis (no. 140) and Bayon (no. 200, part 5) (RCP). Caesalpinus's priority is still maintained by Italian sources.

FABRICIUS (HIERONYMUS) ab Aquapendente, 1533?–1619

160 De venarum ostiolis, 1603. Facsimile ed., with introduction, translation and notes by K. J. Franklin. *Springfield, Illinois, Charles C. Thomas, 1933.* [xi], 98 pp. Illus, port. facsims, bibliog. (ftn. refs). 8vo, 25 cms.

Biographical notice pp. 7–18, the early history of work on venous valves pp. 19–24, the theatre of the school of anatomy in Padua pp. 25–30, bibliographical note on first edition pp. 31–36, translation pp. 41–66, facsimile pp. 67–94.

Fabricius, professor at Padua and one of Harvey's teachers, had discovered the valves in the veins in 1574 and demonstrated them in 1578. Harvey was much influenced by Fabricius in developing his conception of the circulation.

History

HECKER (JUSTUS FRIEDRICH CARL) 1795–1850

161 Die Lehre vom Kreislauf vor Harvey. Eine historische Abhandlung. *Berlin, Friedrich August Herbig, 1831.* i–iv, 5–32 pp. 8vo, 19 cms.

Manuscript notes in German. A very scarce essay on the pre-Harveian history of the circulation, perhaps the earliest monograph on the subject.

After Harvey

PRIMEROSE (JAMES) *c.* 1598–1659

162 Exercitationes, & animadversiones in librum Guilielmi Harveii, medici & anatomici in Collegio Londinensi Regii, de motu cordis et circulatione sanguinis. [*Lugduni Batavorum, ex officina Joannis Maire, 1647*]. 84 pp. 4to, 20 cms.

Abstracted from *Recentiorum disceptationes de motu cordis, sanguinis, et chyli, in animalibus* (Keynes 6).

Primerose of Hull, born in France, had studied in Paris and was acquainted with Riolan. His adverse views on Harvey were first published in 1630 in London and it is alleged that he wrote it in a fortnight (Bayon's *William Harvey, physician and biologist,* (see no. 200) part 2, pp. 85–6). It is a defence of Galen's doctrines and "abounds in obstinate denials, sometimes of what may be called perversions, of statements involving matters of fact . . ." (Willis's *William Harvey* (see no. 140) pp. 212–3).

DESCARTES (RENÉ) 1596–1650

163 A Discourse of a method for the well guiding of reason and the discovery of truth in the sciences. *London, Dawsons, 1966.* [6] ff., 127 pp. 12mo, 16 cms.

Facsimile reprint of English translation, London, Thomas Newcombe, 1649. First published in French (Paris, 1637).

Descartes accepted Harvey's doctrine of the pathway of the circulation, but he still maintained the old idea of fermentation and expansion of the blood as the propulsive force. The controversy between Descartes and Harvey on the nature of cardiac motions is discussed by R. Toellner in A. G. Debus' *Science, medicine and society.* (London, 1972, vol. 2, pp. 73–89) (RCP).

164 L'Homme . . . et la formation du foetus, avec les remarques de Louis de la Forge. Nouvelle éd. *Paris, Compagnie des Libraires, 1729.* [5] ff., 78, 148 pp., [6] ff. Illus (folding plates). 8vo, 17 cms.

Dedicatory letter by editor, Clerselier, friend of Descartes. Pp. 97–148 "Version de la préface que Monsieur Schuyl a mise au devant de la version latine [Leyden, 1662] qu'il a faire du Traité de l'homme de René Descartes".

Autograph (stamp): Dr G. Durante (?: unclear).

This book, the first French edition of which was published in 1664, is described by Sir M. Foster as the "first text-book of physiology, written after the modern fashion though in a popular way", (see no. 194, p. 58).

SAINT-GERMAIN (BERTRAND DE)

165 Descartes considéré comme physiologiste et comme médecin. *Paris, Victor Masson, 1869.* xi, 532 pp. Bibliog. (ftn refs). 8vo, 23 cms.

Contains a good account of 16th century medicine up to the discovery of the circulation; analyses Descartes' ideas and his support of the Harveian doctrine.

VALÉRY (PAUL) 1871–1945

166 The Living thoughts of Descartes. (The Living Thoughts Library). *London, Cassell, 1948.* viii, 133 pp. Port., bibliog. 8vo, 19 cms.

Contains *Discourse on the method* (pp. 35–93) in which Descartes deals with the circulation.

SORBIÈRE (SAMUEL) 1610–1670

167 Discours sceptique sur le passage du chyle et sur le mouvement du cœur, où sont touchees quelques difficultés sur les opinions des veines lactees & de la circulation du sang. [*anon.*], *Leyde, l'imprimerie de Jean Maire, 1648.* 154 pp. 12mo, 13 cms.

Provenance: "Ex libris Gomari [?] de Lieu [?] ven huus" 1649; other unclear writing.

This very rare book, cited by Weil (no. 203) and by Keynes (see no. 128, p. 452) was exhibited at the Royal College of Physicians in 1957. Published anonymously, it is listed under the works of Sorbière in N. F. J. Eloy *Dictionnaire historique de la médecine* (Mons, 1778. 4 vols). It is in the form of a letter to Dr du Prat and pp. 56–154 contain a discussion of the circulation between the author and friends. Sorbière was a strong partisan of the Harveian doctrine. He studied medicine in Paris and Holland, and visited England in 1663 but fell into disfavour on account of a published version of his visit, and returned to France. He also wrote a work on transfusion of blood from animals to man.

RIOLAN (JEAN) 1580–1657

168 Manuel anatomique et pathologique ou abregé de toute l'anatomie, & des usages que l'on en peut tirer pour le connaissance & pour la guerison des maladies. Augmenté de la sixième partie, sur les mémoires & livres imprimez de l'autheur, des traitez des veines lactées, de la circulation du sang, des ongles, des poils, des valvules des veines, et de l'anatomie pneumatique. *Paris, Gaspar Meturas, 1653.* [20] ff., 760 pp., [6] ff. 8vo, 15 cms.

This edition of Riolan's handbook contains his last word in his dispute with Harvey who never replied to it. It is cited by Weil (no. 203), and according to him, the book is very rare. Pp. 696–738 comprise Riolan's *Discours contenant le jugement general du Sieur Riolan, touchant le mouvement du sang, tant aux brutes, qu'aux hommes, tiré de la réponse qu'il a faite à Slegel et les utilitez de la circulation.*

WALAEUS (JOHANNES DE) 1604–1649

169 Medica omnia (quae hactenus inveniri potuere) ad chyli et sanguinis circulationem eleganter concinnata. In quibus multa nova, plurima renovata, utilia vero universa, non minus perspicue, quam breviter proponuntur. Atque adeo quidquid vel in insti-

tutione nervosum, vel in praxi salubre desiderati possit; solide hic, & sincere explicatur. Ab oblivionis injuria vindicare, & in lucem nunc primum proferre, voluit C. Irvinus, philosophices ac chirurgices magister Edinburgensis. *Londini, excudebat J. C. & prostant venales apud T. Davies & T. Sadler, 1660.* [8] ff., 288 pp. 8vo, 18 cms.

Wing W293. Pp. 219–88 Johannis Walaei Epistolae duae: de motu chyli et sanguinis: ad Thomam Bartholinus, Casp [aris] filium (with own title-page). Text foxed.

The first London edition of Walaeus's letters which were printed with Harvey's *De motu cordis* for the first time in 1643, and in the first London edition of 1660 (see no. 82). A French edition was published in 1647. Walaeus was a benevolent critic of Harvey.

BARTHOLINUS (THOMAS) 1616–1680

170 Epistolarum medicinalium à doctis vel ad doctos scriptarum, centuria I & II. Cum indicibus necessariis. *Hafniae, impensis Petrus Haubold, 1663.* [10] ff., 739, [1] pp., [18] ff. Illus. (2 full-page and 6 smaller woodcuts in text). 8vo, 16 cms.

Autograph: C. Mauvezin (? commune de Mauvezin, Hautes-Pyrénées).

Thomas Bartholinus, like his father Caspar (1585–1629), became professor of medicine at Copenhagen after studying at Leyden, Paris, Montpellier and Padua. He wrote several works on the lymphatics. The series of 200 letters to eminent men include letters to Harvey (pp. 105–7) and others on the circulation. (See Dalton, *Doctrines of the circulation*, 1884, pp. 216–18, (no. 192), for review of Bartholinus's *Institutiones anatomicae*).

FROMMANN (JOHANN CHRISTIAN), praeses, *b. c.* 1640

171 Exercitationem medicam, de haemorrhoidibus ad circulationem sanguinis Harvejanam accommodatum . . . praeses Joh. Christianus Frommann . . . ac respondens Johannes Roederus. *Coburgi, typis Ducalibus exscripsit Johannes Conradus monachus, 1669.* [2] ff., 44 pp. 4to, 20 cms.

A very early work accepting Harvey's view of the circulation.

HILL (OLIVER) *b.* 1630?

172 The fifth Essay of D.M., a Friend of truth and physick, against the circulation of the blood. Showing its absurdity and impossibility, and the cause of pulsation; and of the motion is (*sic*) seen by means of the microscopes in the blood, and its vessels. [i.e. first part]. [*anon.*]. *London, Edward Evetts, 1700.* 88 pp. 8vo, 18 cms.

Wing H2005, Osler 744. This first part is anonymous. This copy lacks leaf A2 (pp. 3–4) which presumably carried a dedication (catchword "To" at the bottom of p. 2): this has been cut out. The copy in the Royal College of Physicians library also lacks A2, and the dedication is not mentioned by Osler. The type decreases in size at p. 84 and still further at the end, p. 88, as noted by Osler.

[*and*] The second part of the book against the circulation of the blood. And the first part having shew'd the absurdity, nonsense, and impossibility of that blind hypothesis. This shews the true cause of the motion is (*sic*) seen in the blood; and of the pulsation of the heart and arteries, by set times or intervals: by a way more agreeable to reason and to nature than any grounded and built upon that supposition. To wit, by the heat of life kindling in the left ventricle, and breaking out into flames and flashes, like the lightning, (which shines but from time to time) and making a puff and blast: the first

whereof swells the heart; and the other moves the blood. By Oliver Hill. *London, I. Dawks, 1701.* [2] ff., 16, 89–158 pp., [1] f. 8vo, 18 cms.

This part has a dedication "To the learned gentlemen of the house in Warwick-Lane" (i.e. the Royal College of Physicians of London) signed by Oliver Hill. Osler has collective title-page for the two parts which is lacking in this copy. The British Library has a third part dated 1701.

A curious diatribe against the circulation with liberal citations from the Scriptures. The author is the same Oliver Hill who was admitted to St. John's College, Cambridge, in 1648 aged 18 and became F.R.S. in 1676. Thomas Birch describes Hill's disputing the use of quicksilver and spirits of wine in the making of baroscope (*History of the Royal Society*, 1757, vol. 3, p. 360), his claims to generate animals from maydew and wash them out of their cells by black pepper in distilled water (pp. 366–7), and his dispute with Hooke in which he maintained "that there was no such thing as gravity in air" (p. 371) although his experiment to prove it failed (p. 374). Hill alludes to this and to his diatribe against circulation of the blood at the beginning of his book *A Rod for the back of fools* . . . London, William Turner, 1702, p. 5 (RCP): "I have silenced *Keith* the Renegado Quaker, who wounded Truth and Scripture through the sides of the Quakers, because I did not find in him the Lips of Knowledge. And I have done the same with the Doctors of Physick,"—the Royal College of Physicians—"in the matter of the Blood's pretended Circulation; and with the Society of the College of *Gresham*,"—the Royal Society—"in the case of their Pressure and Gravitation of Air, and other Errors of theirs." Asked by the Royal Society in February 1678 (Birch, vol. 3, p. 384) for a report on a discourse, he returned the discourse with an impolite sentence in Latin; presumably after this his connection with the Society ceased. The date of his death appears to be unknown.

FOUQUET (Henri) 1727–1806

173 Praelectiones medicae decem, habitae in Ludovicaeo medico Monspeliensi, prò Regia Cathedra vacante per obitum N. D. Gabrielis-Francisci Venel . . . *Monspelii, apud Joannem Franciscum Picot, 1777.* i–xii, 13–110 pp. Bibliog. (ftn. refs). 8vo, 19 cms.

The first two lectures ('De certis & dubiis in systemate Harveiano de circulatione' pp. 13–26, 'De veterum doctrina circà sanguificationem' pp. 27–40) deal with Harvey and the circulation.

Autograph: D. C. Francisco Seysiriat ab auctore colendissimo offertur hoc opusculum.

Fouquet practised at Montpellier where he was elected professor at the age of 60. He is best known for his *Essai sur le pouls* (see nos. 37–8).

EWING (Alexander)

174 Observations on the Harveian doctrine of the circulation of the blood, in reply to those lately advanced by George Kerr Esq. *London, Longman, Hurst, Rees, Orme and Brown, T. and G. Underwood; Edinburgh, W. Blackwood; Aberdeen, A. Brown, 1817.* [vi], xviii, 251 pp. Bibliog. (ftn. refs). 8vo, 20 cms.

Presentation copy to Dr. P. Blaikie, M.D.; R. Maitland to P. Jamieson April 1871 (possibly Patrick Jamieson, a Peterhead doctor).

A defence of Harvey in reply to George Kerr's essay, *Observations on the Harveian doctrine of the circulation of the blood*. London, Longman [and others], 1816. Callisen gives a list of reviews, one of which (*Edinburgh medical and surgical Journal*, 1817, **13**, 501–7), covers Ewing's defence also. A second edition of Kerr (London, J. Callow, 1819) is in the Royal College of Physicians' library.

COXE (John Redman) 1773–1863

175 An Inquiry into the claims of Doctor William Harvey to the discovery of the circulation of the blood; with a more equitable retrospect of that event. To which is added, an introductory lecture, . . . in vindication of Hippocrates from the sundry charges of

ignorance preferred against him by the late Professor Rush. *Philadelphia, E. L. Carey & A. Hart, J. G. Auner, 1834.* xxvi, 27–258 pp. Bibliog. 8vo, 22 cms.

Pp. i–iv wanting—? first leaf (blank) and half-title. Text foxed.

Coxe's *Inquiry* is an anti-Harveian work analysing Harvey's *De motu cordis* in detail and citing contemporary writers. The appendix contains a remarkably comprehensive bibliography of early works on the circulation, and gives the first reference in English to Maurocordato, later cited by Bayon (see no. 200). An Italian translation of Maurocordato is now in R.C.P. library (*Pneumaticum instrumentum circulandi sanguinis sive de motu et usu pulmonum.* Firenze, 1965).

MEAD (ALFRED)

176 A Book for the public. New discovery. The causes of the circulation of the blood; and the true nature of the planetary system. Proposing, also, a natural adjustment of the measures of time and space, for parliamentary adoption; and shewing how the above discovery may be applied to the further prolongation of health and life. *London, A. Mead [privately printed], 1848.* 61, [1] pp. 8vo, 22 cms.

A curious work explaining the circulation by physical principles and a discussion on the nature and properties of light.

JEŽEK (F.)

177 Umsturz der Harvey'schen Lehre vom Blutkreislaufe und Erklärung der natürlichen Blutbewegung. *Leipzig, Peter Hobbing, 1892.* vii, 61 pp. Illus. 8vo, 25 cms.

Ježek was a very late opponent of Harvey and claimed that the lungs and not the heart should be regarded as the main cause of the circulation. (See Wilson no. 246 and Carson no. 253).

Harveian Orations

Selected Harveian Orations, delivered at the Royal College of Physicians of London, dealing with Harvey and the history of the circulation. For other Harveian Orations, see nos. 178–90, 666, 689, 719, 877, 882, 1005, 1014, 1112.

A complete list of Harveian Orators since 1657, with their subjects is maintained at the College, together with a complete set of those published. The manuscript of some unpublished orations is also available, either in the original or photocopied. The most complete list of orators to be published is to be found in Wm Munk's *Roll of the Royal College of Physicians of London* (London, 1878–1968. 5 vols); see vol. 3, pp. 360–4, vol. 4, pp. 612–14; vol. 5, pp. 470–1.

The content of the orations, with other miscellaneous facts about them, has been the subject of comment in *Bibliotheca Osleriana* (Oxford, 1929, p. 83), *British medical Journal*, 1947, **2**, 622–3, and RCP *College Commentary*, 1972, **7**, 14–16.

OGLE (JOHN WILLIAM) 1824–1905

178 The Harveian Oration 1880, with additional notes and an appendix. *London, [privately printed], 1881.* [iii], 209 pp. Port., bibliog. (ftn. refs). 8vo, 23 cms.

The frontispiece is a plate of Harvey with the two children of Charles I at the Battle of Edge Hill, 1642.

Contains much information on Harvey and the circulation. In appendix p. 166, details of Marshall Hall (1790–1857) and resuscitation from drowning.

JOHNSON (Sir GEORGE) 1818–1896

179 The Harveian Oration delivered at the Royal College of Physicians June 24, 1882. *London, Smith, Elder, 1882.* 64 pp. Illus., bibliog. (ftn. refs). 8vo, 18 cms.

Deals with Italian claims for Caesalpinus as discoverer of the circulation, mainly advanced in *La Scoperta della circolazione del sangue* (Milano, 1876) by Professor Giulio Ceradini (1844–1894).

BRUNTON (Sir THOMAS LAUDER) 1844–1916

180 Modern developments of Harvey's work: the Harveian Oration 1894 delivered before the Royal College of Physicians, October 18th, 1894. *London, Macmillan, 1894.* 35 pp. Bibliog. (ftn. refs). 8vo, 22 cms.

PAYNE (JOSEPH FRANK) 1840–1910

181 Harvey and Galen: the Harveian Oration delivered before the Royal College of Physicians October 19, 1896. *London, Henry Frowde, 1897.* 52 pp. Bibliog. 8vo, 23 cms.

Important historical work on Galen's doctrines of the circulation.

MOORE (Sir NORMAN) 1847–1922

182 The Harveian Oration delivered before the Royal College of Physicians of London on October 18, 1901. *London, John Murray, 1901.* 59 pp. Bibliog. (ftn. refs). 8vo, 22 cms.

Deals with Harvey's friends and contemporaries.

OSLER (Sir WILLIAM) 1849–1919

183 The Growth of truth as illustrated in the discovery of the circulation of the blood: being the Harveian Oration delivered at the Royal College of Physicians, London, October 18, 1906. *London, Henry Frowde, 1907.* 44 pp. 8vo, 23 cms.

Third impression, originally published 1906. A classic oration in Osler's best style.

CRAWFURD (Sir RAYMOND HENRY PAYNE) 1865–1938

184 On forerunners of Harvey in antiquity: the Harveian Oration for 1919 delivered before the Royal College of Physicians of London on St. Luke's day (October 18th). *London, Adlard & West Newman, 1919.* 40 pp. 8vo, 20 cms.

Autograph: Charles Singer (1876–1960, M.D., D.Litt., D.Sc., F.R.C.P., M.R.C.S., F.S.A.). Covers Aristotle, Erasistratus and Galen.

LANGDON-BROWN (Sir WALTER LANGDON) 1870–1946

185 The Background to Harvey: the annual Harveian Oration delivered before the Royal College of Physicians on October 19th, 1936. *London, British Medical Association, 1936.* 21 pp. 8vo, 22 cms.

Reprinted from *British medical Journal*, 1936, 2, 793–9.

YOUNG (Sir ROBERT ARTHUR) 1871–1959

186 The Pulmonary circulation—before and after Harvey: the Harveian Oration, 1939, delivered at the Royal College of Physicians on December 15th, 1939. *London, Headley, [1940?].* 32 pp. Bibliog. 8vo, 22 cms.

A valuable history of the pulmonary circulation, citing English translation of Ibn-an-Nafis.

HUNTER (Donald) *b.* 1898

187 Harvey and his contemporaries: the Harveian Oration for 1957. *London, Lancet, 1957.* 28 pp. Bibliog. 8vo, 22 cms.

Reprinted from *Lancet*, 1957, **2**, 811–19.

KEYNES (Sir Geoffrey Langdon) *b.* 1887

188 Harvey through John Aubrey's eyes: the 254th Harveian Oration delivered at the Royal College of Physicians, 17 October 1958. *London, Lancet, 1958.* 23 pp. Bibliog.

Reprinted from *Lancet*, 1958, **2**, 859–65, with additions.

THOMSON (Sir Arthur Peregrine) *b.* 1890

189 The Consummation of William Harvey: the Harveian Oration 1961. *London, British Medical Association, 1961.* 22 pp. Bibliog. 8vo, 22 cms.

Reprinted from *British medical Journal*, 1961, **2**, 1303–09.

"The most important Harveian oration for very many years." D.E.B. (pencilled note on fly-leaf). Deals with the work of Harvey's successors on the circulation and respiration.

BEDFORD (Davis Evan) *b.* 1898

190 Harvey's third circulation: De circulo sanguinis in corde: the Harveian Oration of 1968. *London, British Medical Association, 1968.* [ii], 15 pp. Bibliog. 8vo, 22 cms.

Reprinted from *British medical Journal*, 1968, **4**, 273–7.

Deals with the history of the coronary circulation.

History and Bibliography

FLOURENS (Marie Jean Pierre) 1794–1867

191 Histoire de la découverte de la circulation du sang. 2ᵉ éd. *Paris, Garnier frères, 1857.* 284 pp. Bibliog. (ftn. refs). 12mo, 18 cms.

Provenance: unidentified foreign bookplate.

First edition, 1854. The classical French history of the discovery of the circulation.

DALTON (John Call) 1825–1889

192 Doctrines of the circulation: a history of physiological opinion and discovery, in regard to the circulation of the blood. *Philadelphia, Henry C. Lea's son, 1884.* i–xi, [12]–296 pp. Bibliog. (ftn. refs). 8vo, 21 cms.

Presentation copy: "Viva Sherman, from my uncle J. C. Dalton, 1884".

A valuable history of the discovery of the circulation from Aristotle to Harvey. The appendix gives lengthy quotations from early Greek and Latin texts. This book has now become scarce.

JOHNSON (Sir George) 1818–1896

193 A Defence of Harvey as the discoverer of the circulation of the blood in reply to Prof. Scalzi, of Rome. *London, Smith, Elder, 1884.* [ii], 23 pp. 8vo, 18 cms.

Publisher's catalogue (2 pp.) bound in. This *Defence* was written in reply to Scalzi's defence of Caesalpinus as the discoverer of the circulation of the blood, a view which Johnson had previously rejected in his Harveian Oration of 1882 (see no. 179). Professor Francesco Scalzi (1821–1889) was a supporter of Johnson's previous opponent Ceradini (see no. 179), and had written *Andrea Cesalpino, scopritore della circolazione del sangue* (Roma, 1876) previous to the address attacked by Johnson.

George Johnson is best known for his work on Bright's disease (see no. 722) and the arteriolar lesions ("Lumleian lectures on the muscular arterioles...", *British medical Journal*, 1877, **1**, 443–7, 473–5, 503–5, 539–40, 577–80), and for his paper on gallop rhythm ("A Clinical lecture on triple pericardial friction-sound, and on reduplication of the first sound of the heart" in his *Medical lectures and essays*. London, Churchill, 1887, pp. 521–40; reprinted with slight amendments from *Lancet*, 1876, **1**, 697–701).

FOSTER (Sir MICHAEL) 1836–1907

194 Lectures on the history of physiology, during the sixteenth, seventeenth and eighteenth centuries. (Cambridge Natural Science Manuals. Biological Series). *Cambridge, University Press, 1901.* [ix], 310 pp. Port., bibliog. 8vo, 23 cms.

Contains an important history of the circulation from Vesalius to Malpighi, with translated passages from Colombo, Servetus and Caesalpinus.

STIRLING (WILLIAM) 1851–1932

195 Some apostles of physiology, being an account of their lives and labours; labours that have contributed to the advancement of the healing art as well as to the prevention of disease. *London, privately printed by Waterlow & Sons, 1902.* [iv], iv, 129 pp. Illus, ports, facsims. Folio, 34 cms.

The biographies cover the discovery of the circulation and its physiology before and after Harvey, and include among others Vesalius, Servetus, Fabricius, Casserius, Gaspare Aselli, Harvey, Thomas Bartholinus, Borelli, Malpighi, Descartes, Stensen, Nehemiah Grew, Frederik Ruysch, Leeuwenhoek, Willis, Vieussens, Lower, Mayow, Boerhaave, René A. F. De Réaumur, Haller, John Hunter, Spallanzani, Priestley, and Hales.

JACQUINOT (LOUIS) *b.* 1879

196 Histoire de la découverte de la circulation à Lyon. (Thesis, Lyon, No. 122, 1904). *Lyon, R. Schneider, 1904.* 155 pp. Diagr., bibliog. 4to, 26 cms.

The author seeks to prove that Honoré Fabri (1607–1688), professor of philosophy at the College of the Trinity at Lyon for fifty years, taught the circulation publicly prior to Harvey's *De Motu Cordis*, but did not publish it until 1666 in his *Tractatus Duo*. Even Coxe, an anti-Harveian, ridicules this claim. Includes some interesting details of Servetus.

SINGER (CHARLES JOSEPH) 1876–1960

197 The Discovery of the circulation of the blood. (Classics of Scientific Method). *London, G. Bell, 1922.* x, 80 pp. Illus, ports, facsims, bibliog. 8vo, 19 cms.

PARSONS (EMILY WINIFRED)

198 The Circulation of the blood. (Sheldon Books of Popular Science). *London, Sheldon Press, 1934.* 204 pp. Illus, diagrs. 8vo, 19 cms.

A popular work on the circulation with a chapter on the historical aspects.

ASCHOFF (KARL ALBERT LUDWIG) 1866–1942

199 Über die Entdeckung des Blutkreislaufs: eine Stellungnahme zum Streit um William Harvey und ein Ausblick auf die spätere Entwicklung der Geschichte der Medizin. (Freiburger Forschungen zur Medizingeschichte Heft 1). *Freiburg im Breisgau, Hans Speyer Verlag, Hans Ferdinand Schulz, 1938.* 47, [1] pp. 8vo, 22 cms.

Gives full citations of pertinent passages from Servetus, Colombo, Caesalpinus and Harvey.

BAYON (HENRY PETER GEORGE) 1876–1952

200 William Harvey, physician and biologist: his precursors, opponents and successors [in 5 parts].

Reprinted from *Annals of Science*, 1938, **3**, 59–118 (parts 1 and 2), 435–56 (part 3); 1939, **4**, 65–106 (part 4), 329–89 (part 5). Illus, ports, facsims, bibliog. 8vo, 25 cms.

Part 5 wanting in this copy, which includes his "William Gilbert (1544–1603), Robert Fludd (1574–1737), and William Harvey (1578–1657) as medical exponents of Baconian doctrines". (reprinted from *Proceedings of the Royal Society of Medicine*, 1938–9, **32**, 31–42 (*Section of the History of Medicine*, pp. 1–12). Bibliog.).

Autographs of H. J. Norman (1881–1948) and Charles Singer (1876–1960); also autograph letters from the author to Dr. Hubert James Norman and one from Charles Singer to Norman.

The most comprehensive bibliographical reference work on the history of the circulation. Part 1 covers the significance of Harvey's achievement in discovering the circulation of the blood, the first favourable mention by Robert Fludd, and the position of *De motu cordis* in experimental medicine and *De generatione* and modern biology. Part 2 outlines the reception of the Harveian circulation, consequent discoveries of the lymphatic system (Aselli, Pecquet, Rudbeck, Bartholinus) and the capillaries (Malpighi, van Leeuwenhoek, Spallanzani), literary references and very late opposition. Other parts cover Harvey's precursors: Galen, Ibn an-Nafis, Mondini de Luzzi (1270–1324), Leonardo da Vinci, Berengario da Carpi (1470–1530), François Rabelais (c. 1483–1553), Vesalius (part 3); Servetus and his followers in Italy, Poland and Hungary, Colombo and Juan Valverde de Hamusco (part 4); Ulisse Aldrovandi (1522–1605), Volcker Coiter (1534–?1574), Caesalpinus, Fabricus ab Aquapendente, Paolo Sarpi (1552–1623), and Giovanni Nardi (*d.* 1655) and claims of anticipation (part 5).

HERPIN (ALEXANDRE) 1880–

201 La Querelle de la découverte de la circulation. *Paris, J. B. Baillière, 1943.* 69 pp. 8vo, 22 cms.

Contains a useful account of Descartes on the circulation.

LATRONICO (NICOLA) and others

202 Il cuore nella storia della medicina. (Monografie Cardiologiche n. 4). [*Milano, Recordati, 1953*]. 144, [3] pp. Illus, ports, facsims, bibliog. 8vo, 25 cms.

Deals with Malpighi, Valsalva, Morgagni, Lancisi, Albertini, etc. Profusely illustrated.

WEIL (ERNST) 1891–1965

203 The Echo of Harvey's *De motu cordis* (1628) 1628–1657.

Reprinted from *Journal of the History of Medicine and allied Sciences*, 1957, **12**, 167–74. Bibliog. Marginal notes by DEB referring to books in the library.

A valuable bibliography of early works on the circulation after *De motu cordis*. Dr. Weil was not only the author of papers on the history of medicine and science, but was also an antiquarian bookseller in this field.

DOBY (Tibor) *b.* 1914

204 Discoverers of blood circulation from Aristotle to the times of Da Vinci and Harvey. Preface by John F. Fulton. (The Life of Science Library no. 40). *London, New York & Toronto, Abelard-Schuman, 1963.* [xvii], 285 pp. Illus, ports, tables, bibliog. 8vo, 22 cms.

A lively history of the discovery of the circulation before and after Harvey.

PAGEL (Walter) *b.* 1898

205 William Harvey's biological ideas: selected aspects and historical background. *Basel, New York, S. Karger, 1967.* 394 pp. Illus, ports, facsims, bibliog. 8vo, 25 cms.

An exhaustive analysis of the history of the circulation, liberally annotated and illustrated.

MATTIOLI (Mario)

206 La Scoperta della circolazione del sangue. *Napoli, Edizioni Scientifiche Italiane, 1972.* [v], 351, [1] pp. Illus, ports, facsims, bibliog. 8vo, 25 cms.

Inserted a letter of thanks to the author via the publisher.

EARLY WORKS ON THE HEART AND CIRCULATION AFTER HARVEY

Early works on the heart and circulation after Harvey deal with the discovery of the lymphatics; the earliest works on heart disease such as Annibale Albertini (no. 207), Bulgezio (no. 211), Alos (no. 222) and Senac (no. 247), Marshall Hall (no. 258) and Haller (nos. 241–2) contain good accounts of the peripheral circulation. Latin texts such as those of Chirac, Scaramucci, Maurocordato, Bohn, Brun, etc. are now virtually unobtainable, but Sprengel-Jourdan (no. 1026) vol. 4, covers these authors.

ALBERTINI (Annibale) *fl.* early 17th cent.

207 De affectionibus cordis libri tres . . . [Ed. 3]. *Caesenae, apud Nerium, 1648.* [16] ff., 335 pp. 8vo, 23 cms.

Pp. 5–12, 229–36 are misbound, but the text is complete. Purchased in 1970 from R. D. Gurney for £60.

According to Paul White (see no. 357), this is the earliest work on heart disease, the first edition (Venice, 1618) being pre-Harveian. The second edition was published at Caesena, 1626. It is cited by Forbes, Dezeimeris, Eloy and Haller, went through at least three editions and was evidently well regarded. Little is known of the author who lived at Caesena. He deals with anatomy, physiology, palpitation, syncope and lipothymia.

PECQUET (Jean) 1622–1674

208 Experimenta nova anatomica, quibus incognitum hactenus chyli receptaculum, & ab eo per thoracem in ramos usque subclavios vasa lactea deteguntur. Ejusdem Dissertatio anatomica de circulatione sanguinis, & chyli motu. *Hardervici, apud Joannem Tollium, 1651.* [11] ff., 204 pp. Illus (plates). 12mo, 13 cms.

Pp. 41–204 *Dissertatio anatomica . . .* with own half-title. Published in the same year as Paris first edition of Pecquet.

[*and*] VESLING (JOHANN) 1598–1649

Syntagma anatomicum... *Francofurti, sumptibus Johannis Beyeri, 1641.* [12] ff., pp. 1–194. 12mo, 13 cms.

Illustrated title-page cropped. Some pages misnumbered.

[*and*] FOLLI (CECILIO) 1624–1686

Sanguinis a dextro in sinistrum cordis ventriculum defluentis facilis reperta via, cui non vulgaris in lacteas nuper patefactas venas animadversio praeponitur. *Francofurti, sumptibus Ioannis Beyeri, 1641.* [1] f., pp. 195–[243]. Illus.

[*and*] NICOLAUS, Rheginus, *c.* 1280–*c.* 1350

De nupero Botalianorum invento, quo viam sanguinis e dextro in sinistrum cordis ventriculum afferunt. Cl[audii] Galeni Pergameni sententia. Abhinc mille quingentis annis monumentis literum publicato. [Interprete Nicolao Regio Calabro]. *Francofurti, sumptibus Joannis Beyeri, 1641.* pp. 244–54.

Title-page should perhaps have been printed on p. 245.

[*and*] BOTALLO (LEONARDO) *c.* 1519–*c.* 1587

De via sanguinis a dextro in sinistrum cordis ventriculum. *Francofurti, sumptibus Joannis Beyeri, 1641.* pp. 255–62.

[*and*] KYPER (ALBERT) *c.* 1605–1655

Medicinam rite discendi et exercendi methodus. *Lugd. Batavorum, apud Hieronymum de Vogel, 1643.* 320, [4] pp. 12mo, 13 cms.

A composite volume, now very rare. Bookplate: coat of arms of Trotter of Mortonhall, co. Edinburgh (*cf.* B. M. Franks Collection, nos. 29858–60, etc.).

Jean Pecquet, a French physician, practising at Dieppe and later in Paris, discovered the receptacle of the chyle and its continuation into the thoracic duct. He showed that Aselli's lacteals pour their contents into the receptacle and the thoracic duct pours its contents into the venous system at the junction of the jugular and subclavian veins.

Vesling met Harvey during his tour with the Duke of Lennox and wrote two letters to Harvey, one criticising Primerose (see no. 162) and Parisanus. At first he expressed doubts about the circulation which were cleared up after he received a reply from Harvey.

Folli and Botallo described patent foramen ovale as the normal pathway through the septum from right to left side of the heart, rather than Galen's invisible pores. Bayon (see no. 200) gives Folli's dates as 1615–1650. Sources also disagree about Botallo's dates.

ENT (Sir GEORGE) 1604–1689

209 Opera omnia medico-physica; observationibus curiosissimis, ratiociniisque solidissimis, ex solidiore & experimentali philosophia petitis... Nunc primum junctim edita... *Lugduni Batavorum, apud Petrum Vander, 1687.* Port. [15] ff., 629, 26 pp. 8vo, 17 cms.

Provenance: Ex libris Ferdinandi Joannis Francisci Schweinitz, Anno 728 (*sic*).

His *Apologia pro circuitione sanguinis* ([9] ff., pp. 1–418) was first published in 1641 and is now very rare. In it Ent defended Harvey against Emilio Parigiano, known as Parisanus, an elderly Venetian physician (*b.* 1567) who had studied under Fabricius at Padua. The original manuscript of this book is in the library of the Royal College of Physicians (MS 129). Sir George Ent, who graduated at Padua in 1636, was a personal friend of Harvey, and persuaded him to publish his *De generatione animalium*, and saw it through the press.

GASSENDI (PIERRE) 1592–1655

210 Petri Gassendi Elegans de septo cordis pervio observatio.

Pp. 362–4 in PINEAU (Severin) *c.* 1550–1619, *De virginitatis notis graviditate et partu . . . Accedunt alia.* Amstelaedami, apud Joannem Ravesteynium, 1663. 394 pp., [17] ff. Illus, tables. 12mo, 14 cms. First published, 1650.

This volume also contains: BUONACCIOLI (Lodovico) *d. c.* 1620 [*De foetus formatione*]. pp. 145–338; PLATER (Felix) 1536–1614. *De origine partium earumque in utero conformatione.* pp. 339–62; SEBITZ (Melchior) 1539–1625. *De notis virginitatis.* pp. 365–94. [17] ff. indexes.

Gassendi, a French prelate and astronomer, observed a case of persistent foramen ovale and opposed the Harveian doctrine in favour of Galen's route through the septum.

BULGEZIO (ATTILO) *d.* in, or before 1657

211 De affectionibus cordis tractatus in tres libros divisus. Quibus accessit De morbis venenatis, venenisq; tractatus generalis. *Patavii, apud Joannem Baptistam Pasquati, 1657.* [4] ff., 143, [1] pp. 4to, 20 cms.

De morbis venenatis . . . (pp. 103–43) has a separate title-page.

One of the earliest separate treatises on heart diseases. The section on the heart comprises (1) Anatomy of heart, arteries and respiration; (2) Palpitations of heart; (3) Syncopes. This rare book, published posthumously (see dedication by the editor, Franciscus Panizzolus), is cited by Sir John Forbes in the bibliography to his translation of Laennec (no. 458) and by Testa (see no. 449).

BETBEDER (PIERRE DE) *fl.* 1666–1689

212 Questions nouvelles sur la sanguification & circulation du sang. Ensemble, un traité des vaisseaux lymphées ou lymphatiques découverts depuis peu. Ouvrage fort curieux à toutes sortes de personnes, & très-utile à ceux qui exercent la medecine. *Paris, Jean d'Houry, 1666.* [8] ff., 152 pp. 12mo, 15 cms.

MS note on fly-leaf. Autographs: Ex libris Petri Le Clerc chirurgi Bezuae manentiae [?] 1742. (i.e. Pierre Leclerc, surgeon at ? Bezu-la-Forêt, Seine Inférieure, Normandy). Bouier (? Jean Bouhier 1673–1746 of Dijon, magistrate, had a famous library, but the ascription seems unlikely).

A rare early work on the circulation, discussing questions which had arisen since Harvey's book. The author had repeated some of Harvey's experiments.

LOWER (RICHARD) 1631–1691

213 Tractatus de corde. Item de motu et colore sanguinis et chyli in eum transitu. *Amstelodami, apud Danielem Elzevirium, 1669.* [8] ff., 232 pp. Illus (folding plates). 8vo, 16 cms.

First Elzevir edition, published in the same year as the London edition. Our copy lacks original plates; replaced by xerox reproductions. Fulton 6 (John F. Fulton. *A Bibliography of two Oxford physiologists, Richard Lower 1631–1691, John Mayow 1643–1679.* Oxford, 1935).

Autograph: Alex[ande]r [Hunter?—this name deleted].

214 *The same.* Early science in Oxford by R. T. Gunther; vol. 9, *De corde* by Richard Lower, London 1669, with introduction and translation by K. J. Franklin. *Oxford, printed for subscribers, 1932.* xxxv, [i], [120] pp., [7] ff., 220 pp., [10] ff. Illus (plates). 8vo, 22 cms.

Biographical notice pp. xv–xxxv, translation [120 pp.] and a facsimile of the *Tractatus.*

Lower came next to Harvey in time and merit as a writer on the heart (Keynes) and his book went through 16 editions. The only translations are into French (Paris 1670) and into English by

Franklin. The Royal College of Physicians has an unpublished translation (MS 402) by N. Peters (1739). Lower first noticed the difference of colour between arterial and venous blood, and by injection showed anastomoses between the coronary arteries.

215 De catarrhis 1672: reproduced in facsimile and for the first time translated from the original Latin, together with a bibliographical analysis, by Richard Hunter and Ida Macalpine. *London, Dawsons, 1963.* xxii, [i], 16, 29 pp. Facsims, bibliog. 8vo, 23 cms.

Biography pp. xi–xv, *De catarrhis:* introduction pp. xix–xxii, facsimile 16 pp., translation and notes pp. 1–13, bibliographical analysis of *Tractatus de corde*, 1672 and *De catarrhis* pp. 15–29.

Signed presentation copy from the translators to DEB 24 March 1970.

De catarrhis was added to the very rare second edition of the *Tractatus* (London, 1670) without its own title-page. A separate copy of *De catarrhis* only, lacking a title page, is in the library of the Royal College of Physicians of London.

MAYOW (John) 1643–1679

216 Medico-physical works: being a translation of *Tractatus quinque medico-physici.* (Alembic Club Reprints no. 17). *Edinburgh and London, E. & S. Livingstone for the Alembic Club, 1957.* xxiv, 331 pp. Illus (plates), port. (frontispiece). 8vo, 19 cms.

Contents: On sal nitrum and nitro-aerial spirit; on respiration; on the respiration of the foetus in the uterus and in the egg; on muscular motion and animal spirits; on rickets; to which is appended a method of treatment.

Bookplate: W. D. Foster, M.D. Cantab.

Mayow showed that only a part of the air was needed for respiration or the burning of a flame, namely nitro-aerial particles, later recognised as oxygen. The *Tractatus* was first published at Oxford in 1674.

BARBETTE (Paul) *fl.* 17th cent.

217 Oeuvres chirurgiques et anatomiques . . . appropriées à la circulation du sang, et autres découvertes des modernes; avec un traité de la peste enrichi d'observations. *Genève, Francois Meige, 1675.* [12] ff., 626 pp., [12] ff. 8vo, 14 cms.

Additional engraved title page.

Barbette practised in Amsterdam where he gained great fame in medicine and surgery. His surgery became a standard work and the early Latin text was translated into Dutch, German, French and English, the first English edition appearing in 1672 and the third in 1676. Barbette's dates do not seem to be definitely known. Although some sources (the earliest traced is the *Surgeon-General's Catalogue*, 2nd series, 1897, vol. 2) give 1629–1699, this appears to be contradicted by this volume, which mentions a widow ("la Veufve du Defunt . . . a esté cause de ce long retard"—l'imprimeur de la traduction latine, au lecteur, f.3r). This is also the basis of "[d. before 1675]" in the Wellcome Historical Medical Library's *Catalogue of printed books*, 1966, vol. 2, p. 97). Barbette was presumably still alive at the time of his *Opera chirurgico-anatomica*, 1672, containing a preface by the author.

BORELLI (Giovanni Alfonso) 1608–1679

218 De motu animalium opus posthumum. *Romae, ex typographia Angeli Barnabo, 1680–81.* 2 tom. Illus. 4to, 23 cms.

Tom. 1, wanting; tom. 2, [2] ff., 520 pp. Illus. (folding plates); the heading of the first page of text reads: Pars secunda de internis animalium motionibus, earumque immediatis causis. Some contemporary MS marginal notes in Latin. Complete set in RCP library.

Borelli, professor of mathematics at Messina and Pisa, was a leading iatro-mathematician. This second part contains his work on the circulation and motion of the heart. Unlike Descartes (nos. 163–4) he accepted Harvey's view of the propulsive power of systole. He studied the mechanics of systole, the force of the heart, and the hydraulics of the flow of blood in the arteries.

MALPIGHI (MARCELLO) 1628–1694

219 De polypo cordis dissertatio. With an English translation *A Treatise on cardiac polyps* by J. M. Forrester. *Uppsala, Almqvist and Wiksells, 1956.* [i], 123–32, 12 pp. 4to, 30 cms.

Facsimile reproduction from Malpighi's *Opera omnia* (Londini, apud Robertum Scott & Georgium Wells, 1686, tom 1, pp. 123–32). Printed for European Congress of Cardiology, Stockholm, 1956.

BLANKAART (STEVEN) 1650–1702

220 Tractatus novus de circulatione sanguinis per tubulos, deque eorum valvulis &c. Ed. 4.

Pp. 301–21 (with own title-page) in his *Anatomia practica rationalis, sive cadaverum morbis denatorum anatomica inspectio. Accedit item Tractatus novus de circulatione sanguinis per tubulos, deque eorum valvulis* &c. Amstelodami, ex officina Corn. Blancardi, 1688. [11] ff., 321, [i] pp., [6] ff. Illus. (frontispiece). 12mo, 14 cms.

Last leaf 'Catalogus operum auctoris hactenus editorum'. Bookplate with the arms of the Comte de Carburi.

Important early treatise on the circulation describing several of the author's experiments. Cited by Bayon (see no. 200, part 2, p. 108) as a pioneer of arterial injections in the study of the circulation. Blankaart (or Stephen Blancard) was a pioneer in arterial injections as a means of investigating the circulation and also published a medical dictionary (Amsterdam, 1679); the English translation (London, 1684) was the first medical dictionary to be published in the British Isles.

LEEUWENHOEK (ANTONI VAN) 1632–1723

221 On the circulation of the blood. Latin text of his 65th letter to the Royal Society (7th Sept., 1688). Facsimile, with intro. by A. Schierbeek. (Dutch Classics on History of Science, vol. 2). *Nieuwkoop, B. de Graaf, 1962.* 33, [1], 165–186, [1] pp. Illus. (folding plate), port. 8vo., 24 cms.

The introduction contains (1) a short history of the discovery of the circulation; (2) the position of Leeuwenhoek in the history of the circulation; (3) biographical data on Leeuwenhoek.

Leeuwenhoek, a draper of Delft, without scientific training, was an ingenious microscopist who confirmed Malpighi's work on the circulation through the lungs; in addition he visualised the red blood corpuscles.

ALOS (JOANNES) *fl.* 17th cent.

222 De corde hominis disquisitio physiologico-anatomica. *Barcinone, Ex typog. Antonii Ferrer, & Balthasaris Ferrer bibliopolarum, per Jacobum Gascon, 1694.* [14] ff., 247 pp. 4to, 21 cms.

Written inside front cover: Jesus Maria Joseph. Purchased from Davis & Orioli in 1955, for £35.

This book, of great rarity, has escaped mention by writers on the history of the circulation except Izquierdo (see no. 100, pp. 207–8). It is cited by Haller (*Bibliotheca anatomica*, 1779, tom. 2, p. 536), and by Hirsch (*Biographisches Lexikon*, 1929, vol. 1, p. 99), and in Chinchilla's history of Spanish medicine (*Anales historicos . . .* 1845, tom. 2, pp. 481–2).

In chapter 20, *De circulari motu sanguinis*, pp. 166–85, the author explains and accepts Harvey's doctrine. He also discussed transfusion of blood. Alos was professor of medicine and first physician to the King of Spain.

PITCAIRNE (ARCHIBALD) 1652–1713

223 Opuscula medica: quorum multa nunc primum prodeunt. Ed. 3, Edimburgensi (*sic*) auctior. *Roterodami, typis Fritsch et Böhm, 1714.* [2] ff., 283, [3] pp. 4to, 23 cms.

Autograph: D'Aumont m.d.m. 1747 (?Arnulphe Daumont, 1720–1800, professor of medicine at the faculty at Valence, contributor to the *Encyclopédie* of Diderot).

The third edition of his *Dissertationes medicae* (Roterodami, 1701).

224 The Works of Dr. Archibald Pitcairn (*sic*), wherein are discovered the true foundation and principles of the art of physic: with cases and observations upon most distempers and medicines. Done from the Latin original, with some account of the author's life prefixed. There is also added, His method of curing the small-pox, written in the year 1704 for the use of the noble and honourable family of March. *London, E. Curll, J. Pemberton and W. Taylor, 1715.* [1] f., xvi pp., [6] ff., i–vi, 7–275 pp. 8vo, 20 cms.

Autograph: N. Ashby.

Consists for the most part of translations of the dissertations published in his *Opuscula medica* including the dissertation on the circulation of the blood through the small vessels, originally published in 1693. Pitcairne, a defender of Harvey, also discussed the ideas of Hippocrates on the circulation. A celebrated Scottish physician, he became professor of medicine at Leyden in 1692. This first English edition is very rare.

VIEUSSENS (Raymond de) 1641–1716

225 Novum vasorum corporis humani systema. *Amstelodami, apud Paulum Marret, 1705.* [24] ff., 260 pp. 8vo, 16 cms.

Garrison and Morton 2729. Engraved additional title page. Title page in black and red.

Leaf 2 (with engraved arms of Guido C. Fagon, to whom the book is dedicated) wanting. Autograph: ex libris J.B.S [—; name erased] medicinae alumni in universitate monspeliensi anno 1791. This book is now very rare.

226 Oeuvres françoises de M. Vieussens, dediées à nos seigneurs des états de la Province de Languedoc. [*Toulouse, Jean Guillemette, 1715.*] 2 tom. Illus (folding plates). 4to, 28 cms.

Tom. 1 contains *Traité nouveau de la structure et des causes de mouvement naturel du cœur*, ([16] ff. (including collective title-page), 141, [1] pp., [4] ff. Illus. (folding plates)); and *Traité nouveau de l'oreille divisé en deux parties.* ([6] ff., 102 pp., [3] ff. Illus (plates)); tom. 2 contains *Traité nouveau des liqueurs du corps humain.* ([6] ff. (including collective title-page), 388 pp., [8] ff.).

Book-stamp: Grande Bibliothèque de Toulouse. Purchased from Thiébaud, 1950. See letter from Louis Deglaude inserted.

227 Experiences et reflexions sur la structure et l'usage des viscères; suivies d'une explication physico-méchanique de la pluspart des maladies. *Paris, Jean Thomas Hérissant, 1755.* [2] ff., xxxviii, 483, [4] pp. Illus (folding plate). 12mo, 17 cms.

Bookplate (armorial): Antoine Louis (surgeon, 1723–1792).

KELLETT (CHARLES ERNEST) *b.* 1903

228 Raymond de Vieussens' experiments and reflexions. (Lecture, History of Clinical Sciences Series). *Los Angeles, University of California, 1961.* [i], 13 pp. Port., facsims. 8vo, 24 cms.

MAJOR (RALPH HERMON) 1884–1970

229 Raymond Vieussens and his treatise on the heart. *New York, Paul B. Hoeber, 1932.* [10 pp.]. Illus, ports, facsims, bibliog. 4to, 28 cms.

Reprinted from *Annals of medical History*, 1932, n.s. **4**, 147–54.

Vieussens, professor of medicine at Montpellier and physician to St. Eloys Hospital, gained an international reputation by his *Neurographia universalis* (1685) and made many important contributions to the anatomy and pathology of the heart, describing the coronary arteries, the intra-mural circulation of the myocardium, and cases of mitral stenosis and aortic incompetence. Like Descartes (nos. 163–4) he still accepted the Galenic doctrine of expansion of the blood by innate heat of the heart.

MORLAND (JOSEPH) 1671?–1716

230 Disquisitions concerning the force of the heart, the dimensions of the coats of the arteries and circulation of the blood. *London, John Lawrence, 1713.* [4] ff., 88 pp. Diagrs. 8vo, 18 cms.

A curious work dealing with the physics of the circulation with some historical references. A rare work, not mentioned in reference books. The author was the son of Sir Samuel Morland (1625–1695), diplomatist, mathematician and inventor, whose posthumous work *Hydrostatics* he edited in 1697. He graduated M.D. at Leyden 1699, aged 28, and became F.R.S. in 1703. He was surgeon to the Royal Hospital of Invalids at Paris and his *Dissertation on the high operation for the stone* was translated from the French in 1729. According to the unpublished "Register of Fellows" at the Royal Society he died in 1716.

BELLINI (LORENZO) 1643–1704

231 Opuscula aliquot, ad Archibaldum Pitcairnium, Professorem Lugduno-Batavum [*sic*], in quibus praecipue agitur de motu cordis in & extra uterum, ovo, ovi aere & respiratione. De motu bilis & liquidorum omnium per corpora animalium. De fermentis & glandulis, &c. *Lugduni Batavorum, apud vid. & fil. Corn. Boutesteyn, 1714.* [10] ff., 268 pp., [1] ff. Illus. (folding plates). 4to, 20 cms.
Bound with his Exercitationes anatomicae duae de structura et usu renum ut et de gustus organo novissime deprehenso; praemissis ad faciliorem intelligentiam quibusdam de saporibus. Accedunt quaedam renum monstrorum exempla, ex medicorum celebrium scriptis collecta per Gerhardium Blasium. *Lugduni Batavorum, apud Joh. Arnold. Langerack, 1711.* [5] ff., 166 pp. Illus. (folding plates). 4to, 20 cms.

Bellini, professor of anatomy at Pisa, was an iatro-mathematician and a pupil of Borelli. He developed theories concerning the movements of the auricles and ventricles and the mechanics of the peripheral circulation. His reputation depends especially on his work on the kidneys (see his *Exercitationes . . . de structura et usu renum* above).

KEILL (JAMES) 1673–1719

232 Tentamina medico-physica, ad quasdam quaestiones quae oeconomiam animalem spectant, accommodata. Quibus accessit Medicina statica britannica. *Londini, apud Geo. Strahan & W. & J. Innys, 1718.* [2] ff., xxiv, 149, [1] f., xiii, [31], 48 pp. Tables, diagrs. 8vo, 20 cms.

Medicina statica britannica (i.e. [1] f., xiii, [31], 48 pp.) has own title-page; [31] pp. tables.
Arms stamped on front cover: [not identified].
James Keill studied the force of the heart (*Philosophical Transactions*, 1720, **30**, 995–1000) and the weight and velocity of the blood. His work is reviewed at length by Daremberg (*Histoire des sciences médicales*, 1870, tom. 2, pp. 866–74) (see no 1030). English translation in Santorio *Medicina statica*, 1723.

SANTORIO (SANTORIO) 1561–1636

233 Medicina statica: being the aphorisms of Sanctorius translated into English, with large explanations. To which is added Dr. Keil's *Medicina statica britannica*, with comparative remarks and explanations as also Medico-Physical essays on I. Agues. II. Fevers. III. An elastic fibre. IV. The gout. V. The leprosy. VI. Kings-evil. VII. Venereal diseases, by

John Quincy. 3rd ed. *London, W. and J. Newton, E. Bell, W. Taylor & J. Osborn, 1723.* viii, 344, [18], [vi], 116 pp. Illus (frontispiece, folding plate). 8vo, 20 cms.

Pp. 321–44: *Medicina statica britannica*; being the aphorisms of Dr Keil, explained and compared with the foregoing aphorisms of Sanctorius. First included in the second edition, 1720. *Medico-physical essays* (London, W. and J. Newton, A. Bell, W. Taylor, and J. Osborn, 1724. [vi], 116 pp.) has own title-page.

Autographs: Will[ia]m Hayes, E. Wyvill (possibly Edward Wyvill, 1793–1869, of Brasenose College, rector of Spennithorne, Yorkshire? There is a Reverend William Ambrose Hayes of Worcester College (B.A. 1879, M.A. 1883), son of Thomas, a clergyman of Bracewell in Yorkshire. The Yorkshire connection is conjectural; there are several graduates of the name William Hayes).

MALOUIN (CHARLES) 1695–before 1718

234 Traité des corps solides, et des fluides, ou examen du mouvement du sang, de celui du cœur, des artères, et des autres vaisseaux du corps humain, selon les loix de la mécanique de la physique & de la médecine . . . *Paris, Jouenne, 1718.* [8] ff., 135, [1] pp., [3] ff. 12mo, 13 cms.

Autograph: Le Maiguez, Doct. Med.

An early work on haemodynamics and role of the heart, arteries and veins in the circulation, published posthumously by the author's brother, Jacques-Laurent Malouin; a French translation of his *De vero et inauditu artificio quo moventur solida, unaque de cordis et cerebri motu* (Caen, 1715).

ROBINSON (BRYAN) 1680–1754

235 A Treatise of the animal oeconomy. *Dublin, George Greirson, 1732.* iv, 283, [1] pp. Illus (folding plate), tables. 8vo, 21 cms.

Our imprint reads "Dublin, printed by and for George Greirson, at the Two Bibles in Essex Street, M,DCC,XXXII". Greirson was first a bookseller (1709–15) but later printer (1715–33?). There is also a "London" imprint (in the library of the Royal College of Physicians) with the addition to the title "viz. Of the motion of the fluids through the vessels. Of muscular motion, the motion of the blood, and respiration. Of secretion. Of the discharges of human bodies". The imprint reads "Dublin, printed by George Greirson, for C. Rivington, at the Bible and Crown in St. Paul's Churchyard, London, M.DCC.XXXII". This address is that of Charles Rivington (1668–1752) bookseller.

Autographs: Fran[cis?] Duany. Ex libris [Catt?] Money. Book-stamp: Western Medical and Chirurgical Society; presentation plate from Mr Greetham?, November 24, 1846.

236 A Continuation of a Treatise of the animal oeconomy. To which is added A Letter to Dr. Cheyne. Containing an account of the motion of water through orifices and pipes; and an answer to Dr. Morgan's remarks on the first part of this treatise. *Dublin, George Ewing and William Smith, 1737.* [3] ff., 339–491 pp., [1] f. (errata), 55, [1] pp. 8vo, 21 cms.

Both *A Continuation* (1737) and *A Letter to Dr. Cheyne* (1735, i.e. 55, 1 pp.) have their own separate title-pages. The latter title concludes (after Dr. Morgan's) "remarks on Dr. Robinson's *Treatise of the animal oeconomy*".

An early work on haemodynamics and metabolism. Robinson applied Newtonian principles to the investigation of animal motion, and predicted the pulse rate from the length of the body. His book was widely quoted by Haller, Sprengel and Daremberg.

George Cheyne, M.D., 1671–1743, was a student of Archibald Pitcairne. Thomas Morgan, M.D., *d.* 1743, was formerly a minister dismissed for his deist views.

HALES (STEPHEN) 1677–1761

237 Statical essays: containing [vol. 1] vegetable staticks; or, an account of some statical experiments on the sap of vegetables. Being an essay towards a natural history of vegetation: of use to those who are curious in the culture and improvement of gardening, &c. Also a specimen of an attempt to analyse the air, by a great variety of chymico-statical experiments, which were read at several meetings before the Royal Society. 3rd ed., with amendments. [Vol. 2] Haemastatics; or an account of some hydraulic and hydrostatical experiments made on the blood and blood-vessels of animals. Also an account of some experiments on stones in the kidneys and bladder; with an enquiry into the nature of those anomalous concretions. To which is added, an appendix, containing observations and experiments relating to several subjects in the first volume. The greatest part of which were read at several meetings before the Royal Society. With an index to both volumes. 2nd ed., corrected. *London, W. Innys and R. Manby, T. Woodward, and [vol. 1 only] J. Peele, 1738–40.* 2 vols. Illus (plates), tables. 8vo. 20 cms.

Vol. 1: [3] ff., xiv, 376 pp.; vol. 2: [5] ff., xxii, [xxvi], 354, [xxii] pp. Garrison and Morton 765.

Vegetable staticks first published 1727, 2nd ed. 1731 with *Haemastatics*, first published 1733 under collective title *Statical essays*. Imprimatur of Royal Society facing title page of vol. 2, following title-page in vol. 1. The *Statical essays* were translated into German, French and Italian.

Stephen Hales, vicar of Teddington, had no medical qualifications but was one of the first to study haemodynamics by animal experiment. He recorded the arterial and venous pressures in horses and estimated the cardiac output and the velocity of the blood flow.

CLARK-KENNEDY (ARCHIBALD EDMUND) *b.* 1893

238 Stephen Hales, D.D., F.R.S.: an eighteenth century biography. *Cambridge, Cambridge University Press, 1929.* xii, 256 pp. Illus, ports, facsims, bibliog. (ftn. refs). 8vo, 22 cms.

LANCISI (GIOVANNI MARIA) 1654–1720

239 De motu cordis et aneurysmatibus opus postumum in duas partes divisum. *Neapoli, excudebat Felix Carolus Musca, 1738.* [2] ff., xxviii, 219 pp. Illus (plates). 4to, 23 cms.

Engraved title-page in red and black type.

Autograph: D. Georgius Manis [?] Cavallero Reg. Societ. Hispalens. alumno. [Hispalensis, of Hispalis = Seville?].

240 *The same.* Aneurysms: the Latin text of De aneurysmatibus opus posthumum. Rome, 1745. Revised, with translation and notes by [Mrs] Wilmer Cave Wright. (New York Academy of Medicine Library, History of Medicine Series no. 10). *New York, Macmillan, 1952.* xxxv , 362 pp. Facsim., bibliog. (notes). 8vo, 22 cms.

Latin text and English translation on facing pages.

Lancisi, physician to Pope Innocent XI, made many important contributions to the heart, injected the coronary arteries with mercury, described coronary calcification, and cases of sudden death. He also described cardiac syphilis and distension of the jugular veins in dilatation of the right ventricle.

HALLER (ALBRECHT) 1708–1777

241 Dr. Albert Haller's Physiology; being a course of lectures upon the visceral anatomy and vital oeconomy of human bodies;... compiled for the use of the University

of Gottingen . . . *London, W. Innys and J. Richardson, 1754.* 2 vols. Frontis. 8vo, 23 cms.

Vol. 1: viii, lxxxiii, 339 pp.; vol. 2: iv, 468 pp.
In vol. 1 is a long footnote (pp. lx–lxxx), Circulatio Harviana, with cross-references to the lectures. Contains important chapters on the arteries, veins, heart and circulation.

242 Deux memoires sur le mouvement du sang, et sur les effets de la saignée fondes sur des experiences faites sur des animaux. *Lausanne, Marc-Mic. Bousquet, 1756.* [1] f., viii, 343 pp. Frontis. 8vo, 18 cms.

Book-stamp: Bib. du dist[t] d'Amiens.
Haller was a versatile scientist, bibliographer, botanist, anatomist and physiologist. He was professor at Gottingen for 17 years, after which he returned to his native Berne. In these *Memoires* he supported Harvey in regarding the heart as the sole source of the circulation, but he noted the effect of respiration on the jugular veins.

WHYTT (Robert) 1714–1766

243 Essais physiologiques, contenant (1) Des recherches sur les causes du mouvement des fluides dans les très-petits vaisseaux des animaux. (2) Des observations sur la sensibilité & sur l'irritabilité des parties du corps animal, à l'occasion du mémoire de M. Haller sur ce sujet . . . Traduits de l'anglois par M. Thebault. *Paris, Frères Estienne, 1759.* [2] ff., 296 pp. 12mo, 17 cms.

Whytt, professor of medicine at Edinburgh, opposed the doctrines of Haller (nos. 241–2, 897) in favour of those of Stahl. He believed that the vital force of the capillaries oscillated perpetually and independently of the heart and so assisted the circulation. His *Physiological essays* were first published in Edinburgh, 1755.

HEWSON (William) 1739–1774

244 The Works of William Hewson, F.R.S.; ed. with an introduction ["on the life and writings of Hewson, with a history of coagulation of the blood"] and notes by George Gulliver, F.R.S. (Sydenham Society). *London, Sydenham Society, 1846.* lvi, 360 pp. Illus (plates), port., bibliog. (ftn. refs). 8vo, 23 cms.

Provenance: Medical Library, Bath.
Hewson was a pupil of the Hunters and later assisted William Hunter at the Great Windmill Street school. He described the lymphatic system in birds, fish and a turtle, for which he was awarded the Copley gold medal by the Royal Society.

SPALLANZANI (Lazare) 1729–1799

245 Expériences sur la circulation observée dans l'universalité du systême vasculaire; les phénomènes de la circulation languissante; les mouvemens du sang indépendans de l'action du cœur; la pulsation des artères. Ouvrage traduit de l'italien avec des notes, précédé d'un esquisse de la vie littéraire de l'auteur par J. Tourdes . . . *Paris, Maradan, 8 [i.e. 1799–1800].* [2] ff., 410 pp. Illus (frontispiece), bibliog. (ftn. refs). 8vo, 21 cms.

Originally published at Modena in 1773, and translated into French and English (1801.) Spallanzani was a versatile scientist, having been professor of philosophy and belles lettres at Reggio for 6 years, and next professor of natural history at Pavia. He was a great traveller, a pioneer experimental physiologist on digestion, respiration, generation and the circulation. He used the microscope to study the capillary circulation in embryos and various animals. Like Haller, he supported Harvey's view of the primacy of the force of the heart as the cause of the circulation.

WILSON (ANDREW) 1718–1792

246 An Enquiry into the moving powers employed in the circulation of the blood; in a lecture delivered at Newcastle, 28th December, 1773, to a large company of gentlemen of the faculty, and others. *London, E. & C. Dilly, 1774.* [2] ff., 64 pp. 8vo, 24 cms.

This work was translated into Italian in *Opuscoli scelti sulle scienze e sulli arti*, by Carlo Amoretti and Francesco Soave (Milan, 1779, vol. 2, pp. 255–72). Wilson was a Scottish physician who practised at Edinburgh, Newcastle and later at London. He is alleged to have anticipated Carson (see no. 253) in describing the role of the lungs and atmospheric pressure in the circulation, and certainly regarded the force of the heart as of little importance beyond the main arteries, and believed that cardiac diastole was an active suction.

SÉNAC (JEAN BAPTISTE) 1693–1770

247 Traité de la structure du cœur, de son action et de ses maladies. 2e éd. *Paris, Mequignon l'ainé, 1783.* 2 tom. Illus (folding plates), port. (frontispiece). 4to, 27 cms.

Tom. 1: xii, 532 pp. Includes portrait and plates; tom. 2: [iv], 611 pp. Bookplate and book-stamp: Brighton and Sussex Medico-Chirurgical Society, 1847.

Sénac, physician to Louis XV, wrote the first text-book on the anatomy, physiology and diseases of the heart. He was above all an astute clinician, observing the heaving apex beat, throbbing of the neck arteries, and pulsation of the jugular veins in dilation of the right heart. He recognised ossification of the coronary arteries, irregularities of the heart. First edition published in 1749.

DEGRIS (GEORGES) 1874–?

248 Étude sur Sénac, premier médecin de Louis XV (1693–1770). *Paris, L. Boyer, 1901.* 78 pp. Bibliog. 8vo, 24 cms.

M.D. thesis, Paris, 1901, no. 458.

CRUIKSHANK (WILLIAM CUMBERLAND) 1745–1800

249 Anatomie des vaisseaux absorbans du corps humain. Traduit de l'anglais par M. Petit-Radel. *Paris, Froullé, 1787.* xxii, 406, [2] pp. Illus (folding plates). 8vo, 20 cms.

Last two pages approbation.

Cruikshank, who was physician to Samuel Johnson, succeeded Hewson (see no. 244) as William Hunter's assistant at the Great Windmill Street school and later took charge of it with Matthew Baillie. He was a pioneer worker on the anatomy of the lymphatics and published his *Anatomy of the absorbing vessels of the human body* (London, 1786) (RCP) one year prior to this French translation.

ZULIANI-GIBELLINI (FRANCESCO) 1743–1806

250 De quibusdam cordis affectionibus ac praesertim de ejusdem, ut ajunt, prolapsu specimen observationibus innixum. *Brixiae, edente Nicolao Bettoni, 1805.* [ii], ix, 157 pp. Bibliog. (ftn. refs). 4to, 25 cms.

YOUNG (THOMAS) 1773–1829

251 The Croonian Lecture. On the functions of the heart and arteries.

Extracted from *Philosophical Transactions of the Royal Society*, 1809, **99**, 1–31. 4to, 29 cms.

Thomas Young, described by Garrison (Garrison and Morton 1486) as one of the greatest men of science of all time, was a pioneer in optics and the wave theory of light. He was also an accomplished Egyptologist and decipherer of the hieroglyphics. In his Croonian Lecture he clarified the physical laws governing the circulation of the blood.

LEGALLOIS (JULIEN JEAN CÉSAR) 1770–1814

252 Expériences sur le principe de la vie, notamment sur celui des mouvemens du cœur, et sur le siège de ce principe; suivies du rapport fait à la première classe de l'Institut sur celles relatives aux mouvemens du cœur. *Paris, D'Hautel, 1812.* [v], xxiv, 365, 16 pp. Illus. (folding plate). 8vo, 21 cms.

Garrison and Morton 928. Last 16 pp. 'Catalogue des livres qu'on trouve chez D'Hautel'.

Presentation copy to M. Thénard (possibly the chemist Louis-Jacques Thénard, 1777–1857, later a baron).

Legallois studied medicine at Caen, became involved in political troubles and later settled in Paris. He was one of the first physiologists to use experimental methods and concluded that the spinal cord and sympathetic nerves supplied the stimulus to the power of the heart and to respiration. The library's copy is a very rare first edition. An English translation was published in Philadelphia, 1813.

CARSON (JAMES) 1752–1843

253 An Inquiry into the causes of respiration; of the motion of the blood; animal heat; absorption; and muscular motion; with practical inferences. 2nd ed. *London, Longman, Rees, Orme, Brown, Green & Longman, 1833.* xvii, 447 pp. Illus (plates.) 8vo, 22 cms.

Pp. 415–47 comprise a reprint of his Edinburgh thesis *Disputatio physiologica inauguralis de viribus quibus sanguis circumvehitur.* (Edinburgi, excudebant Adamus Neill et socii, 1799.) First edition (Liverpool, 1815) published with title *An Inquiry into the causes of the motion of the blood.*

Carson, originally a minister of the church, studied medicine at Edinburgh and later practised at Liverpool. He was elected F.R.S. in 1837. His M.D. thesis was not regarded favourably, but later he supported his views by experiments showing the importance of the elastic function of the lungs and atmospheric pressure in promoting the venous return to the heart. He suggested artificial pneumothorax as a therapeutic measure in 1822, but his attempt to carry it out failed owing to pleural adhesions.

COHEN OF BIRKENHEAD (HENRY COHEN) baron, *b.* 1900

254 James Carson, M.D., F.R.S., of Liverpool. (Faculty of the History of Medicine and Pharmacy. Gideon de Laune Lecture, 1962).

Reprinted from *Medical History*, 1963, **7**, 1–12. Illus, port., facsims, bibliog.

Presentation copy to DEB from author with a letter. Contains a full bibliography of Carson's publications.

SARLANDIÈRE (JEAN BAPTISTE) 1787–1838

255 Mémoire sur la circulation du sang, éclairée par la physiologie et la pathologie. *Paris, Cordier, 1822.* 63 pp. Illus (folding plate), bibliog. (ftn. refs). 8vo, 21 cms.

A rare early work in the history of the circulation, defending Caesalpinus as its discoverer, and supporting Bichat and others on the vital force of the capillaries in the circulation.

BARRY (Sir DAVID) 1780–1835

256 Recherches expérimentales sur les causes du mouvement du sang dans les veines. Mémoire lu a l'Académie des Sciences le 8 Juin 1825 avec le rapport de M. le baron Cuvier et M. le professeur Dumeril. *Paris, Crevot, 1825.* 74 pp. Illus. (plate). 8vo, 20 cms.

Plate wanting.

BARRY (Sir David)

257 Experimental researches on the influence exercised by atmospheric pressure upon the progression of the blood in the veins, upon that function called absorption, and upon the prevention and cure of the symptoms caused by the bites of rabid or venomous animals . . . with an appendix, containing the original reports of Baron Cuvier and of Professors Dumeril and Laennec . . . *London, Thomas and George Underwood, 1826.* xvi, 175 pp. Illus. (plate). 8vo, 22 cms.

Lacks plate and half title-page.

Barry, surgeon to the Forces, made experiments on horses, dogs, and donkeys, before a distinguished audience including Laennec, Cruveilhier, Edwards and Legallois. Laennec, in whose wards Barry studied the pulsation of the jugular veins, signed a report on the experiments. Barry showed the influence of respiration on filling the veins. He mentions the work of Carson in Liverpool (see no. 253).

HALL (Marshall) 1790–1857

258 A Critical and experimental essay on the circulation of the blood; especially as observed in the minute and capillary vessels of the batrachia and of fishes. *London, Sherwood, Gilbert & Piper, [1837].* [i], xviii, 187, 16 pp. Illus (plates). 8vo, 23 cms.

Last 16 pp. publisher's catalogue, April 1844.

Apparently originally published by R. B. Seeley, 1831. *Callisen*, Bd. 28, p. 359 gives a new edition by the publishers of our copy as 1837.

Marshall Hall was a successful practitioner, a prolific writer, and a keen investigator. He was a pioneer in the study of reflex action, of resuscitation after drowning, and described sudden death from arrest of the coronary circulation. The present work contains a review of the peripheral circulation and his own experimental observations.

VOLKMANN (Alfred Wilhelm) 1800–1877

259 Die Hämodynamik nach Versuchen von A.W.V. *Leipzig, Breitkof & Härtel, 1850.* viii, 484 pp. Illus (including folding plates), tables, diagrs, bibliog. 8vo, 23 cms.

Garrison and Morton 771. Book-label. Henri Anière, bookseller, Paris.

Contains a chapter on the pulse (chapter 14, Vom Pulse, pp. 407–45).

MAREY (Etienne Jules) 1830–1904

260 Physiologie médicale de la circulation du sang, basée sur l'étude graphique des mouvements du cœur et du pouls artériel, avec application aux maladies de l'appareil circulatoire. *Paris, Adrien Delahaye, 1863.* viii, 568 pp. Illus, diagrs. (sphygmograph tracings), bibliog. (ftn. refs). 8vo, 23 cms.

Signed presentation copy to Dr Bastien (could this be Henry Charlton Bastian, 1837–1915; probably, too early).

Marey, a French physiologist was a pioneer in the study of the circulation by graphic methods, and devised a clinical sphygmograph and the first polygraph. With Chauveau he was the first to perform cardiac catheterisation on living horses, and by means of his cardiac sound he recorded the intracardiac pressures in right and left ventricles and the right atrium. (See also his larger work on the circulation, no. 59).

TEXT-BOOKS AND SOME IMPORTANT CONTRIBUTIONS, 1800–1920

with some important later works

The clinical era in cardiology starts with the use of percussion, and the treatises of Corvisart, Allan Burns, Testa and Kreysig appeared prior to Laennec's *Auscultation médiate* (1819), after which rapid advances in physical diagnosis were made. The best guide to progress in the 19th century is provided by the text-books then current. In this section British text-books are followed by American, French, German, and Italian, etc. works.

Of English text-books, Hope's is the most important, but much can be learned about current practice from some of the lesser known treatises; for example, Dobell described an early cardiac bed, Fothergill, Balfour and Wardrop deal especially with the gouty heart, and Fuller, Semple and Shapter give excellent reviews of current knowledge. Of Irish text-books, those of Stokes, Hayden and Bellingham contain lengthy accounts of the fatty heart.

Among French writers, Forget is credited with establishing the back-pressure theory as a general principle in all forms of heart disease. Huchard and Germain Sée were early exponents of the coronary theory of angina in France, and Merklen's lectures, much praised by Vaquez, are still worth reading.

German treatises contain valuable and extensive bibliographies. Kreysig's is the most important prior to auscultation, after which von Dusch's was the most popular work and his diagrams have been reproduced in many other works even into the present century. Zehetmayer gave the first account of the genu-pectoral posture in pericardial effusion, and Friedreich and Fraentzel provide early accounts of left heart failure. The most extensive bibliography of cardiology is that given by Edens.

British

DAVIS (JOHN FORD) 1773–1864

261 An Inquiry into the symptoms and treatment of carditis; or, the inflammation of the heart; illustrated by cases and dissections. *London, Longman, Hurst, Rees, and Orme, 1808.* xvi, 190 pp. Bibliog. (ftn. refs). 8vo, 17 cms.

Davis was physician to the General Hospital at Bath, where this book was printed by Wood and Cunningham. The term carditis was applied largely to cases of pericarditis in older literature, with fever, tachycardia and cardiac pain. Though a colleague suggested that his cases were varieties of rheumatic heart disease, he rejected this, but subsequently (1832) he wrote on pericarditis and rheumatism of the heart. His book was widely quoted in contemporary literature, and is cited by Forbes in his bibliography, accompanying his translation of Laennec (no. 458).

262 A Second inquiry respecting pericarditis, or rheumatism of the heart. *Bath, J. Upham, 1832.* 20 pp. 12mo, 17 cms.

Presentation copy from the author. Provenance: Ex libris Medicae Societatis Edinensis (book-stamp).

BURNS (ALLAN) 1781–1813

263 Observations on some of the most frequent and important diseases of the heart; on aneurysm of the thoracic aorta; on preternatural pulsation in the epigastric region; and on the unusual origin and distribution of some of the large arteries of the human body. Illustrated by cases. *Edinburgh, Thomas Bryce; London, John Murray, J. Callow, 1809.* vi, 322 pp. 8vo, 23 cms.

Garrison and Morton 2738. Autograph: John Gillies (1792–1834, M.D. Edinburgh 1817, traveller and botanist).

264 *The same;* with an introduction by Dickinson W. Richards. (New York Academy of Medicine Library. History of Medicine Series no. 21). *New York, London, Hafner, 1964.* x, vi, 322 pp. 8vo, 21 cms.

Facsimile reprint of 1809 edition.

265 *The same.* Osservazioni sopra alcune più frequenti ed importanti malattie del cuore, sull'aneurisma dell'arco dell'aorta e sulla non naturale pulsazione nella regione epigastrica. *Milano, Giuseppe Buocher, 1816.* [iii], 228 pp. 8vo, 23 cms.

Autograph: W[illia]m M'Tyer (M.D. Glasgow, M.R.C.S.E., M.F.P.S.G. Practitioner at Maybole, Ayrshire, *d.* 1878). Bookplate: Terence East (Charles Frederick Terence East, 1894–1967, M.A., D.M., F.R.C.P.).

Besides the Italian, a German translation was published in 1813. His book became one of the standard works on the heart prior to Laennec's discovery, alongside those of Corvisart (nos. 360–65), Kreysig (no. 416) and Testa (no. 449).

Allan Burns, lecturer on surgery and anatomy at Glasgow, worked in his brother's dissecting room, but not having a university degree was unable to practise at Glasgow. However, he obtained the clinical notes of the cases he dissected and his treatise attempts to correlate the anatomical findings with symptoms, on the lines of Morgagni. The section on diseases of the coronary arteries and syncope anginosa (chapter 7) established the ischaemic theory of anginal pain. His views on the physiology of the circulation, like Wardrop's, were at variance with Harvey's. His book on the surgical anatomy of the head and neck gained him an international reputation as an anatomist. Biography by J. B. Herrick (*Bulletin of the Society of medical History of Chicago*, 1928–35, **4**, 457–83) (RCP).

CUMING (THOMAS) 1798–1887

266 A Case of diseased heart, with observations.

Pp. 319–34 in *Dublin Hospital Reports and Communications in Medicine and Surgery*. Dublin, Hodges and M'Arthur, 1822. Vol. 3 (ix, 500 pp.). Bibliog. (ftn. refs). 8vo, 22 cms.

Provenance: Corfu Medical Book Society; Aldershot Military Medical Book Club (book-stamp).

This is an early account of aortic incompetence with post-mortem, prior to Corrigan's (see no. 270) or Hodgkin's. Cuming describes visible pulsation of the arteries, the vibrating pulse, angina pectoris, and terminal left heart failure. Probably the first case of angina pectoris due to aortic disease in which coronary arterial disease was specifically excluded.

BEDFORD (DAVIS EVAN) *b.* 1898

267 An Early account of aortic incompetence by Thomas Cuming (1798–1887).

Reprinted from *Medical History*, 1967, **11**, 398–401. Bibliog. Contains a biographical sketch.

ADAMS (ROBERT) 1791–1875

268 Cases of diseases of the heart accompanied with pathological observations.

Pp. 353–453 in *Dublin Hospital Reports and Communications in Medicine and Surgery*. Dublin, Hodges and M'Arthur, 1827. Vol. 4 (xi, 599 pp.). 8vo, 22 cms. Garrison and Morton 2745.

Provenance: Ionian Military Medical Library. Aldershot Military Medical Book Club (book-stamp).

Adams was surgeon to the Jervis Street Infirmary, Dublin, and President of the Royal College of Surgeons of Ireland. His paper of 100 pages includes the first description of Adams-Stokes syndrome, a good account of mitral stenosis with arrhythmia, and cases of ruptured heart, ossific aortic and coronary disease.

ELLIOTSON (JOHN) 1791–1868

269 On the recent improvements in the art of distinguishing the various diseases of the heart, being the Lumleyan (*sic*) Lectures delivered before the Royal College of Physicians in the year 1829. *London, Longman, Rees, Orme, Brown, and Green, 1830.* [i], 35, pp. [8] ff. Illus (8 plates with descriptions on 8 facing leaves), bibliog. (ftn. refs). Folio, 44 cms.

Elliotson, physician to St. Thomas's Hospital, and later professor of medicine at University College, was unrivalled as a clinical teacher in his time and one of the first to teach stethoscopy, but fell into disrepute when he adopted mesmerism and phrenology in his teaching. These Lumleian Lectures contained much that was new at this date on murmurs and valvular disease. The book is now very rare; the engravings are by Skelton who did the engravings for Baillie's *Morbid anatomy* (2nd ed., see no. 901).

CORRIGAN (Sir DOMINIC JOHN) 1802–1880

270 On permanent patency of the mouth of the aorta, or inadequacy of the aortic valves.

Pp. 225–45 in *Edinburgh medical Journal*. Edinburgh, Adam Black, 1832. Vol. 37 (x, 450 pp.). Illus. (plate with 3 figures), bibliog. (ftn. refs). 8vo, 22 cms.

Garrison and Morton 2748. Plate bound upside down and facing p. 224.

Corrigan's classical account of aortic incompetence. The volume also includes a review (pp. 385–408) of the first edition of Hope's *Treatise on the diseases of the heart and great vessels*. For papers on the history of aortic incompetence, see no. 999.

HOPE (JAMES) 1801–1841

271 A Treatise on the diseases of the heart and great vessels, and on the affections which may be mistaken for them: comprising the author's view of the physiology of the heart's action and sounds, as demonstrated by his experiments on the motions and sounds in 1830, and on the sounds in 1834–5. 3rd ed. *London, John Churchill, 1839.* xxxvi, 639 pp. Illus (plates), bibliog. (ftn. refs). 8vo, 23 cms.

Illustrated publisher's catalogue for 1840 (16 pp.) bound in at front.

The first edition, 1832, was reviewed in *Edinburgh medical Journal*, 1832, **37**, 385–408 (no. 270): "In conclusion, the treatise of Dr Hope is at present the best in the English language on the subject of diseases of the organs of circulation". The second edition appeared in 1835.

272 *The same.* Von den Krankheiten des Herzens und der grossen Gefässe. Uebersetzung aus dem Englischen: mit einem Vorworte, Anmerkungen und Zusätzen herausgegeben von Dr. Ferd. Wilh. Becker. *Berlin, Theod. Christ. Friedr. Enslin, 1833.* xxx, 505 pp. Illus. (plate), bibliog. (ftn. refs). 8vo, 21 cms.

Contemporary marginal notes in German. Autograph: Dr. Friedrich Roth.

HOPE (JAMES)

273 *The same*. Tratto delle malattie del cuore e dei vasi maggiori . . . Traduzione dall'inglese del dottore Francesco Airoldi, fatta sulla terza ed ultima edizione di Londra . . . *Milano, Vincenzo Guglielmini, 1844.* 2 vol. Illus (plates), bibliog. (ftn. refs). 8vo, 22 cms.

Uncut copy in four fascicules with original wrappers. Vol. 1 (fascicules 1–2): [vii], xxii, 326, [5] pp.; vol. 2 (fascicules 3–4): [iv], 413 pp.

Provenance: Biblioteca Ospedale Civile Venezia.

HOPE (ANNE), formerly FULTON, 1809–1887

274 Memoir of the late James Hope, M.D., physician to St. George's Hospital, &c. &c. by Mrs. Hope. To which are added Remarks on classical education, by Dr. Hope; and, Letters from a senior to a junior physician, by Dr. Burder. The whole edited by Klein Grant. 3rd ed. *London, J. Hatchard, 1844.* xv, 365 pp. 8vo, 21 cms.

Autograph: Revd. E. Williams, Priston Rectory [Somerset], 1844.

First edition was published in 1842. Hope began to use the stethoscope about 1820, while a student at Edinburgh, and later spent a year in Paris under Andral and Corvisart. His text-book was a masterpiece far outclassing any previous work on the heart, and represented the consummation of Laennec's discovery in regard to the heart. Hope married Anne Fulton in 1831 and died of tuberculosis aged 39.

DAVIES (THOMAS) 1792–1839

275 Lectures on the diseases of the lungs and heart. *London, Longman, Rees, Orme, Brown, Green & Longman, 1835.* xvi, 512 pp. Tables, 8vo, 23 cms.

Provenance: Fort Pitt Medical Library (book-stamp), purchased 30 Oct. 1837.

German translation, 1836. Davies founded the Royal Hospital for Diseases of the Chest, developed tuberculosis and moved to Paris where he studied at the Necker Hospital under Laennec, graduated M.D. Paris in 1812, and introduced the stethoscope to London where he became assistant physician to the London Hospital.

RAMADGE (FRANCIS HOPKINS) 1793–1867

276 Asthma, its varieties and complications: or, researches into the pathology of disordered respiration; with remarks on the treatment applicable to each variety: illustrated by cases, and plates coloured from nature. Also, A Succinct treatise on the principal diseases of the heart. 2nd ed. *London, Longman, Brown, Green & Longmans, 1847.* xxiii, 484 pp. Illus (coloured plates). 8vo, 23 cms.

Autograph: John Cree Innis [?], 21 Exchange Square, Glasgow.

First edition, 1835. A brief account of current views on heart disease including angina pectoris, and a good account of the nervous heart, palpitation and left chest pain.

LATHAM (PETER MERE) 1789–1875

277 Lectures on subjects connected with clinical medicine comprising diseases of the heart. 2nd ed. *London, Longman, Brown, Green and Longmans, 1846.* 2 vols. Bibliog. (ftn. refs). 8vo, 20 cms.

Vol. 1: xxiii, 374 pp. (Publisher's catalogue, April 1847, [2], 32 pp. bound in at end); vol. 2: xi, 419 pp. (Publisher's catalogue, October 1847, 32 pp. bound in at end).

Autograph: H[enr]y Denne (possibly Henry Denne, F.R.C.S., L.S.A., surgeon of the Kent and Canterbury Hospital until his death in 1875).

The first edition was published in 1836, and a German translation in Leipzig in 1847. Latham's lectures were highly regarded by contemporary writers, and his Harveian Oration (1839) was praised by Sir Thomas Watson for its elegant latinity. His lectures on angina pectoris are especially interesting and include the post-mortem on Arnold of Rugby who died in his first attack and had only one coronary artery. Latham was physician to the Middlesex Hospital, 1815–1824, and later to St. Bartholomew's Hospital, and was known as "Heart Latham".

GRAVES (ROBERT JAMES) 1797–1853

278 Clinical lectures on the practice of medicine. To which is prefixed a criticism by Professor Trousseau. Reprinted from the second edition, ed. by the late Dr. Neligan. *London, New Sydenham Society, 1884.* 2 vols. Tables, bibliog. (ftn. refs). 8vo, 23 cms.

Vol. 1: xxiv, 673 pp.; vol. 2: xii, 651 pp.

Graves, one of those who made the Dublin School of Medicine famous, gives a good account of pericarditis (vol. 2, pp. 170–207) and of Graves' disease (exophthalmic goitre; palpitation of the heart with enlargement of the thyroid gland, vol. 2, pp. 220–3. See also Garrison and Morton 3815). Like Stokes, especially (see no. 470) he was a pioneer in the use of the stethoscope in Dublin. The second edition of Graves' book was published in 1848, the first edition (*A System of clinical medicine*) in 1843 (Garrison and Morton 2218).

STOKES (WILLIAM) 1804–1878

279 Observations on some cases of permanently slow pulse.

Pp. 73–85 in *Dublin quarterly Journal of medical Science*. Dublin, Hodges and Smith, 1846. Vol. 2 (viii, viii, x, 606 pp.). Illus, ports, bibliog. (ftn. refs). 8vo, 21 cms. Garrison and Morton 2756.

280 Diseases of the heart and aorta. *Dublin, Hodges & Smith, 1854.* xvi, 689 pp. Bibliog. (ftn. refs). 8vo, 23 cms.

Garrison and Morton 2760. Autograph: H[enr]y Denne, 1862.

281 *The same.* Traité des maladies du cœur et de l'aorte. Ouvrage traduit, avec l'autorisation de l'auteur, par le Dr. Sénac. *Paris, Adrien Delahaye, 1864.* xix, 716 pp. Bibliog. (ftn. refs). 8vo, 22 cms.

MULCAHY (RISTEARD)

282 "Diseases of the heart and aorta" by William Stokes (1854). A modern clinical review.

Reprinted from *Irish Journal of medical Science*, 1955, no. 350, February, 53–66. Presentation copy from the author.

STOKES (Sir WILLIAM) 1839–1900

283 William Stokes: his life and work (1804–1878) by his son, William Stokes. (Masters of Medicine Series). *London, T. Fisher Unwin, 1898.* 256 pp. Ports, bibliog. 8vo, 20 cms.

Publisher's catalogue (12 pp.) bound in at end. Bibliography of Stokes' works pp. 243–7. Autograph: M. D. Genney (or Jenner?).

Stokes qualified in Edinburgh and while still a student there wrote the first treatise on the use of the stethoscope in English in 1825 (no. 470 and note). He was physician to the Meath Hospital, Dublin, a friend of Graves and a pioneer in the diagnosis of diseases of the heart and lungs. His text-book on heart disease gained him an international reputation and German (1855), Italian

(1858) and French (1864) editions were published. Unlike most of his contemporaries, he was not predominantly interested in physical signs, and regarded the state of the myocardium as more important than that of the valves and was obsessed with fatty heart as a form of myocardial disease so that it became a fashionable diagnosis. He is remembered especially for the Adams-Stokes syndrome and Cheyne-Stokes breathing. He was physician to the Queen in Ireland and honoured by the Ordre pour le Mérite by the German Emperor.

ORMEROD (Edward Latham) 1819–1873

284 Observations on the clinical history and pathology of one form of fatty degeneration of the heart: being the substance of a paper read before the Brighton and Sussex Medico-Chirurgical Society, Oct. 4, 1849. *London, Wilson and Ogilvy, 1849.* 33 pp. Illus, tables, bibliog. (ftn. refs). 8vo, 21 cms.

Reprinted from *London medical Gazette*, 1849, **44**, 739–44, 787–93, 831–7, 873–9, 917–22.

Author's presentation copy to Dr. G. Johnson (possibly George, later Sir George Johnson, M.D., F.R.C.P., F.R.S., 1818–1896).

An important paper on fatty heart, mentioning coronary disease as one of the causes. Ormerod was a pathologist at St. Bartholomew's Hospital and later practised at Brighton where he became physician to the Sussex County Hospital.

BELLINGHAM (O'Bryen) 1805–1857

285 Course of lectures on diseases of the heart; delivered at St. Vincent's Hospital [Dublin] during the session 1849–50.

In *London medical Gazette, or Journal of practical Medicine*. London, Longman, Brown, Green & Longmans, 1850. Vol. 10 ([i], 1137 pp.). 8vo, 22 cms.

His text-book published in the year of his death was based on these lectures on pp. 1–8, 89–94, 177–83, 265–71, 353–9, 441–4, 529–33, 617–22, 726–30. Bellingham was surgeon to St. Vincent's Hospital, Dublin, and an authority on aneurysm, treating popliteal aneurysm by continuous digital compression maintained by relays of students. His accounts of paracentesis of the pericardium and rheumatic heart disease are of historical interest.

286 A Treatise on diseases of the heart. *Dublin, Fannin, 1857.* xix, 623 pp. Illus. (frontispiece), tables, bibliog. (ftn. refs). 8vo, 22 cms.

Provenance: book-stamp, Middlesex Hospital Library.

MULCAHY (RISTEARD)

287 O'Bryen Bellingham—a centenary tribute.

Reprinted from *Journal of the Irish Medical Association*, 1957, **41**, 180–3. Presentation copy.

WALSHE (Walter Hayle) 1812–1892

288 A Practical treatise on the diseases of the heart and great vessels, including the principles of their physical diagnosis. 4th ed. *London, Smith, Elder, 1873.* [i], xii, 582 pp. Illus, tables, diagrs (sphygmogram tracings), bibliog. (ftn. refs). 8vo, 23 cms.

The first edition was published as *A Practical treatise on diseases of the lungs and heart, including the principles of physical diagnosis*, London, Taylor, Walton & Maberly, 1851 (Garrison and Morton 2757); 2nd ed. 1854. The third edition was divided into two parts: *A Practical treatise on the diseases of the lungs . . .* 3rd ed. 1860 (4th ed. 1871), and the 3rd ed., 1862, of the above volume.

REYNOLDS (Sir JOHN RUSSELL) 1828–1896

289 Walter Hayle Walshe, M.D.: a biographical sketch. *London, J. & A. Churchill, 1893.* 26 pp. 8vo, 23 cms.

Reprinted with additions from *Lancet*, 1892, **2**, 1535–8.

Walshe was physician to University College Hospital, professor of morbid anatomy and later of clinical medicine. He had studied in Paris under Louis and Andral before taking his degree in Edinburgh. His text-book, like that of von Dusch (no. 424), was a popular reference work on physical signs and diagnosis. He mentioned erosion of the ribs in coarctation of the aorta for the first time in any text-book, and was one of the first to recognise the presystolic character of the direct mitral murmur in mitral stenosis.

WARDROP (JAMES) 1782–1869

290 On the nature and treatment of the diseases of the heart: containing also an account of the musculo-cardiac, the pulmo-cardiac, and the veno-pulmonary functions. *London, John Churchill, 1851.* viii, i–vi, 7–587 pp. Illus, bibliog. (ftn. refs). 8vo, 23 cms.

Publisher's catalogue (32 pp.), March 1852, bound in at end.

The first part of this treatise dealing with the pathological physiology of the circulation was first published in London in 1837 (*On the nature and treatment of diseases of the heart; with some new views on the physiology of the circulation*, part 1); no more were published, although French and German editions followed. The full treatise appeared in 1851, with a second edition in 1859. Wardrop, who was surgeon to King George IV and attended him in his last illness, diagnosed as gouty heart, was an authority on aneurysm and on ophthalmic surgery and pathology.

O'FARRELL (PATRICK THEODORE JOSEPH) 1889–1968

291 An Early Victorian surgeon-cardiologist (James Wardrop, 1782–1869).

Reprinted from *Irish Journal of medical Science*, 1956, no. 366, June, 271–5. Author's presentation copy.

GAIRDNER (Sir WILLIAM TENNANT) 1824–1907

GIBSON (GEORGE ALEXANDER) 1854–1913

292 Life of Sir William Tennant Gairdner . . . with a selection of papers on general and medical subjects. *Glasgow, James Maclehose, 1912.* xi, 817 pp. Illus, ports, bibliog. 8vo, 24 cms.

This volume contains Gairdner's papers on dilated heart, cardiac murmurs, tricuspid obstruction, aneurysm of the aorta, etc., and a bibliography of his writings (pp. 799–809).

Gairdner, professor of medicine at Glasgow, is best known for his description of angina sine dolore (in Sir J. R. Reynolds' *System of medicine*. London, 1877, vol. 4, pp. 535–600, especially pp. 554, 566) (RCP), and the auriculo-systolic murmur of mitral stenosis (*Edinburgh medical Journal*, 1861, **7**, 438–53) (RCP).

MARKHAM (WILLIAM ORLANDO) 1818–1891

293 Diseases of the heart: their pathology, diagnosis and treatment. 2nd ed. *London, J. Churchill, 1860.* xvi, 276 pp. Bibliog. (ftn. refs). 8vo, 21 cms.

First edition, 1856. Markham was physician to St. Mary's Hospital and later editor of the *British medical Journal*. He translated Skoda's book on auscultation and percussion in 1853.

FULLER (HENRY WILLIAM) 1820–1873

294 On diseases of the heart and great vessels: their pathology, physical diagnosis, symptoms and treatment. *London, John Churchill, 1863.* viii, 247 pp. Tables, bibliog. (ftn. refs). 8vo, 23 cms.

Publisher's catalogue ([2], 32 pp.), April 1865, bound in.

Separate publication of those parts of his *On diseases of the chest* (1862) which relate to diseases of the heart and great vessels (*Preface*, p.v.).

Fuller, physician to St. Georges Hospital, gave a useful review of contemporary knowledge prior to the more important works of Gibson, Bramwell and Sansom. A German edition was published in Berlin, 1864.

BLAKISTON (PEYTON) 1801–1878

295 Clinical observations on diseases of the heart and thoracic aorta. *London, Longman, Green, Longman, Roberts and Green, 1865.* xii, 316 pp. Bibliog. (ftn. refs). 8vo, 22 cms.

Book-plate (armorial): Thomas Lewis (Sir Thomas Lewis, cardiologist, author of several books in this catalogue).

Blakiston first entered the church; when he developed tuberculosis, he was treated by Louis in Paris where he studied auscultation. He became physician to the Birmingham General Hospital, and a colleague of Hodgson, and published a book on chest diseases and auscultation in 1848. His book is mentioned by Austin Flint (see no. 351, p. 149).

PEACOCK (THOMAS BEVILL) 1812–1882

296 On some of the causes and effects of valvular disease of the heart: being the Croonian Lectures of the Royal College of Physicians for 1865. *London, John Churchill, 1865.* viii, 114 pp. Illus, tables, bibliog. (ftn. refs). 8vo, 23 cms.

Publisher's catalogue, October (1880!), (16 pp.) bound in at end.

297 On the prognosis in cases of valvular disease of the heart. *London, J. & A. Churchill, 1877.* 55 pp. Illus, tables, bibliog. (ftn. refs). 8vo, 23 cms.

Publisher's catalogue, July 1877 (24 pp.), bound in at end. Revised reprint of a paper in *St. Thomas's Hospital Reports*, 1871, **2**, 233–58.

Peacock was physician to St. Thomas's Hospital and the London Hospital for Diseases of the Chest. He is best known for his work *Malformations of the human heart* (no. 795).

WATERS (ALDERMAN THOMAS HOUGHTON) 1826–1912

298 On diseases of the chest: being contributions to their clinical history, pathology, and treatment. 2nd ed. *Philadelphia, Lindsay & Blakiston, 1874.* xiii, 431 pp. Illus (plates). 8vo, 23 cms.

J. & A. Churchill's catalogue, Oct. 1873 [24] pp., bound in at end. Part I, Diseases of the lungs (pp. 1–279). Part II, Diseases of the heart (pp. 281–431).

Signature: Henry March, 1874; book-label: Library of James P. Marsh, no. 1185.

Waters was physician to the Liverpool Royal Infirmary and professor of medicine at University College, Liverpool. His book comprises a series of lectures covering the heart sounds, pericarditis, valvular disease, sudden death and aneurysm. This edition, printed in Liverpool, was also published in London by Churchill, who published the first edition in 1868.

MYERS (ARTHUR BOWEN RICHARDS) 1838–1921

299 On the etiology and prevalence of diseases of the heart among soldiers. The "Alexander" Prize Essay). *London, J. Churchill, 1870.* vii, 94 pp. Tables, diagrs (tracings). 8vo, 23 cms.

Garrison and Morton 2768. Publisher's catalogue, April 1870 (40 pp.), bound in at end.

Myers, assistant surgeon to the Coldstream Guards, wrote this classic account of the soldier's heart and attributed aneurysm to tight equipment, but dealt with syphilis, tobacco, etc. Now a very rare book.

DOBELL (HORACE BENGE) 1828–1917

300 On Affections of the heart and in its neighbourhood: cases, aphorisms and commentaries. *London, H. K. Lewis, [1872] (reprinted 1876).* [xv], 124, [2] pp. Illus, bibliog. (ftn. refs). 8vo, 23 cms.

Last 2 pp. "Works by Dr Dobell" (advertisement). A list of new books published by H. K. Lewis, August 1876 ([2], 20, [2] pp.) is bound in.

Provenance: book-stamp for duplicates sold: Manchester Medical Society; autographs: E[rnest] Bosdin Leech (1875–1950, M.A., M.D., F.R.C.P.); A. H. Holmes (Arthur Hillyard Holmes, 1889–1954, M.B., Ch.B., F.R.C.P.).

Dobell was physician to the Royal Chest Hospital, and his book is of interest as showing an early cardiac bed, and dealing with clubbing of the fingers.

FOTHERGILL (JOHN MILNER) 1841–1888

301 The Heart and its diseases, with their treatment; including the gouty heart. 2nd ed. *London, H. K. Lewis, 1879.* xii, 516, [4] pp. Illus, tables, diagrs, bibliog. (ftn. refs). 8vo, 23 cms.

Last 4 pp. "Works by the same author", etc. Publisher's catalogue ([2], 20 pp.) also bound in. Autograph: Morison July 6th [18]81.

Fothergill was physician to the West London and Victoria Park Hospitals. Like Balfour, he pays tribute to Von Dusch's text-book (see no. 424). His chapter on the gouty heart was entitled "Combined heart and kidney disease" in the first edition (1872), and refers to elderly patients "pestered with gout and ultimately slain with heart disease".

SHAPTER (THOMAS) 1809–1902

302 Notes and observations on diseases of the heart and of the lungs in connexion therewith. *London, J. & A. Churchill, 1874.* xv, 237 pp. Bibliog. (ftn. refs). 8vo, 23 cms.

Publisher's catalogue (24 pp.), June 1875, bound in at end.

Shapter was physician to the Royal Devon and Exeter Hospital and gives a useful account of the general outlook on heart disease at this period.

HAYDEN (THOMAS) 1823–1881

303 The Diseases of the heart and of the aorta. *Dublin, Fannin, 1875.* xii, 1232 pp. Illus, tables, diagrs, bibliog. (ftn. refs). 8vo, 22 cms.

Provenance: East Kent and Canterbury Medical Library, December 1880.

Hayden was physician to the Mater Misericordiae Hospital, Dublin and his bulky book, now rather rare, gives an excellent account of aneurysm and fatty heart, then a popular diagnosis in Dublin. It contains many detailed case reports of interest.

SEMPLE (ROBERT HUNTER) 1814–1891

304 A Manual of the diseases of the heart, their pathology, diagnosis prognosis and treatment. *London, J. & A. Churchill, 1875.* viii, 296 pp. Bibliog. (ftn. refs). 8vo, 23 cms.

Publisher's catalogue (24 pp.), June 1875, bound in at end.

Author's presentation copy (June 1875) to the Society of Apothecaries of London (presentation bookplate; book-stamp).

Semple was physician to the Bloomsbury and Eastern Dispensaries in London. His book provides a most useful historical review of contemporary cardiology and a discussion of bleeding and depletive therapy.

BALFOUR (GEORGE WILLIAM) 1823–1903

305 Clinical lectures on diseases of the heart and aorta. 3rd ed. *London, Adam & Charles Black, 1898.* xxi, 479 pp. Illus, tables, diagrs (sphygmograph tracings), bibliog. (ftn. refs). 8vo, 23 cms.

4 pp. publisher's advertisements bound in.

The first edition was published in 1876, the second in 1882, and in this third edition the text is largely rewritten with additions.

306 The Senile heart: its symptoms, sequelae and treatment. *London, Adam & Charles Black, 1894.* ix, 300 pp. Illus, diagrs (sphymograph tracings), bibliog. (ftn. refs). 8vo, 20 cms.

Deals with the gouty heart and gouty diathesis. He mentions cardiac ischaemia, but favours the neuralgic origin of anginal pain.

SIBSON (FRANCIS) 1814–1876

307 Collected works . . . ed. [with "a short account of the life and writings of Dr. Sibson"] by William M. Ord. *London, Macmillan, 1881.* 4 vols. Illus, tables, diagrs, bibliog. (ftn. refs). 8vo, 23 cms.

Vol. 1, xliii, [i], 403 pp. (biography pp. xix–xliii); vol. 2, viii, 432 pp.; vol. 3, viii, 415 pp.; vol. 4, viii, 539 pp.

Deals with topographical anatomy of heart. Vols 3 and 4 contain his important accounts of pericarditis, adherent pericardium and endocarditis from Reynolds's *System of medicine*, 1877, vol. 4, pp. 186–528. (RCP)

SANSOM (ARTHUR ERNEST) 1838–1907

308 The Lettsomian Lectures on the treatment of some of the forms of valvular disease of the heart, delivered before the Medical Society of London. *London, J. & A. Churchill, 1883.* [iii], 93 pp. Illus, diagrs, bibliog. (ftn. refs). 8vo, 18 cms.

Publisher's catalogues ([i], 16 pp.) bound in at end.

309 The Diagnosis of diseases of the heart and thoracic aorta. *London, Charles Griffin, 1892.* xxiii, 567 pp. Illus, tables, diagrs, bibliog. 8vo, 24 cms.

Publisher's catalogue (32 pp.) bound in at end. Most chapters have bibliographies.

A standard work on diagnosis and physical signs in heart disease, which includes a long section on the sphygmograph, apex cardiogram, and venous pulse. Sansom, who was physician to the London Hospital, introduced a new pleximeter and was the first to describe the mitral origin of the split second sound in mitral stenosis (opening snap).

BRAMWELL (Sir Byrom) 1847–1931

310 Diseases of the heart and thoracic aorta. *Edinburgh, Young J. Pentland, 1884.* xvi, 783 pp. Illus, diagrs (sphygmograph tracings), tables, bibliog. (ftn. refs). 8vo, 24 cms.

Publisher's catalogue, July 1888, included ([1], 23 pp.). Autograph: J. A. Taylor, March 22nd 1889. Gives a full account of the pulse, sphygmograph, and apex tracing.

RUSSELL (William) 1852–1940

311 Investigations into some morbid cardiac conditions, including the "Cartwright" Prize Essay on "The Heart in debility". *Edinburgh, Bell & Bradfute, 1886.* ix, 148 pp. Illus, diagrs. 8vo, 20 cms.

Russell was lecturer on pathology at Edinburgh. This work deals with functional murmurs in anaemia and vegetative endocarditis.

GIBSON (George Alexander) 1854–1913

312 Cheyne-Stokes respiration. *Edinburgh, Oliver and Boyd, 1892.* [vii], 133 pp. Diagrs, bibliog. (ftn. refs). 8vo, 22 cms.

Author's presentation copy.
A valuable historical account with a comprehensive bibliography of Cheyne-Stokes breathing in the footnotes.

313 Diseases of the heart and aorta. (Pentland's Medical Series, vol. 6). *Edinburgh and London, Young J. Pentland, 1898.* xxi, 932 pp. Illus., tables, diagrs, bibliog. 8vo, 24 cms.

Publisher's catalogue (32 pp.) bound in. Extensive bibliography (pp. 888–914).
Gibson, physician to the Edinburgh Royal Infirmary, described the continuous Gibson murmur of patent ductus arteriosus. His text-book gives a very good review of contemporary cardiology with a full bibliography to each chapter, and an early x-ray of dextrocardia. His account of angina pectoris is historically important.

FOXWELL (William Arthur) 1853–1909

314 Essays in heart and lung disease. *London, Charles Griffin, 1895.* xiv, 476 pp. Illus, tables, diagrs, bibliog. (ftn. refs). 8vo, 22 cms.

Arthur Foxwell, physician to the Queen's Hospital, Birmingham, wrote especially on anaemic murmurs.

BROADBENT (Sir William Henry) 1835–1907 and
BROADBENT (Sir John Francis Harpin) 1865–1946

315 Heart disease: with special reference to prognosis and treatment. *London, Baillière, Tindall and Cox, 1897.* x, 11–331 pp. Illus, diagrs (sphygmograph tracings). 8vo, 22 cms.

Publisher's catalogue (32 pp.) bound in. Autograph: Lewis Hickey, Wyngan, January 1899, from Dr. G. V. Gilray.
"For the most part a reproduction of lectures on 'Prognosis in Valvular Disease of the Heart' delivered before the Harveian Society in 1884, and of the Lumleian Lectures at the Royal College of Physicians on 'Prognosis in Structural Diseases of the Heart' delivered in 1891." (*Preface*).

316 *The same.* 3rd ed. *London, Baillière, Tindall & Cox, 1900.* xiii, 420 pp. Illus, diagrs, bibliog. (ftn. refs). 8vo, 22 cms.

Contains additional chapters on acute diseases of the heart, endocarditis, pericarditis, myocarditis and aneurysm of the aorta.

The publication of a second edition has not been traced; a fourth edition appeared in 1906. The first, third and fourth editions were published in America at the same time. A German translation was published in 1902.

317 Selections from the writings medical and neurological of Sir William Broadbent . . . ed. by Walter Broadbent . . . (Oxford Medical Publications). *London, Frowde and Hodder & Stoughton, 1908.* viii, 444 pp. Illus, bibliog. 8vo, 23 cms.

Publisher's catalogue (Spring list 1908 of medical works "including those formerly published by Young J. Pentland", 32 pp.) bound in at end. "In the choice of Authors and Subjects, the publishers have had the advantage throughout of the advice and assistance of Wm. Osler, MD, FRS."

Contains papers on angina and pseudo-angina pectoris, hypertension and aneurysm. Extensive bibliography of Broadbent's papers pp. 431–9.

BROADBENT (MARY ETHEL)

318 Life of Sir William Broadbent . . . ed. by his daughter, M. E. Broadbent. *London, John Murray, 1909.* xi, 306 pp. Port. (frontispiece). 8vo, 23 cms.

Broadbent, physician to St. Mary's Hospital, studied in Paris and learned percussion from Piorry. His book on the pulse (1890, see no. 62), his text-book and paper on adherent pericardium (see no. 317, pp. 21–5) all became standard works. Broadbent's sign, however, was first described by his son, Walter Broadbent in 1895. For long Broadbent's three stages of mitral stenosis (cf. no. 317, pp. 12–13) became current teaching. He died of bacterial endocarditis.

CHAPMAN (Charles Williams) 1843–1941

319 Heart disease in childhood and youth. With two appendices; with an introduction by Sir Samuel Wilks. 2nd ed. *London, Medical Publishing Co., 1903* [143] pp. [various paging]. Illus, diagrs. 8vo, 20 cms.

Autograph: W. Strugnell (Walter Thomas Strugnell, M.D., M.R.C.S., L.S.A. *d.* 1927?).

First edition, 1900. Chapman was physician to the Heart Hospital, London, and this book deals mainly with rheumatic heart disease.

320 The Heart and its diseases: a handbook for students and practitioners. *Edinburgh, E. & S. Livingstone, 1927.* xii, 216 pp. Illus, diagrs, bibliog. (ftn. refs). 8vo, 19 cms.

OSLER (Sir William) 1849–1919

321 On the so-called Stokes-Adams disease (slow pulse with syncopal attacks, etc.). *London, Lancet, 1903.* 30 pp. Diagr. (sphygmograph tracing), bibliog. (ftn. refs). 8vo, 22 cms.

Reprinted from *Lancet*, 1903, **2**, 516–24.

LINDSAY (James Alexander) 1856–1931

322 Lectures chiefly clinical and practical on diseases of the lungs and heart. *New York, William Wood, 1904.* viii, 447 pp. Bibliog. (ftn. refs). 8vo, 23 cms.

Book-stamp: Public Library, Hutchinson, Kansas; autograph: W. H. Kirkpatrick M.D.

Lindsay was professor of medicine at Belfast.

STEELL (Graham) 1851–1942

323 Text-book on diseases of the heart . . . with an appendix on the volume of blood in relation to heart disease by J. Lorrain Smith. (Publications of the University of Man-

chester no. 20; Medical Series no. 7). *Manchester, University Press, 1906.* xiii, 389 pp. Illus, diagrs. 8vo, 19 cms.

Publisher's catalogue (8 pp.) bound in at end.

A cardiac classic, important in relation to mitral disease, alcoholic heart disease, etc. Graham Steell was physician to the Manchester Royal Infirmary and the leading cardiologist in the North of England at this time; he is best remembered for the Graham Steell murmur of relative pulmonary incompetence.

POYNTON (Frederic John) 1869–1943

324 Heart disease and thoracic aneurysm. (Oxford Medical Publications). *London, Henry Frowde, Hodder & Stoughton, 1907.* x, 310 pp. Illus, diagrs. 8vo, 19 cms.

Publisher's catalogue (16 pp.) bound in at end.

Poynton was physician to University College Hospital and to Great Ormond Street Hospital. He pioneered research in rheumatic heart disease in children. When a Fellow of the Royal College of Physicians, he once captained Somerset County Cricket Club.

MACKENZIE (Sir James) 1853–1925

325 Diseases of the heart. (Oxford Medical Publications). *London, Henry Frowde, Hodder & Stoughton, 1908.* xix, 386 pp. Illus, diagrs (sphygmograph tracings), bibliog. 8vo, 25 cms.

Publisher's catalogue (32 pp.) bound in at end. "In the choice of Authors and Subjects the publishers have had the advantage throughout of the advice and assistance of William Osler, M.D., F.R.S."

Provenance: presented "by a humble gastro-enterologist Tommy Hunt, Feb. 1962" (Thomas Cecil Hunt, C.B.E., D.M., F.R.C.P., M.R.C.S., *b.* 1901).

This copy of the first edition is in perfect condition.

326 *The same.* 3rd ed. (Oxford Medical Publications). *London, Henry Frowde, Hodder & Stoughton, 1914.* xxiii, 502 pp. Illus, diagrs (sphygmograph tracings). 8vo, 25 cms.

A second impression of the third edition. Second edition, London, 1910; third edition, 1913; fourth edition, 1925.

This book revolutionised cardiology in English speaking countries and gained for Mackenzie an international reputation. It was translated into French, German, Italian and Russian.

327 Principles of diagnosis and treatment in heart affections. *London, Henry Frowde, Hodder & Stoughton, 1916.* viii, 264 pp. Illus, diagrs (sphygmograph tracings). 8vo, 22 cms.

Book-stamp: Medical Society of London.

328 *The same.* Fourth impression. *London, Henry Frowde, Hodder & Stoughton, 1918.* viii, 264 pp. Illus, diagrs (sphygmograph tracings). 8vo, 22 cms.

Autograph: Frank Hiam, Middlesex Hospital, London W.1; and, 10 Newland, Northampton (Frank Hiam, M.R.C.S., L.R.C.P., L.D.S., R.C.S., dental surgeon).

This book was much reprinted, and was translated into German, Italian, Russian and Polish. The second edition was published in 1923; the third in 1926.

329 The Soldier's heart. *London, British Medical Association, 1916.* 11 pp. 8vo, 23 cms.

Includes Wilson (Robert McNair) 1882–1963. The Irritable heart of soldiers pp. 9–11; the whole reprinted from *British medical Journal*, 1916, 1,117–20.

MONTEITH (WILLIAM BLACK RANKIN)

330 Bibliography, with synopsis of the original papers, of the writings of Sir James Mackenzie, M.D., F.R.C.P., LL.D., F.R.S.; ed. by W. B. R. Monteith. *London, Humphrey Milford, Oxford University Press, 1930.* 99 pp. 8vo, 22 cms.

WILSON (ROBERT MACNAIR) 1882–1963

331 The Beloved physician, Sir James Mackenzie: a biography. *London, John Murray, 1927.* x, 316 pp. Port. (frontispiece). 8vo, 23 cms.

Autograph: In remembrance, to Lady Berry from Frances Mackenzie (wife of Sir James Mackenzie, and formerly Frances Bellamy Jackson). Lady Berry may be the first wife of the surgeon, Sir James Berry (1860–1946); she died in 1934.

MacNair Wilson was medical correspondent to *The Times* for 30 years; after the 1914 war, he became assistant to Mackenzie and wrote *The Nervous heart*, 1919 (no. 970).

SAWYER (Sir JAMES) 1844–1919

332 Points of practice in maladies of the heart: Lumleian Lectures at the Royal College of Physicians. *Birmingham, Cornish Bros., 1908.* 96, viii pp. Bibliog. (ftn. refs). 8vo, 20 cms.

Autograph: W. Strugnell, May 1909.

Sawyer was physician to the Queen's Hospital, and professor of medicine at Birmingham.

ALLBUTT (Sir THOMAS CLIFFORD) 1836–1925 and
ROLLESTON (Sir HUMPHRY DAVY) 1862–1944

333 A System of medicine by many writers; ed. by Sir Clifford Allbutt and Humphry Davy Rolleston. Vol. 6: Diseases of the heart and blood-vessels. *London, Macmillan, 1909.* xvi, 861 pp. Illus, tables, diagrs, bibliog. 8vo, 23 cms.

This volume contains important contributions by Newton Pitt on right-sided valvular disease, by Osler on Adams-Stokes disease, by Douglas Powell on angina pectoris, and by Allbutt on aortic disease and functional disorders of the heart. Each section contains a valuable bibliography.

BROCKBANK (EDWARD MANSFIELD) 1866–1959

334 The Diagnosis and treatment of heart disease; practical points for students and practitioners. 6th ed. *London, H. K. Lewis, 1930.* xiv, 240 pp. Illus, diagrs. 8vo, 19 cms.

Brockbank maintained that the crescendo presystolic murmur occurred in the presphygmic period of early systole. The first edition was published in 1911.

MOON (ROBERT OSWALD) 1865–1953

335 The Prognosis and treatment of diseases of the heart. *London, Longmans, Green, 1912.* xi, 111 pp. Bibliog. (ftn. refs). 8vo, 20 cms.

Moon was physician to the National Heart Hospital and a classical scholar.

COWAN (JOHN MARSHALL) 1870–1947

336 Diseases of the heart; with chapters on the electro-cardiograph by W. T. Ritchie . . . and the ocular manifestations in arterio-sclerosis by Arthur J. Ballantyne. *London,*

Edward Arnold, 1914. xx, 438 pp. Illus, diagrs, tables, bibliog. (chapters, ftn. refs). 8vo, 23 cms.

Provenance: Medical Society of London (book-stamp).

This became the standard English text-book after Mackenzie's (see nos. 325–6). Later editions of the book were written with W. T. Ritchie. Cowan was physician to the Glasgow Royal Infirmary, an early worker with the polygraph and electrocardiograph, a founder member of the Cardiac Club, and physician to King George V and Edward VIII, in Scotland.

COWAN (John Marshall) 1870–1947 and
RITCHIE (William Thomas) 1873–1945

337 Diseases of the heart . . . with a chapter on the ocular manifestations of arterial disease by Arthur J. Ballantyne. 2nd ed. *London, Edward Arnold, 1922.* xvi, 605 pp. Illus, tables, diagrs, bibliog. (ftn. refs).

338 *The same.* 3rd ed. *London, Edward Arnold, 1935.* xvi, 631 pp. Illus, tables, diagrs, bibliog. 8vo, 24 cms.

Considerable bibliography (646 references).

SUTHERLAND (George Alexander) 1861–1939

339 The Heart in early life. (Oxford Medical Publications). *London, Henry Frowde, Hodder & Stoughton, 1914.* xvi, 211 pp. Diagrs (polygraph tracings). 8vo, 20 cms.

Sutherland, who was a paediatrician and physician to the Paddington Green Children's Hospital, was an early worker with the polygraph and on rheumatic heart disease.

LEWIS (Sir Thomas) 1881–1945

340 Lectures on the heart . . . *New York, Paul B. Hoeber, 1915.* [vii], 124 pp. Illus, diagrs (sphygmograph tracings). 8vo, 22 cms.

Publisher's catalogues (9, [1], 14 pp.) bound in at end.

Five lectures delivered in America "comprising the Herter Lectures (Baltimore), a Harvey Lecture (New York) and an address to the Faculty of Medicine at McGill University (Montreal)"—*title-page.*

341 The Soldier's heart and the effort syndrome. *London, Shaw, [1918].* xi, 144 pp. Tables. 8vo, 22 cms.

342 Diseases of the heart described for practitioners and students. (Department of Clinical Research, University College Hospital, London). *London, Macmillan, 1933.* xx, 297 pp. Illus, tables, diagrs. 8vo, 23 cms.

Second edition, 1937.

343 *The same.* 3rd ed. *London, Macmillan, 1942.* xx, 297, [1] pp. Illus, tables, diagrs. 8vo, 23 cms.

Bookplate: Medical Women's Federation Reference Library, presented by Dr. A. M. C. Macpherson, Aug. 1942.

Sir Thomas Lewis, physician to University College Hospital, became the pre-eminent authority on cardio-vascular disease in the first half of the 20th century. He was the editor of *Heart*, founded in 1908, later succeeded by *Clinical Science*. He identified auricular fibrillation, and his work *The*

Mechanism and graphic registration of the heart beat (3rd ed., no. 526) first published in 1911 as *The Mechanism of the heart beat*, went through three editions. After this, he became interested in peripheral vascular disease and the blood vessels of the skin. He is renowned not only for his researches, but ability to interpret scientific methods in simple terms applicable to the bedside, as exemplified by his *Clinical disorders of the heart beat* (various edition, no. 527–9) and later by his *Diseases of the heart*, a classic text-book. Like Mackenzie, he died from myocardial infarction.

PRICE (FREDERICK WILLIAM) 1873–1957

344 Diseases of the heart: their diagnosis, prognosis and treatment by modern methods. 2nd ed. *London, Humphrey Milford, Oxford University Press, 1927.* xvi, 534 pp. Illus, tables, diagrs (tracings), bibliog. (ftn. refs). 8vo, 23 cms.

First edition, 1918 (RCP). Price was physician to the National Heart Hospital, and one of the first to confine his practice to cardiology. Like Sir James Mackenzie before him, he practised from no. 133 Harley Street.

Later Works

BRAMWELL (JOHN CRIGHTON) 1889–1976

345 Heart disease: the principles of diagnosis and treatment. *London, Edward Arnold, 1932.* vii, 244 pp. Illus, tables, diagrs, bibliog. (ftn. refs). 8vo, 22 cms.

Publisher's catalogue [8] pp. bound in at end.

BRAMWELL (JOHN CRIGHTON) 1889–1976 and
KING (JOHN THEODORE) *b.* 1889

346 The Principles and practice of cardiology. (Oxford Medical Publications). *London, Humphrey Milford, 1942.* viii, [i], 509 pp. Illus, tables, diagrs, bibliog. 4to, 26 cms.

EVANS (WILLIAM) *b.* 1895

347 Cardiology. *London, Butterworth, 1948.* xi, 310, 20 pp. Illus, tables, diagrs. 8vo, 25 cms.

Last 20 pp. index. Profusely illustrated.
Evans was physician to the London and National Heart Hospitals and a renowned teacher. He published his autobiography (*Journey to Harley Street*) (RCP) in 1968.

WOOD (PAUL HAMILTON) 1907–1962

348 Diseases of the heart and circulation. (The "Practitioner" Series). *London, Eyre & Spottiswoode for the Practitioner, 1950.* xxxi, 589 pp. Illus, tables, diagrs, bibliog. (chapter refs). 8vo, 25 cms.

349 *The same.* 2nd ed. *London, Eyre & Spottiswoode, 1956.* xxxix, 1005 pp. Illus, tables, diagrs (tracings), bibliog. (chapter refs). 8vo, 25 cms.

Signed by the author and with his notes for the third edition published posthumously in 1968. Given to DEB by the author's wife.

This famous text-book had a profound influence on cardiological practice and teaching in this country and abroad. Wood was a great teacher and clinician and his book shows how technical knowledge can be made effective at the bedside.

350 An Appreciation of mitral stenosis. *London, British Medical Association, 1954.* 68 pp. Tables, diagrs, bibliog. 8vo, 22 cms.

Reprinted from *British medical Journal*, 1954, **1**, 1051–63, 1113–24. Part 1, Clinical features pp.1–36; part 2, Investigations and results pp. 37–68. Presentation copy from the author.

This authoritative account of all aspects of mitral stenosis comprises the lecture delivered before the San Francisco Heart Association on October 29, 1953, and modified for the Strickland Goodall Lecture of the Society of Apothecaries of London, March 24, 1954.

American

FLINT (Austin) 1812–1886

351 A Practical treatise on the diagnosis, pathology and treatment of diseases of the heart. *Philadelphia, Blanchard & Lea, 1859.* xv, 473 pp. Illus. (frontispiece), bibliog. (ftn. refs). 8vo, 24 cms.

Publisher's advertisements and catalogue ([2], 32 pp.) bound in. Autograph: D. H. T. (?) Horner Francis.

Austin Flint, professor of clinical medicine at New Orleans, was an early convert to the stethoscope, and wrote extensively on disease of the lungs and heart. His name is attached to the presystolic murmur in aortic incompetence and his treatise was the first authoritative American book on diseases of the heart (*Preface*, p.v.).

CLARK (Alonzo) 1807–1887

352 Lectures on diseases of the heart, delivered at the College of Physicians and Surgeons, New York. *New York, London, Bermingham, 1884.* 251 pp. Bibliog. (ftn. refs). 12mo, 19 cms.

Bermingham's Medical Library stamped on cover.

An early American text-book comprising 17 lectures delivered at the College of Physicians and Surgeons, New York. With George Philip Cammann (1804–1864) (see *American medical Times*, 1864, **8**, 105–6, 119, 129–31, 143–4), he introduced auscultatory percussion in 1840 (see pp. 33–4; see also Bowditch (no. 483) p. 92).

KEATING (John Marie) 1852–1893 and EDWARDS (William Aloysius) 1860–1933

353 Diseases of the heart and circulation in infancy and adolescence. *Philadelphia, P. Blakiston, 1888.* 215 pp. Illus, tables, diagrs, bibliog. 8vo, 25 cms.

Advertisements and publisher's catalogue ([2] [30] pp.) bound in at end. Provenance: The Library of Nursing.

An early American text-book dealing with congenital heart disease, endocarditis, pericarditis and cardiac neuroses including angina pectoris.

BABCOCK (Robert Hall) 1851–1930

354 Diseases of the heart and arterial system, designed to be a practical presentation of the subject for the use of students and practitioners of medicine. *New York & London, D. Appleton, 1903.* xxi, 853 pp. Illus, diagrs, bibliog. 8vo, 25 cms.

An early American text-book profusely illustrated with sphygmograms, etc. Babcock was professor of medicine at Chicago.

HIRSCHFELDER (ARTHUR DOUGLASS) 1879–1942

355 Diseases of the heart and aorta; with an introductory note by Lewellys F. Barker. 2nd ed. *Philadelphia and London, J. B. Lippincott, 1913.* xxviii, 738 pp. Illus, tables, diagrs, bibliog. 8vo, 25 cms.

Autograph: Lindley Scott, 30 Cadogan Place S.W. (Lindley Marcroft Scott, *d.* 1939, physician in charge of the Heart Section of the Royal Victoria Hospital, Netley).

The first edition was published in 1910. Hirschfelder was professor of medicine at Johns Hopkins University, and his book was the standard American text-book of its time; it was written when the electrocardiograph had only just come into use, and so illustrated profusely with pulse tracings and polygrams. He described the Hirschfelder or *h* wave of the jugular tracing in 1907 at the same time as Gibson. The bibliographies at the end of each chapter are a useful source of current references. Hirschfelder became professor of pharmacology at the University of Minnesota in 1913, a post he held until retirement.

Later Works

CRUMMER (LEROY) 1872–1934

356 Clinical features of heart disease. *London, Henry Kimpton, 1925.* xix, [ii], 353 pp. 8vo, 21 cms.

A chatty little book by the great American bibliophile.

WHITE (PAUL DUDLEY) 1886–1973

357 Heart disease. (Macmillan Medical Monographs). *New York, Macmillan, 1931.* xxi, 931 pp. Illus, tables, diagrs, bibliog. 8vo, 24 cms.

Extensive bibliography pp. 689–877. The second edition appeared in 1937, the third in 1944, and the fourth in 1951.

Paul White's epoch-making book for long remained unrivalled and set a new standard in cardiological text-books.

CHRISTIAN (HENRY ASBURY) 1876–1951

358 The Diagnosis and treatment of diseases of the heart. *New York, Oxford University Press, 1935.* vi, 373 [i.e. 413] pp. Diagrs, bibliog. (chapter refs). 8vo, 24 cms.

Additional pages following 84 (1), 128 (10), 221 (10), 259 (6), 273 (2), 283 (2), 309 (17).

Christian was a leading teacher on cardiology in U.S.A.

STROUD (WILLIAM DANIEL) 1891–1959

359 The Diagnosis and treatment of cardio-vascular disease. 3rd ed. *Philadelphia, F. A. Davis, 1945.* 2 vols. Illus, ports, tables, diagrs, bibliog. (chapter refs). 4to, 27 cms.

Vol. 1, xxxiii, 942, xxxii pp.; vol. 2, xxii, 1001–1775, xxxii pp. Last xxxii pp. index, the same in each volume. Acquired 1946.

First edition, 1940; second edition, 1943. A useful reference work in its time.

French

CORVISART DES MARETS (JEAN NICOLAS) 1755–1821

360 Essai sur les maladies et les lésions organiques du cœur et des gros vaisseaux. Extrait des leçons cliniques de J. N. Corvisart . . . publié, sous ses yeux, par C. E. Horeau. *Paris, de l'imprimerie de Migneret, 1806.* lvi, 484 pp., [1] f. (errata leaf). 8vo, 21 cms.

First leaf (blank?) missing.

The first edition of Corvisart (Garrison and Morton 2737) was written by Horeau from lecture notes, but later editions were by Corvisart himself. Corvisart founded clinical cardiology and introduced percussion into the clinic after translating Auenbrugger's work. He classed cardiac enlargement as active or passive aneurysm of the heart, and recognised the purring tremor as a sign of valvular obstruction but did not listen to the heart. His *Essai* was the first treatise on heart disease to conform to the pattern of a text-book and deal systematically with pericarditis, myocardial disease, carditis and aneurysm. He was physician to Napoleon and a reputed bon viveur.

The second part of his surname appears usually as des Marets or Desmarets, but the forms des Marest (Garrison and Morton) and Desmarest are occasionally found. "Afin de se distinguer des nombreux autres membres titrés de sa famille, et en souvenir de son aieul, Charles de Conzart, Ecuyer, Seigneur des Maretz, qui vivait au XVIIIe siècle, a Thénorgues, Corvisart ajouta à son nom celui de *des Marets*; il le conserva jusqu'en 1790, date à laquelle il l'abandonna pour reprendre son véritable nom" (*Les Biographies médicales*, 1927–28, tom. 1, pp. 101–12).

361 *The same.* 2e éd., corrigée et augmenté. *Paris, H. Nicolle de l'imprimerie de Mame, 1811.* xlvi, 478 pp. 8vo, 23 cms.

362 *The same.* 3me éd., corrigée et augmentée. *Paris, Méquignon-Marvis, 1818.* xxxvi, 489 pp. 8vo, 22 cms.

Binding: half-red niger retaining original paper cover and printed label.

363 *The same.* [3me éd.].

Pp. 1–175 in *Encyclopédie des sciences médicales* . . . , 7e division, [vol. 12], Paris, au Bureau de l'Encyclopédie, 1838. [iii], iii, 670 pp. 8vo, 22 cms.

This volume also contains: AUENBRUGGER (Leopold) 1722–1809. *Nouvelle méthode pour reconnaître les maladies internes de la poitrine par la percussion de cette cavité* . . . ; ouvrage traduit du latin et commenté par J.-N. Corvisart. pp. [177]–347; and BAYLE (Antoine Laurent Jessé) 1799–1858. *Recherches sur la phthisie pulmonaire . . . et Recueil de mémoires et de travaux divers . . .* pp. [349]–656; Tables des matières contenues dans ce volume pp. 657–70.

It is bound with [vol. 4], 1835, [i], xxii, 23–477 pp. This contains SYDENHAM (Thomas) 1624–1689. *Médecine pratique* . . . , traduite par A.-F. Jault, xxii, 23–354 pp. HUXHAM (John) 1692–1768. *Essai sur les fièvres et sur leurs différentes espèces et des dissertations* . . . , pp. [355]–475; Table, p. 477.

Footnote references throughout. *The Encyclopédie des sciences médicales*, written by various authors (rédacteur en chef: Antoine Laurent Jessé Bayle 1799–1858), was published from an office in the Rue Servandoni, Paris, between 1834 and 1846 in 41 volumes. A list of contents is given in the *Index-catalogue of the library of the Surgeon General's Office*, 2nd series, vol. 5, pp. 2–3, but without the titles of the divisions. These can be found in J. C. Brunet's *Manuel du libraire*, tom. 6, pp. 370–1, item 6529.

364 *The same.* A Treatise on the diseases and organic lesions of the heart and great vessels . . . trans. from the French by C. H. Hebb. *London, Underwood & Blacks; Edinburgh, Adam Black, 1813.* xx, xxxvi, 404 pp. 8vo, 22 cms.

Autographs: T. [?] J. [?] Graham 1836 (possibly Thomas John Graham, M.D. Glasgow, F.R.C.P. Edin., M.R.C.S. Eng., of Epsom, Surrey, 1795–1876, author of *Modern domestic medicine* and other works), Parkinson 1945 (Sir John Parkinson, 1885–1976, M.D., F.R.C.P.). Acquired 1947.

Hebb's translation of the second French edition, now very rare. Christopher Henry Hebb, M.R.C.S. (1722–1861) was medical attendant to Lucien Bonaparte, one of the originators of the Provincial Medical Association (now the British Medical Association), and Mayor of Worcester where he practised for many years.

365 *The same*. An Essay on the organic diseases and lesions of the heart and great vessels . . . trans. from the French with notes by Jacob Gates, M.M.S.S., with an introduction by Dr. Dickinson W. Richards. (New York Academy of Medicine Library. History of Medicine Series no. 16). *New York, Hafner, 1962* [x], xii, v–xiv, 15–344 pp. 8vo, 21 cms.

Facsimile reprint of the first American edition (Boston, Bradford & Read; Philadelphia, Anthony Finley, 1812).

Gates's translation of the first French edition antedated Hebb's English translation of the second edition.

366 Aphorismes de médecine clinique; recueillis par F.-V. Mérat, publiés par le docteur Paul Busquet . . . *Paris, Masson, 1929.* [i], 115, [3] pp. 8vo, 23 cms.

Publisher's catalogue, September 1929, (48 pp.) bound in at end. An extract from *Triangle* (Sandoz journal of medical science) 1957, no. 2, 37–9, is inserted. It comprises a transcription of a selection from the aphorisms of Corvisart taken from this book.

These aphorisms recorded from Corvisart's lectures were rediscovered in a manuscript of F. V. Mérat in the library of the Académie de Médecine in Paris and published by Dr. Busquet, the librarian, in 1929.

STOLL (MAXIMILIAN) 1742–1788

367 Aphorismes sur la connaissance et la curation des fièvres . . . traduits en français par J. N. Corvisart, avec le texte Latin. *Paris, Régent et Bernard,* [*et*] *Mequignon, 1797.* xx, 581 pp. 8vo, 21 cms.

Latin text with French translation on the facing page.

DALLY (JOHN FREDERICK HALLS) 1877–1944

368 Life and times of Jean Nicolas Corvisart (1755–1821).

Extracted from *Proceedings of the Royal Society of Medicine,* 1940–41, **34,** 239–46 (Section of History of Medicine, pp. 17–24). Bibliog.

Author's presentation copy with autograph letter.

FERRUS (GUILLAUME MARIE ANDRÉ) 1784–1861

369 Notice historique sur J. N. Corvisart. *Paris, Bechet jeune, 1821.* 32 pp. 8vo, 22 cms.

Rebound three-quarter niger marbled boards by Douron (Grenoble) with original paper covers.

GANIÈRE (PAUL)

370 Corvisart, médecin de Napoleon. *Paris, Flammarion, 1951.* [i], 314, 1 pp. Bibliog. 8vo, 22 cms.

Biography of Corvisart with a bibliography of the author's sources of historical information.

MOREAU DE LA SARTHE (JACQUES LOUIS) 1771–1826

371 Fragmens pour servir à l'histoire des progrès de la médecine en France. *Paris, [Le Moniteur], 1813.* 60 pp. 8vo, 20 cms.

Reprinted from *Le Moniteur*, 1812, nos. 232, 357, 359 and 362. Contemporary review of Corvisart's *Essai*, 2e éd., 1811.

PORTAL (ANTOINE) baron, 1742–1832

372 Sur les anévrismes du cœur, dans lesquels les parois de cet organe, au lieu d'être amincies, ont conservé leur épaisseur ordinaire ou en ont acquis une plus grande. (Lu à l'Académie des Sciences de l'Institut, avril 1817). [*Paris, no publisher, 1817?*] 40 pp. Bibliog. (ftn. refs). 4to, 27 cms.

Published in *Journal universel des sciences médicales*, October 1817, **8**, 5–89; also in *Mémoires du Muséum d'Histoire Naturelle*, 1818, **4**, 62–101 (which thus has the same number of pages as the separate work above—is the latter possibly a reprint from this journal?).

BERTIN (RENÉ JOSEPH HYACINTHE) 1757–1828

373 Traité des maladies du cœur et des gros vaisseaux . . . redigé par J. Bouillaud. *Paris, J. B. Baillière, 1824.* xlviii, 465 pp. Illus (6 folding plates), bibliog. (ftn. refs). 8vo, 21 cms.

Signature: Henry Alford (1806–1898, surgeon 1830–1859, and then consulting surgeon, to the Taunton and Somerset Hospital). Provenance: Taunton and Somerset Hospital Standert (?) Library no. 52.

American edition, Philadelphia, 1833. Bertin, professor and physician to the Cochin Hospital, Paris, described especially cardiac hypertrophy which he classified as concentric, eccentric and simple. He also described the mitral presystolic murmur, and endocarditis, though Bouillaud his interne, who edited the book, was actually responsible for the description of endocarditis.

MUSSO (VICTOR)

374 Essai sur l'étiologie, le diagnostic et les caractères anatomiques des anévrysmes du cœur; thèse presentée et soutenue à la Faculté de Médecine, le 11 juillet 1827, pour obtenir le grade de Docteur en médecine. (Thèse no. 164). *Paris, à l'imprimerie de Didot le jeune, 1827.* 26 pp. 4to, 28 cms.

Autograph: Mr. [?] Recamier (there is a Joseph Claude Anthelme Récamier 1774–1852, membre de l'Académie de Médecine, Paris).

BOUILLAUD (JEAN BAPTISTE) 1796–1881

375 Traité clinique des maladies du cœur, précedé de recherches nouvelles sur l'anatomie et la physiologie de cet organe. *Paris, J. B. Baillière, 1835.* 2 tom. Illus (folding plates), tables, bibliog. (ftn. refs). 8vo, 21 cms.

Tom. 1: xxiii, 534 pp.; tom. 2: [iii], 632 pp. Second edition, 1841.
Autograph: Terence East 1955.

376 *The same. Bruxelles, H. Dumont, 1836.* [i], viii, 9–387 pp. Illus (3 folding plates), bibliog. (ftn. refs). 8vo, 25 cms.

This Brussels edition is a reprint of the first Paris edition in one volume, printed in double columns.

BOUILLAUD (JEAN BAPTISTE)

377 *The same.* Die Krankheiten des Herzens, nach dem Französischen, deutsch bearbeitet und mit Zusätzen herausgegeben von Dr. Alfr. Ferd. Becker. *Leipzig, Gustav Wuttig, 1836–7.* 2 Bände in 1. Bibliog. (ftn. refs). 8vo, 22 cms.

Bd. 1: vi, 298 pp. Bd. 2: [i], 369, [1] pp. German translation of first French edition.

Autograph: Dr. Burk [?]. Book-stamps: Koen[ig] Fried[richs] Univers[ität] zu Halle; duplum Biblioth[ecae] Acad[emiae] Halens[is] vend.

ROLLESTON (JOHN DAVY) 1893–1946

378 Jean Baptiste Bouillaud 1796–1881: a pioneer in cardiology and neurology.

Reprinted from *Proceedings of the Royal Society of Medicine*, 1930–31, **24**, 1253–62 (Section of the History of Medicine, pp. 37–46). Port., bibliog. 4to, 26 cms.

Author's presentation copy.

Bouillaud was interne to Bertin (see no. 373) at the Cochin Hospital, then physician to the Pitié and later to the Charité Hospital where he followed Corvisart and Laennec. The first edition of his treatise was a landmark in cardiology, representing the application of Laennec's auscultation to diseases of the heart. He first described and named endocarditis, first recorded accurate methods of weighing and measuring the heart, and described the *bruit de diable*, and the *bruit de rappel* in mitral stenosis. According to Potain he described gallop rhythm before Traube. He was an inflexible disciple of Broussais and practised bleeding *coup sur coup* for all forms of inflammatory diseases, particularly heart affections, rheumatic fever and pericarditis. His law of coincidence between acute rheumatism, pericarditis and endocarditis (1836) finally established rheumatic heart disease (Maladie de Bouillaud) as a clinical entity.

PIGEAUX (ANTOINE LOUIS JULES) 1807–?

379 Traité pratique des maladies du cœur, contenant des recherches historiques, anatomiques et physiologiques spéciales sur cet organe. *Paris, Just Rouvier, 1839.* [ii], xvi, 768 pp. 8vo, 22 cms.

An early text-book after Corvisart and Laennec, contains 138 pages on pericarditis, and good historical summaries of each condition described; Italian translation, 1841. He also wrote a book on diseases of the arteries (*Traité pratique des maladies des vaisseaux*, Paris, 1843).

GENDRIN (AUGUSTIN NICOLAS) 1796–1890

380 Leçons sur les maladies du cœur et des grosses artères faites à l'Hôpital de la Pitié pendant les années 1840–41 . . . recueillies et publiées sous les yeux par MM. E. Colson et Dubreuil-Hélion. Tom. 1er. *Paris, Germer Baillière, 1841–2.* [iii], vii, 648 pp. 8vo, 22 cms.

Only one volume published. German edition, Leipzig, 1843.

An early work on physical signs and murmurs, with a long section of almost 300 pages on pericarditis.

PIORRY (PIERRE ADOLPHE) 1794–1879

381 Über die Krankheiten des Herzens und der grossen Gefässe, der Arterien, Venen und lymphatischen Gefässe. Aus dem Französischen von Dr. G. Krupp. *Leipzig, Christian Ernst Kollman, 1844.* [iv], 476 pp. 8vo, 22 cms.

Piorry, physician to the Charité Hospital, is best known for his pleximeter and his book on percussion (*De la percussion médiate*. Paris, 1828) (no. 471). His text-book on heart diseases, first published, 1841?, is unimportant, apart from pleximetry. Gustav Krupp of Cassel translated works mainly of French authors such as Piorry, Bouillaud, Chomel, Magendie and Rayer.

ARAN (François Amilcar) 1817–1861

382 Practical manual of the diseases of the heart and great vessels; a work intended to facilitate and extend the study of these diseases; trans. from the French by Wm. A. Harris. *Philadelphia, Ed. Barrington & Geo. D. Haswell, 1843.* 296 pp. 12mo, 17 cms.

Publisher's catalogue, [4] pp., bound in at end.

Signature: John Rose Cormack 1844 (Sir John Rose Baillie Cormack, 1815–1882, the leading physician to the English in Paris). Acquired 1940.

Aran was physician to the St. Antoine Hospital, Paris, and his book (the original French edition of which was *Manuel pratique des maladies du cœur et des gros vaisseaux.* Paris, J. Rouvier, 1842), was popular and much cited at the time. He was one of the first to perform paracentesis of the pericardium successfully and translated Skoda's work on percussion and auscultation into French.

FORGET (Charles Polydore) 1800–1861

383 Précis théorique et pratique des maladies du cœur, des vaisseaux et du sang. *Strasbourg, Ve Berger-Levrault et fils; Paris, C. Reinwald, 1851.* viii, 480 pp., errata leaf. 8vo, 23 cms.

This volume also contains *Du tact médical.* Paris, imprimé par E. Thunot, 1850. 17 pp. Reprinted from *Gazette médicale de Paris*, 1850; pp. 19–24: *Cas d'empoisonnement par l'arsenic, suivi de gangrène dite spontane d'un des membres inférieurs:* lettre à M. Orfila; and *Du mouvement médical au dix-neuvième siècle.* Strasbourg, Derivaux; Paris, J. B. Baillière, 1846. 27 pp.

Forget, professor at Strasbourg, was credited with originating the theory of retrodilatation behind an obstacle to the circulation as a general physiological principle applicable to all forms of heart disease, and in the judgement of his contemporaries he was the man who put the back pressure theory across.

AUBURTIN (Simon Alexandre Ernest) 1825–?1893

384 Recherches cliniques sur les maladies du cœur, d'après les leçons de M. le professeur Bouillaud . . . précédées de considérations de philosophie médicale sur le vitalisme, l'organicisme et la nomenclature médical par M. le professeur Bouillaud . . . *Paris, J. Viat, 1856.* 11, clxxi, 276 pp. Bibliog. (ftn. refs). 8vo, 22 cms.

Considérations . . . by Bouillaud (clxxi pp.); Recherches . . . by Auburtin (273 pp.); Table des matières pp. 275–6.

Auburtin, the son-in-law of Bouillaud, is best remembered for work which helped to establish the principle of cerebral localisation of the nervous system (see Garrison and Morton 1401.1). The date of his death is suggested by the disappearance of his name from the *Annuaire médical* in 1893 (A. M. Latour on Auburtin in *Dictionnaire de biographie française*, Paris 1948, vol. 4, col. 300, quoted in Edwin Clarke and C. D. O'Malley, *The Human brain and spinal cord*, Berkeley, 1968, p. 492).

BLACHE (René Henri) 1839–1908

385 Essai sur les maladies du cœur chez les enfants. *Paris, P. Asselin, 1869.* 224 pp. Bibliog. 8vo, 23 cms.

Author's presentation copy (signature cropped: "Souvenir de l'aute[ur], [?] René B[lache]).

Deals with pericarditis, endocarditis, myocarditis and hypertrophy in children. Contains a valuable bibliography on congenital and rheumatic heart disease (pp. 217–22) covering 1816–1868.

BUCQUOY (Marie Edme Jules) 1829–1920

386 Leçons cliniques sur les maladies du cœur, professées à l'Hotel-Dieu de Paris. 4me éd. *Paris, V. Adrien Delahaye, 1879.* [iii], 169 pp. Illus, diagrs (tracings), bibliog. (ftn. refs). 8vo, 23 cms.

Publisher's catalogue, (10 pp.) bound in at end.

Signature (badly written): P. L. Sifflet [?], externe des hôpitaux.

First edition, 1873? Bucquoy was physician to the Cochin Hospital and his lectures ran through four editions dealing particularly with mitral stenosis, aortic valve disease, asystole, therapeutics and rheumatic pericarditis.

DUFRESSE DE CHASSAIGNE (Jean Eugène) fl. 1834–77

387 Du traitement et de la guérison de l'anévrisme du cœur. *Paris, Asselin, 1877.* [v], x, 421, [1] pp. Bibliog. 8vo, 23 cms.

Of some historical interest, reviewing heart sounds, rheumatic heart disease and cardiac dilatation. Hirsch's *Biographisches Lexikon* has misspelt the author's name as Dufresne.

ALVARENGA (Pedro Francisco da Costa) 1826–1883

388 Leçons cliniques sur les maladies du cœur, principalement au point de vue de la valeur séméiologique du retard du pouls, du double souffle et de la double vibration des artères, des effets sur ces phénomènes de la compression simple et combinée faite tantôt avec le stéthoscope sur le point ausculté, tantôt avec les doigts en amont et en aval de ce point . . . traduit du portugais par le docteur E. Bertherand. *Lisbonne, imprimerie de l'Académie Royale des Sciences, 1878.* xviii, 361 pp. Tables, diagrs (tracings), bibliog. 8vo, 22 cms.

Bookplate (crest): Dr. Angus Fraser's bequest (to the Aberdeen Medico-Chirurgical Society. Angus Fraser, 1838–1912, was consulting physician to Aberdeen Royal Infirmary). Book-stamp: The Aberdeen Medico-Chirurgical Society.

Twenty-four lectures delivered at the S. Jose Hospital, Lisbon. Alvarenga, although professor of medicine at Lisbon, is included in this section as he had studied in Paris under Piorry; he was, especially concerned with the signs and murmurs of aortic incompetence, displacement of the heart and cyanosis. Several of his many works (see the bibliography of his works before the title-page) on the heart were translated into French.

PAUL (Charles Théodore Constantin) 1833–1896

389 Diagnostic et traitement des maladies du cœur. 2e éd. *Paris, Asselin et Houzeau, 1887.* xx, 974 pp. Illus, tables, bibliog. (ftn. refs). 8vo, 23 cms.

First edition 1883 (Garrison and Morton 2789), English translation 1884.

390 *The same.* Diagnosis and treatment of diseases of the heart. (Wood's Library of Standard Medical Authors). *New York, William Wood, 1884.* vii, 335 pp. Illus, tables, diagrs (tracings), bibliog. (ftn. refs). 8vo, 24 cms.

Translation of the first French edition of 1883.

Autograph: A. W. Williams (probably Arthur Wynn Williams, 1819–1886, physician of the Samaritan Free Hospital for Women and Children and author of many treatises). Book-stamp: Library of J. W. Brown, M.D. (James William Brown, 1897–1958, M.D., F.R.C.P.).

Paul, physician to the Lariboisière Hospital, was especially concerned with anaemic murmurs and devised a new plan of estimating the size of the heart by percussion.

PETER (Charles Félix Michel) 1824–1893

391 Traité clinique et pratique des maladies du cœur et de la crosse de l'aorte. *Paris, J. B. Baillière, 1883.* xii, 844 pp. Illus (incl. plates), diagrs (tracings), bibliog. (ftn. refs). 8vo, 23 cms.

Autograph: Dr. Delezenne (perhaps Camille Delezenne, 1868–1932, membre de l'Académie de Médecine, Paris).

Peter, physician to the Charité Hospital and professor at the Faculty, was a great clinician and man of letters. He was a foremost advocate of the neuralgic and neuritic theory of angina pectoris and an opponent of the ischaemic theory advocated by his contemporary, Germain Sée (see no. 395).

[PARIS THESES]

392 [A collection of five theses on heart disease]. 1887–1893. Various paging. 8vo, 24 cms.

From the library of F. P. Weber (signature: Frederick Parkes Weber, 1863–1962, M.D., F.R.C.P.).

The contents are:

WEBER (Charles Alfred)

Contribution à l'étude anatomo-pathologique de l'artério-sclérose du cœur (scléroses du myocarde). *Paris, G. Steinheil, 1887.* 151 pp. Illus (2 plates), bibliog. (ftn. refs).

Originally Paris thesis 1887, no. 341. Signed presentation copy by the author to Dr. F. P. Weber.

FAURE-MILLER (Roland) 1861–?

Contribution à l'étude clinique des cardiopathies artérielles à type myo-valvulaire. *Paris, Octave Doin, 1892.* 131 pp. Diagrs (tracings), bibliog. (ftn. refs).

Title-page folded to preserve author's signed presentation "to Dr F. P. Weber with best regards". Originally Paris thesis 1892, no. 333.

COURTADE (Denis) 1857–?

Contribution à l'étude thérapeutique de la digitale dans les affections organiques du cœur. *Paris, G. Steinheil, 1888.* [3]–138 pp. Tables, diagrs (tracings).

Originally Paris thesis 1888, no. 68.

GIOCANTI (Jacques-Francois) 1860–?

Contribution à l'étude de l'arythmie cardiaque consécutive aux lésions du myocarde. *Paris, G. Steinheil, 1892.* 109 pp. Diagrs (tracings), bibliog. (ftn. refs).

Originally Paris thesis 1892, no. 323.

KORTZ (Henri) 1864–?

Les maladies de l'aorte et du système artériel dans leurs rapports avec la tuberculose pulmonaire. *Paris, G. Steinheil, 1893.* 112 pp. Bibliog.

Originally Paris thesis 1892, no. 55.

393 HUCHARD (Henri) 1844–1910

Traité clinique des maladies du cœur et de l'aorte. 3me éd. *Paris, Octave Doin, 1899–1905.* 3 tom. Illus, tables, diagrs (tracings), bibliog. (ftn. refs). 8vo, 25 cms.

Tom. 1: 1899. [iii], ii, 574 pp.; tom. 2: 1899. [iii], 589 pp.; tom. 3: 1905. [iii], ii, 1007 pp. First edition, *Maladies du cœur et des vaisseaux*, Paris, 1889; second edition, 1893 (RCP).

HUCHARD (Henri)

394 Six leçons cliniques sur les maladies du cœur. *Paris, J. B. Baillière, 1907.* [i], 216 pp. Bibliog. 8vo, 23 cms.

Huchard, physician to the Necker Hospital, was a foremost teacher in Paris at the end of the century, and a great authority on angina pectoris and arteriosclerosis. He was a powerful advocate of the coronary theory of angina pectoris and assembled 185 *pièces justificatives* as published examples of angina pectoris associated with coronary disease. He also recognised a stage of presclerosis in which hypertension preceded arterio-sclerosis.

395 SÉE (Germain) 1818–1896

Traité des maladies du cœur, étiologie et clinique. (Médecine Clinique, tom. 7–8). *Paris, Lecrosnier et Babé, L. Bataille, 1889–93.* 2 tom. Illus, diagrs (incl. tracings). 8vo, 23 cms.

Tom. 1 (Étiologie et clinique) was published by Lecrosnier and Babé, Paris, 1889. [iii], 646 pp.; tom. 2 (Thérapeutique physiologique du cœur) by L. Bataille, Paris, 1893. [iii], iii, 472 pp.

Tom. 2 author's presentation copy "a mon ami Straus" (Isidore Straus, 1845–1896, M.D. 1868, professor of the Paris Faculty of Medicine 1888—see Bianchon (no. 998) pp. 431–7. Port., bibliog.).

Germain Sée was physician to the Beaujon Hospital and professor of therapeutics. He was the first physician to set up his own laboratory in the hospital where he tested various drugs and performed ligation of the coronary arteries in animals. He was one of the first to adopt the ischaemic theory of angina pectoris and a pioneer in the use of salicylates.

WEILL (Edmond) 1858–1924

396 Traité clinique des maladies du cœur chez les enfants. *Paris, Octave Doin, 1895.* viii, 390 pp.. Bibliog. (ftn. refs). 8vo, 25 cms.

Weill was professor at Lyon and his treatise deals with endocarditis, pericarditis, and congenital heart disease. He advocated prolonged salicylate therapy in rheumatic heart disease.

BARIÉ (Ernest) 1848–1931

397 Traité pratique des maladies du cœur et de l'aorte. Préface par le professeur Potain. 3me éd. *Paris, Vigot frères, 1912.* xi, 1125 pp. Illus, diagrs (tracings), bibliog. (ftn. refs). 8vo, 25 cms.

Publisher's catalogue (14 pp.) bound in at end. The first edition was published in 1900.

Barié was physician to the Laennec Hospital, Paris, a renowned teacher and author of many papers on all aspects of cardiology, notably on pulmonary incompetence. His treatise is a most systematic work with a historical preface to each section, and an extensive bibliography given as footnotes.

GALLAVARDIN (Louis Bénédict) 1875–1957

398 La Dégénérescence graisseuse du myocarde considérée comme surcharge graisseuse de la fibre cardiaque. *Paris, J. B. Baillière, 1900.* [i], 7–186 pp. Illus (plate), bibliog. (ftn. refs). 8vo, 25 cms.

Has cancelled title-page with blank conjugate leaf, possibly explained by use of sheets from Lyon thesis, no. 155 published in the same year, and for which preliminary leaves were allowed for but never printed. For biographical notes see no. 641.

399 Le Rétrécissement mitral oedémateux.

Reprinted from *Journal de Médecine de Lyon*, 1934, **15**, 609–23. Bibliog.

VAQUEZ (Louis Henri) 1860–1936

400 Collection of 15 offprints including early papers on blood-pressure in eclampsia and lead poisoning. 1904–1909.

La Tension artérielle dans le saturnisme aigu et chronique. *Paris, imprimerie de la Semaine médicale, 1904.* 19 pp. 8vo, 22 cms.

Reprinted from *Semaine médicale*, Paris, 1904, **24**, 385–7. Signed presentation copy.

Hypertension.

Extract from *Congrès français de médecine*, 7e session, Paris, 1904 . . . Rapports etc. Paris, Masson, 1904–1905, tom. 1, pp. 338–96. Illus (on one plate), diagrs (incl. tracings), bibliog. (ftn. refs). 8vo, 25 cms. Signed presentation copy to Dr. Parkes Weber. (Frederick Parkes Weber, 1863–1962.)

Tipped inside an extract "7 französicher Kongress für innere Medizin, abgehalten zu Paris vom 24–28 Oktober 1904" *Muenchener medizinische Wochenschrift* 29. November 1904, no. 48, S.2165–6. A description of the first part of the congress.

Des états anémiques.

Reprinted from *Archives générales de médecine*, Paris, 1905, **1**, 967–80. Bibliog. (ftn. refs); also reprinted in *Bulletin du laboratoire de biologie appliquée*, Paris, 1905, **3**, no. 5, p. 1; no. 6, p. 4. Signed presentation copy.

Des effets mécaniques de l'hypertension sur le système cardio-aortique. *Paris, imprimerie de la Semaine médicale, 1905.* 21 pp. 8vo, 23 cms.

Reprinted from *Semaine médicale*, Paris, 1905, **25**, 217–20. Signed presentation copy.

Le traitement de la phlébite des membres. *Paris, imprimerie de la Semaine médicale, 1905.* 26 pp. 8vo, 22 cms.

Reprinted from *Semaine médicale*, Paris, 1905, **25**, 349–52. Signed presentation copy.

Études sur la rétention et l'élimination des chlorures au cours de cardiopathies: considérations pathogeniques et thérapeutiques, par MM. Vaquez et Digne. *Paris, imprimerie de la Cour d'Appel, 1905.* [i], 26, 23, 12 pp. Tables, bibliog. (ftn. refs). 8vo, 24 cms.

First published as three papers (first part, 26 pp., De l'asystolie survenant au repos.—Role de la rétention chlorurée dans la pathogenie de l'insuffisance cardiaque; second part, 23 pp., Du mode d'élimination du chlorure de sodium chez les cardiaques en dehors des périodes d'asystolie; third part, 12 pp., La Cure de déchloruration au cours des maladies du cœur) in *Bulletins et Mémoires de la Société médicale des Hôpitaux de Paris*, 1905, 3e série, **22**, 613–20, 658–80 and 714–26 respectively. The last part was also published in *Tribune médical*, Paris, 1905, **37**, 517–20.

[1] De la tension arterielle pendant la grossesse et les suite de couches. [2] Valeur diagnostique et pronostique de l'élévation de la pression artérielle au cours de l'éclampsie puerpérale. [3] Sur un cas d'éclampsie survenue un mois après l'accouchement. *Paris, la Société [d'Obstétrique de Paris], 1906.* 11 pp. Bibliog. (ftn. refs). 8vo, 25 cms.

Three papers reprinted under one cover from *Bulletin de la Société d'Obstétrique de Paris*, 1906, **9**, 30–33, 34–37, 38–40 respectively. The first paper was also published in *Tribune médical*, Paris, 1906, **38**, 213. Signed presentation copy.

VAQUEZ (Louis Henri)

400 (*cont.*) Action des rayons X sur l'organisme malade. *Bordeaux, Bureaux des Archives d'Electricité médicale, 1906.* 7 pp. 8vo, 25 cms.

Reprinted from *Archives d'Electricité médicale*, Bordeaux, 1906, **14**, 699–705. Signed presentation copy.

Des "épistaxis" méningées au cours des maladies hypersensitives, par MM. Vaquez et Esmein. [*Paris, Société médicale des Hôpitaux de Paris, 1906*]. 6 pp. 8vo, 25 cms.

Reprinted from *Bulletins et Mémoires de la Société médicale des Hôpitaux de Paris*, 1906, 3e série, **23**, 1189–96. Also published in *Tribune médical*, Paris, 1906, **37**, 709. Signed presentation copy.

Pouls lent d'origine myocarditique (Herzblock), par MM. Vasquez et Esmein. [*Paris, Société médicale des Hôpitaux de Paris, 1907*]. 12 pp. Diagrs (tracings), bibliog. (ftn. refs). 8vo, 24 cms.

Reprinted from *Bulletins et Mémoires de la Société médicale des Hôpitaux de Paris*, 1907, 3e série, **24**, 78–90. Autograph of Vaquez. "Un cas de maladie de Stokes-Adams provoquée par une lésion systematisée du myocarde, siégeant sur le trajet du faisceau de His, et de nature syphilitique". A similar (or possibly the same) case was reported by Vaquez and Esmein in Maladie de Stokes-Adams par lésion scléro-gommeuse du faisceau de His (Herzblock), *Presse médicale*, Paris, 1907, **15**, 57–9.

Éclampsie puerpérale et tension artérielle. *Paris, imprimerie de la Semaine médicale, 1907.* 34 pp. Bibliog. (ftn. refs). 8vo, 22 cms.

Reprinted from *Semaine médicale*, Paris, 1907, **27**, 121–6. Author's signed copy.

Action pharmacodynamique et thérapeutique des nitrites. *Paris, J. B. Baillière, 1908.* 17 pp. Diagrs (tracings), bibliog. (ftn. refs). 8vo, 23 cms.

Reprinted from *Archives des Maladies du Cœur, des Vaisseaux et du Sang*, 1908, **1**, 3–19. Author's signed presentation copy. Vaquez was the first editor of *Archives des Maladies du Cœur*, which he started in January 1908.

Les Injections intra-veineuses de strophantine dans le traitement de l'insuffisance cardiaque, par MM. Vaquez et Leconte. [*Paris, Société médicale des Hôpitaux de Paris, 1909*]. 18 pp. Tables, diagrs, bibliog. (ftn. refs). 8vo, 24 cms.

Reprinted from *Bulletins et Mémoires de la Société médicale des Hôpitaux de Paris*, 1909, 3e série, **26**, 662–79. Also published in *Journal médical français*, Paris, 1909, **3**, 272–6. Author's signed presentation copy.

Battements de cœur et arythmies. *Paris, imprimerie de la Semaine médicale, 1909.* 19 pp. Diagrs (tracings). 8vo, 24 cms.

Reprinted from *Semaine médicale*, Paris, 1909, **29**, 493–6. 2 copies, both signed by the author.

Pathogénie de la tachycardie paroxystique: étude historique et critique. *Paris, J. B. Baillère, 1909.* 26 pp. Illus, diagrs (tracings), bibliog. 8vo, 23 cms.

Reprinted from *Archives des Maladies du Cœur, des Vaisseaux et du Sang*, Paris, 1909, **2**, 609–34. Author's signed presentation copy.

Un Cas de tachycardie paroxystique avec lesion du "faisceau primitif du cœur", par MM. H. Vaquez et Ch. Esmein. [*Paris, Société médicale des Hôpitaux de Paris,1909*]. 8 pp. Illus, diagrs (tracings), bibliog. (ftn. refs). 8vo, 25 cms.

Reprinted from *Bulletins et Mémoires de la Société médicale des Hôpitaux de Paris*, 1909, 3e série, **28**, 814–21. Presentation copy.

401 Maladies du coeur. (Nouveau traité de médecine et de thérapeutique, tom. 23). *Paris, J. B. Baillière, 1921.* viii, 788 pp. Illus, diagrs (incl. tracings), bibliog. 8vo, 25 cms.

Publisher's catalogue ([4] pp.) bound in at end. Extensive references at ends of chapters. Tipped in on half-title page an obituary from *British medical Journal*, 1936, **1**, 865. (A fuller obituary appeared later, pp. 1262–3).

402 *The same.* Diseases of the heart; trans. and ed. by George F. Laidlaw [with an] introduction by William S. Thayer. *Philadelphia & London, W. B. Saunders, 1924.* [4]–743 pp. Illus, diagrs (incl. tracings), bibliog. 8vo, 25 cms.

This American edition was revised by Vaquez with a new preface. Extensive bibliographies.

CLERC (ANTONIN PIERRE) 1871–1954

403 Henri Vaquez (1860–1936). *Paris, Masson, 1936.* 15 pp. Port. 8vo, 22 cms.

Reprinted from *La Presse médicale*, 1936, **44**, 1041–3. Author's presentation copy.

[*and*] LAUBRY (CHARLES) 1872–1960

Henri Vaquez (1860–1936).

Reprinted from *Bulletin de l'Académie Nationale de Médecine*, 1958, **142**, 846–54. Presentation copy "For Dr Bedford".

Vaquez, a disciple of Potain, was the dominant authority on heart disease on the continent of Europe in the early part of the century. He was physician to the Pitié Hospital and professor of medicine at the Faculty. In his early days he worked at haematology and in 1899 described splenomegalic polycythaemia (Maladie de Vaquez). He was a pioneer with Bordet in the radiology of the heart and orthodiagraphy, an early worker on the arrhythmias with the polygraph and electrocardiograph, and published many important papers on all aspects of cardiology with his various assistants. His text-book was for long the standard work on heart disease in France and abroad.

RÉNON (Louis Pierre) 1863–1922

404 Conférences pratiques sur les maladies du cœur et des poumons. *Paris, Masson, 1906.* vi, 382, [1] pp. Bibliog. (ftn. refs). 8vo, 23 cms.

Publisher's catalogue, December 1905, (32 pp.) bound in at end.
Author's presentation copy to a Dr. Philippeaux (?).

Rénon was physician to the Pitié Hospital and his book contains fifteen lectures on the heart, dealing with chlorides and low chloride diet, aneurysm, etc. He describes aneurysmal cachexia, sometimes described as aneurysmal phthisis (not uncommon in those days), and the pleural complications of heart disease. These conferences, comparable with Merklen's *Leçons* (see no. 405), were valuable original contributions to cardiology at the time, and were cited by Allbutt.

MERKLEN (Marie Joseph Félix Pierre) 1852–1906

405 Leçons sur les troubles fonctionnels du cœur (insuffisance cardiaque – asystolie,) publiées par Jean Heitz. *Paris, Masson, 1908.* viii, 428 pp. Illus, port. (frontispiece); diagrs, bibliog. (ftn. refs). 8vo, 23 cms.

Merklen, physician to the Laennec Hospital was described by Vaquez as the perfect physician whose lectures contained more substantial marrow than the long treatises of his contemporaries, and even today they make delightful reading. He was a supporter of Lauder Brunton's theory of distension of the left ventricle as a cause of anginal pain and gave a classical description of left heart failure following angina pectoris. He was an early advocate of the salt-free diet in heart failure.

LECLERQ (ARTHUR) 1856–?

406 Les Maladies du cœur et de l'aorte et leur traitement. *Paris, Octave Doin, 1919.* 552 pp. Illus, diagrs. 8vo, 20 cms.

Later Works

LAUBRY (CHARLES) 1872–1960

407 Leçons de sémiologie cardio-vasculaire: les troubles fonctionnels. *Paris, Octave Doin, 1924.* [iii], ii, 496 pp. Diagrs (incl. tracings). 8vo, 25 cms.

Comprises Laubry's characteristic teaching on cardiovascular symptomatology.

408 Maladies du cœur et des vaisseaux ... avec la collaboration de Daniel Routier, J. Walser, Ed. Doumer. (Nouveau traité de pathologie interne, tom. 3, 1ére partie). *Paris, Gaston Doin, 1930.* vii, 1246 pp. Illus, diagrs (incl. tracings). 4to, 28 cms.

409 Appareil circulatoire. (Collections des Initiations Médicales). *Paris, Masson, 1935.* 186 pp. Illus, diagrs (tracings). 8vo, 20 cms.

Publisher's catalogue, March 1935 (48 pp.) bound in at end.

Author's presentation copy to DEB with a letter, 21st June, 1937, and a menu card of the National Hospital for Diseases of the Heart dinner, at the Café Royal, to Laubry on the occasion of the St. Cyres Lecture 10 June, 1937, to which he refers in his letter. Also a card dated 13 January (no year). Two other letters to DEB relate to Laubry's supposed death during the war (see also note at no. 97). One from J. D. Rolleston (John Davy Rolleston, 1873–1946, M.A., D.M., F.R.C.P., F.S.A., dated 14 April, 1941 says, "I am sorry that the only information I can give you about him is the single line: 'In Nantes verstarb der bekannte Herzspezialist Prof. Laubry', which appeared in the *Schweizerische medizinische Wochenschrift* of January 25, p. 44." The other is from Laubry himself, the first letter of the war announcing that he was alive, dated 29 March 1945: "Voici plus de six mois que nous avons recuvré(!) la liberté et je ne vous ai pas donné de mes nouvelles—pas signe de vie après que le bruit de ma mort est parvenu jusqu'en Angleterre: je vous en fais tout mes excuses, mais soyez tranquille, je ne vous ai pas oubliés."

CLERC (ANTONIN PIERRE) 1871–1954

410 Précis de pathologie médicale: tom. 4. Cœur, par A. Clerc; vaisseaux, par A. Clerc et N. Deschamps. *Paris, Masson, 1931.* viii, 1298 pp. Illus, diagrs (incl. tracings). 8vo, 20 cms.

Publisher's catalogue, August 1930 (48 pp.) bound in at end. Clerc's presentation copy to DEB, 1931.

411 *The same.* Pathologie médicale du cœur et des vaisseaux. 3me éd. *Paris, Masson, 1955.* 2 tom. Illus, diagrs. 8vo, 25 cms.

Tom. 1: Cœur ([v], 1014 pp.) written with Claude Macrez; tom. 2: Vaisseaux ([v], 561 pp.) with P. Noël Deschamps. Presentation copy to DEB signed on back end-paper of tom. 1 by Suzanne Clerc, Pierre Noël Deschamps, C[laude] M[acrez].

An excellent handbook of cardiology. First edition 1931, 2nd edition 1940, both written with Pierre Noël Deschamps (*b.* 1891) as tom. 4 of the series *Précis de pathologie médicale* under the title *Cœur: vaisseaux.* "Cette [3me] édition entièrement refondue de l'ancien *Précis des maladies du cœur et des vaisseaux* est en réalité un nouveau livre" (*Preface*).

412 Titres et travaux scientifiques. *Paris, G. Steinheil, 1931.* 143 pp. Illus, diagrs (incl. tracings), bibliog. 8vo, 25 cms.

Maladies de l'appareil circulatoire, pp. 81–114.

ROGER (GEORGES EUGÈNE HENRI) 1860–1946, and others

413 Nouveau traité de médicine, [par] G. H. Roger, [Georges] Fernand [Isidor] Widal, [et] P[ierre] J[oseph] Teissier, Fascicule 10. Pathologie de l'appareil circulatoire (cœur et vaisseaux). *Paris, Masson, 1933.* 3 tom. Illus, tables, diagrs (incl. tracings), bibliog. (ftn. refs). 4to, 26 cms.

Library lacks tom. 3 (Vaisseaux). Tom. 1: xi, [iii], 991 pp.; tom. 2: [iii], 780 pp.

The editorship of this work was done by P. J. Teissier (1864–1932), who had to give up through prolonged ill-health, and died before the work was published. The rest of the editing was done by René Lutembacher (*b.* 1884, see no. 535), who had already made important contributions to the work (see the editor's preface in tom. 1). The names of the various contributors are given on the title-page of each volume. The plan of the whole series and names of all contributors are found in the xi pp. preceding the title-page of tom. 1.

FROMENT (ROGER) *b.* 1907

414 Étude clinique des maladies du cœur. [2e éd]. (Collection scientifique lyonnaise des cœurs et conferences). *Lyon, Librarie scientifique médicale, [1946].* 334 pp. Illus, diagrs (tracings). 8vo, 25 cms.

Presentation copy to DEB from Gallavardin, March 1946.

A well illustrated summary of contemporary cardiology, first published 1943. Froment succeeded Gallavardin at Lyon.

415 Précis de clinique cardio-vasculaire. *Paris, Masson, 1962.* [iv], 839 pp. Illus, diagrs (incl. tracings). 8vo, 25 cms.

Author's presentation copy to DEB, acquired 1962.

German

KREYSIG (FRIEDRICH LUDWIG) 1770–1839

416 Die Krankheiten des Herzens systematisch bearbeitet und durch eigene Beobachtungen erläutert. *Berlin, Maurer, 1814–1817.* 3 Theile in 4 Bände. Illus (plates), tables (plates), bibliog. (ftn. refs). 8vo, 21 cms.

Band 1 (xxiv, 392 pp.) 1814, contains "Erster allgemeine Theil welcher die Pathologie und Diagnostik enthält." Band 2 (vi, 455, [3] pp.), 1815, contains "Zweiter Theil. Erste Abt. Welcher die nähere Diagnose der Herzkrankheiten, die Erkenntniss und Behandlung der dynamischen und die speciellere Pathologie der organischen Herzkrankheiten enthält." Band 3 (vi, 457–879, [6] pp.), 1816, contains "Zweiter Theil. Zweite Abt., welche die Erkenntniss und Behandlung der besondern organischen und mechanischen Krankheiten des Herzens enthält." This copy also has the dedication and "Inhalt des dritten Theiles" (pp. iii–viii) belonging to Band 4, and included in its collation. Band 4 (viii, 415, [5] pp.) contains "Dritter Theil, Fälle von Herzkrankheiten, Zusätze und Register enthaltend." Index of author's cited, pp. 399–415.

Autograph: Dr. Burk [?].

From 1800 until Laennec's discovery of auscultation, there were only four major text-books on heart disease, that of Burns (1809, nos. 263–5) in England, of Corvisart (1806, nos. 360–65) in France, of Testa (1811) in Italy, and of Kreysig (1814–1817) in Germany. It is a prolix and tedious work, with long sentences and as Herrick (no. 1010, pp. 79–83) states, was based more on research in the library than in the ward. Nevertheless, it has its strong points such as advocating digitalis, and sound views on angina pectoris and coronary disease; Kreysig's wide review of the literature provides a good picture of cardiology at the time.

ZEHETMAYER (FRANZ) 1813–1846

417 Die Herzkrankheiten. Leitfaden zum Selbstunterrichte für Ärzte. *Wien, Braumüller & Seidel, 1845.* xxviii, 411 pp. 8vo, 22 cms.

Cited as an important work of the Vienna school in Skoda's day. It deals with physical examination, heart sounds, arterial and venous pulses, etc. It is noteworthy as giving the first description of squatting or the knee-elbow posture in pericardial effusion. Zehetmayer, professor in Vienna, also wrote *Grundzüge der Perkussion und Auskultation und ihrer Anwendung auf die Diagnostik der Brustfell- und Lungenkrankheiten, als Leitfaden zum Selbstunterrichte für Aerzte* for the same publisher in 1843 (2nd edition 1845; 3rd edition, 1854; Italian translation, Padova, tip. Bianchi, 1854).

TRAUBE (LUDWIG) 1818–1876

418 Über den Zusammenhang von Herz-und Nieren-Krankheiten. *Berlin, August Hirschwald, 1856.* [iii], 81 pp. 8vo, 22 cms.

Provenance (book-stamp): Carl [Karl] Ernst Emil Hoffmann, Dr. Med. (of Basel, anatomist, 1827–1877). Signature: [unreadable], 1879.

A classic work on hypertensive heart disease prior to the sphygmomanometer, a selective translation of which is included, with other works by Traube, in Ruskin's *Classics of hypertension* (no. 763, pp. 186–212). Traube "developed by 1856 the association of contracted kidneys with hypertrophy of the left ventricle. Although, like Bright, he noted in his cases increased arterial pulse tension, and, thanks to von Graefe, haemorrhagic retinitis, he interpreted the hypertrophy of the left heart as primarily compensatory to the decreased renal capillary blood perfusion . . . *Pulsus alternans* was incidentally discovered by Traube in his studies of pulsus bigeminus" (Ruskin, *op. cit.*, p. 186).

419 Die Symptome der Krankheiten des Respirations- und Circulations-Apparats. Vorlesungen gehalten an der Friedrichs-Wilhelms-Universität zu Berlin. *Berlin, August Hirschwald, 1867.* [viii], 168 pp. 8vo, 24 cms.

Lectures given in Berlin dealing with pulse and respiration rate, oedema, etc. Traube studied percussion under Skoda in Vienna and became a great authority on physical diagnosis. He was physician to the Charité Hospital, Berlin, and later professor of medicine.

BAMBERGER (HEINRICH VON) 1822–1888

420 Lehrbuch der Krankheiten des Herzens. *Wien, Wilhelm Braumüller, 1857.* viii, 459 pp. Bibliog. 8vo, 22 cms.

Autographs: A. Gusserow (possibly Adolf Ludwig Sigismund Gusserow, 1836–1906, M.D. 1859, professor of obstetrics at Utrecht 1867, Zürich 1867–1872, Strasbourg 1872–1878 and then Berlin); Erich Meyer 1918 (? Erich Meyer 1874–1927, author of the haematological work *Ueber das Verhalten und den Nachweiss des Schwefelwasserstoffes im Blute*, Halle, 1898. The name is, however, quite common).

One of the standard early German text-books on the heart, and one of Bamberger's chief works. Having graduated M.D. in Prague in 1847, he spent some time under Skoda (no. 479) and Rokitansky (nos. 799, 905). At the time of writing the *Lehrbuch* he was professor at Würzburg, but in 1872 he became professor in Vienna.

HAMERNÍK (JOSEF) 1810–1887

421 Das Herz und seine Bewegung. Beiträge zur Anatomie, Physiologie und Pathologie des Herzens, des Herzbeutels und des Brustfelles. *Prag, H. Dominicus, 1858.* xxv, 240 pp. 8vo, 23 cms.

Hamerník was professor of auscultation and percussion and of respiratory and circulatory diseases at Prague.

FRIEDREICH (NIKOLAUS) 1825–1882

422 Krankheiten des Herzens. 2e Aufll. (Handbuch der speciellen Pathologie und Therapie... herausgegeben von Rud[olf] Virchow, 5e Band, 2e Abt.). *Erlangen, Ferdinand Enke, 1867.* [iv], 334, v–vi pp. Diagrs (tracings), bibliog. 8vo, 24 cms.

Friedrich was professor at Heidelberg, and first documented the hereditary spinal ataxia often known as Friedreich's ataxia (Uber die degenerative Atrophie der spinalen Hinterstränge, *Archiv fur pathologische Anatomie*, 1863, **26**, 391–419, 433–59, etc.). According to Balfour (no. 505, pp. 14–15), Friedreich (in the first edition of this work, 1861, p. 366) seems to have been the earliest German physician to adopt the view that "in stenosis of the left auriculo-ventricular orifice the murmur is sometimes only audible during the time of the active contraction of the auricle".

423 *The same.* Traité des maladies du cœur, par A. (*sic*) Friedreich; traduit de l'allemand sur la 2e éd. par les docteurs Lorber et Doyon. *Paris, Adrien Delahaye, 1873.* [vii], 592 pp. Bibliog. 8vo, 23 cms.

DUSCH (THEODOR) Freiherr von, 1824–1890

424 Lehrbuch der Herzkrankheiten. *Leipzig, Wilhelm Engelmann, 1868.* viii, 380 pp. Illus, diagrs (tracings), bibliog. 8vo, 24 cms.

Manuscript notes in German.

Von Dusch was professor at Heidelberg and his *Lehrbuch* with its closely printed pages has a valuable bibliography (pp. 363–74). It is an exhaustive compendium on diagnosis which, according to Balfour, in the preface to his *Clinical lectures on the diseases of heart and aorta* (no. 305, p. xiv), had no equal in any language at the time. On p. 214 von Dusch following Friedreich describes the presystolic murmur as a well-known indication of mitral stenosis.

STEFFEN (JOHANN THEODOR AUGUST) 1825–1910

425 Klinik der Kinderkrankheiten. Band 3: Krankheiten des Herzens. *Berlin, August Hirschwald, 1889.* viii, 427 pp. Tables, diagrs (tracings), bibliog. (ftn. refs). 8vo, 24 cms.

Deals with heart disease in children including congenital heart disease. Steffen was the son of Wilhelm August Steffen (1792–1874) of Stettin, known for his work on the cholera epidemic in that town in 1831. Steffen himself was a paediatrician, and the above work is a continuation of *Klinik der Kinderkrankheiten: Krankheiten der Lunge und Pleura.* Berlin, August Hirschwald, 1865–70. 2 Bande.

FRAENTZEL (OSCAR MAXIMILIAN VICTOR) 1838–1894

426 Vorlesungen über die Krankheiten des Herzens. *Berlin, August Hirschwald, 1889–1892.* 3 Bande in 2. Bibliog. (ftn. refs). 8vo, 25 cms.

Band 1: Die idiopathischen Herzvergrösserungen. 1889. xii, 252 pp.; Band 2: Die Entzündungen des Endocardiums und des Pericardiums. 1891. x, 283 pp.; Band 3: Schluss. 1892. viii, 108 pp. (with index for all three volumes).

Autograph and book-stamp: Dr. Holniger ("Nervenarzt, Halle").

Fraentzel was assistant to Traube (nos. 418–9). He had a career in military medicine and became professor at the Charité Hospital in Berlin. His special interests were heart and lung diseases (especially tuberculosis). Of his *Vorlesungen* above, his obituary in the *Lancet* (1894, **2**, 765) says that they "are characterised by a clearness of style and soundness of judgment that renders them of great value."

KREHL (LUDOLF VON) 1861–1937

427 Die Erkrankungen des Herzmuskels und die nervösen Herzkrankheiten. 2e Aufll. *Wien und Leipzig, Alfred Holder, 1913.* viii, 578 pp. Bibliog. (chapters, ftn refs). 8vo, 25 cms.

Autograph: Rudolf Kaufmann (1871–1927, the Viennese cardiologist, author of a long series of papers on various aspects, interested in pharmacological side of cardiology. His heart hospital—Herzstation—was originally for soldiers during the First World War). This copy presented to DEB at Vienna Herzstation 1929, by Dr. Hugo Roesler, Kaufmann's pupil. First edition, 1901.

Krehl, professor at Heidelberg, was an authority on myocardial disease and gives a good early account of cardiac infarction.

BASCH (SAMUEL SIEGFRIED KARL) Ritter von, 1837–1905

428 Allgemeine Physiologie und Pathologie des Kreislaufs. *Wien, Alfred Holder, 1892.* viii, 186 pp. Illus, diagrs (tracings). 8vo, 25 cms.

A few manuscript notes in English. Autograph: F. P. Weber, 1892 (from the library of Frederick Parkes Weber, 1863–1962, M.A., M.D., F.R.C.P., F.S.A.).

A very important account of left heart failure and of its pulmonary changes, "lung stiffness", etc. Von Basch graduated M.D. Vienna in 1861 and went to Mexico where he became physician to the Emperor Maximilian. In May 1867 he was taken prisoner at the battle of Queritaro. He was present when the Emperor was executed by a firing squad of the victorious revolutionaries, and accompanied the body to Europe, and published his *Erinnerungen aus Mexico*, Leipzig, 1868. At Leipzig he worked on the influence of the splanchnic nerve on the distribution of blood in the body and experimentally with animals on changes of the circulation, seeking to bring these observations into line with those observed in human disease. After 1878 as professor of experimental pathology at Vienna, he devoted much attention to the study of cardiac dyspnoea and cardiac asthma. Von Basch pioneered the routine recording of blood pressure in clinical cardiology. Actually Potain's much simpler sphygmomanometer soon came into use.

BAUER (KARL JOSEPH VON) 1845–1912 and BOLLINGER (OTTO VON) 1843–1909

429 Über idiopathische Herzvergrösserung. Festschrift . . . des . . . Dr. Max von Pettenkofer, verfasst von . . . Dr. Jos. Bauer und . . . Dr. O. Bollinger. *München, J. F. Lehmann, 1893.* 103 pp. Illus (plate), bibliog. 4to, 26 cms.

Early works on idiopathic hypertrophy and the Munich beer drinkers' heart.

HORVATH (ALEXIS) 1836–?

430 Über die Hypertrophie des Herzens aus den Vorlesugen über allgemeine Pathologie. *Wien und Leipzig, Wilhelm Braumüller, 1897.* iv, 259 pp. Bibliog. (ftn. refs). 8vo, 26 cms.

An important early work on cardiac hypertrophy with account of early theories. Alexis Horvath is the form of the author's name used in translations. The strict translation of the name is Khorvat and his Russian forenames Aleksiei Nikolayevich (see *Index-catalogue of the Library of the Surgeon-General's Office*, 2nd series, vol. 8, p. 631). The original Russian book, transliterated *O hipertrofii serdtsa* (*iz lektsiy po obshtshei patologii*), was published in Kazan, where Horvath was professor, in 1896.

ROSENBACH (OTTOMAR) 1851–1907

431 Die Krankheiten des Herzens und ihre Behandlung. *Wien und Leipzig, Urban & Schwarzenberg, 1897.* xvi, 1128 pp. Bibliog. (ftn. refs). 8vo, 25 cms.

Contains headed notepaper of "Prof. Dr. A. Hoffmann", Düsseldorf, 190–. Garrison and Morton 2799.

Rosenbach, professor in Berlin, was probably the first to associate tabes accompanied by aortic incompetence with syphilis. This copy and the copy at the library of the Wellcome Institute for the History of Medicine have the date 1897. The *Index-catalogue of the library of the Surgeon-General's Office*, the British Museum *Catalogue of printed books* and Garrison and Morton all have 1893–1897. It is probable therefore that this work was issued in parts starting in 1893, the title-page, contents and foreword (xvi pp.) being printed last.

ALBRECHT (EHRENFRIED) 1864–?

432 Der Herzmuskel und seine Bedeutung für Physiologie, Pathologie, und Klinik des Herzens. Ein Versuch zur Entwickelung einer allgemeinen Pathologie und Symptomatologie der Herzmuskelerkrankungen auf anatomischer Grundlage. *Berlin, Julius Springer, 1903.* xv, 590, [1] pp. Illus (7 folding plates), bibliog. (ftn. refs). 8vo, 23 cms.

This is a classic work on the heart muscle. Albrecht with Horvath (no. 430) introduced the injury theory of hypertrophy, later supported by Eyster (no. 890).

DE LA CAMP (OSKAR) 1871–1925

433 Experimentelle Studien über die acute Herzdilatation.

Reprinted from *Zeitschrift für klinische Medizin*, 1904, **51**, 1–79. Tables, diagrs, bibliog. (ftn. refs). An important work on acute dilatation.

PAL (JACOB) 1863–1936

434 Gefässkrisen. *Leipzig, S. Hirzel, 1905* [v], 275 pp. Illus, diagrs (tracings), bibliog. 8vo, 23 cms.

Garrison and Morton 2713. Deals with vascular crises in abdomen, chest, brain and limbs, in reference to angina pectoris and other clinical syndromes. A much quoted work in its time, with an alphabetical bibliography (pp. 262–70). Pal was professor at the Allgemeines Krankenhaus in Vienna.

ROMBERG (ERNST VON) 1865–1933

435 Lehrbuch der Krankheiten des Herzens und der Blutgefässe. 4e und 5e Aufl. *Stuttgart, Ferdinand Enke, 1925.* xv, 833 pp. Illus, diagrs (incl. tracings), bibliog. 8vo, 25 cms.

Publisher's catalogue (4 pp.) bound in at end.

First edition, 1906; second edition, 1909 (RCP); third edition, 1921. Especially valuable for the extensive bilbiographies at end of each chapter. Romberg was professor and director of the Munich University Medical Clinic.

JÜRGENSEN (THEODOR VON) 1840–1907, and others

436 Diseases of the heart, by Th. v. Jürgensen, L. v. Schrötter [and] L. Krehl; ed. with additions by George Dock; authorised translation from the German, under the editorial

supervision of Alfred Stengel. *Philadelphia & London, W. B. Saunders, 1908.* 848 pp. Illus, tables, diagrs, bibliog. 8vo, 25 cms.

Publisher's catalogue (16 pp.) bound in at end. Bibliographies at the end of many sections and copious footnote references.

Part of *Nothnagel's Encyclopaedia of practical medicine.* The section on angina pectoris by Krehl is historically important and includes Nothnagel's vaso-motor angina. Note occlusion of coronary arteries, p. 699. A very complete contemporary review of heart disease with historical data.

GEIGEL (RICHARD) 1859–1930

437 Lehrbuch der Herzkrankheiten. *München und Wiesbaden, J. F. Bergman, 1920.* vii, 316 pp. Illus, diagrs (incl. tracings). 8vo, 25 cms.

Publisher's catalogue (4 pp.) bound in at end.

Geigel was professor at Würzburg.

Later Works

HOCHHAUS (HEINRICH) 1858–1916

438 Die Krankheiten des Herzens und der Gefässe: ein kurzgefasstes praktisches Lehrbuch... bearbeitet und herausgegeben von Dr. G. Liebermeister. *Berlin, Julius Springer, 1922.* vi, 313 pp. Illus, diagrs (incl. tracings), bibliog. 8vo, 25 cms.

Published posthumously from Hochhaus's manuscript by Gustav Liebermeister (1879–1943). Hochhaus was professor and director of the Augusta Hospital at Cologne.

WASSERMANN (SIGMUND) 1877–196–?

439 Neue klinische Gesichtspunkte zur Lehre vom Asthma cardiale. *Berlin [und] Wien, Urban & Schwarzenberg, 1926.* [vii], 168 pp. Illus, diagrs (incl. tracings), bibliog. (ftn. refs). 8vo, 25 cms.

A pioneer work on left heart failure dedicated to Wenckebach, the author's teacher.

BRUGSCH (THEODOR KARL LOUIS) 1878–1963

440 Lehrbuch der Herz- und Gefässerkrankungen einschliesslich der Diagnostik der Kreislaufserkrankungen und der speziellen Prognostik der Herzkranken. *Berlin, Georg Stilke, 1929.* xvi, 694 pp. Illus, tables, diagrs (incl. tracings), bibliog. (ftn. refs). 8vo, 25 cms.

Publisher's catalogue (2 pp.) bound in at end.

A very comprehensive account of heart disease and of prognosis and treatment. The author was professor at Halle.

EDENS (ERNST) 1876–1944

441 Die Krankheiten des Herzens und der Gefässe. *Berlin, Julius Springer, 1929.* viii, 1057 pp. Illus, tables, diagrs (incl. tracings), bibliog. 4to, 26 cms.

Edens was professor at Munich and his text-book is of especial value for its comprehensive bibliography of 246 pages which gives many of the German editions of English and French works.

WENCKEBACH (KAREL FREDERIK) 1864–1940

442 Herz- und Kreislaufinsuffizienz: ein kurzes System der Störungen im Kreislaufapparat. (Medizinische Praxis, Band 12). *Dresden und Leipzig, Theodor Steinkopff, 1931.* x, 120 pp. Illus, diagrs. 8vo, 23 cms.

Publisher's announcement (2 pp.) bound in at end. Second edition 1934, reprinted 1942.

This great Dutch cardiologist graduated M.D. at Utrecht in 1888, and his cardiological researches began while still there. His first full-length work *Die Arhythmie als Ausdruck bestimmter Funktionsstörungen des Herzens* (Leipzig, W. Engelmann 1903) brought him international recognition. His numerous honours and researches will be found in obituaries (e.g. *British Heart Journal*, 1941, **3**, 141–4). He was professor at Groningen (1901), Strasbourg (1911) and Vienna (1914–1929) and his forenames are often found as Karl Friedrich from his German writings. Three eponymous terms are named after him. A short biography, with a bibliography of 120 references, *Karel Frederik Wenckebach (1864–1940): een korte schets van zijn leven en werken* has been written by Dr. G. A. Lindeboom (Haarlem, Bohn, 1965) (RCP). For his St. Cyres lecture, see no 987.

SCHERF (DAVID) *b.* 1899

443 Klinik und Therapie der Herzkrankheiten und der Gefässerkrankungen; Vorträge für praktische Ärzte. 3^e^ Aufl. *Wien, Julius Springer, 1936.* viii, 290 pp. Diagrs (incl. tracings). 8vo, 21 cms.

Publisher's catalogue (2 pp.) bound in at end. First and second editions, 1935.

SCHERF (DAVID) *b.* 1899 and BOYD (LINN JOHN) *b.* 1895

444 Cardio-vascular diseases: their diagnosis and treatment. *London, William Heinemann, 1939.* xii, 458 pp. Diagrs. 8vo, 22 cms.

Acquired in Johannesburg Dec. 1943. This revised English version of the original German work was a very popular text-book in its day.

Scherf (M.S. 1922, M.D. 1923, Privat docent 1935–7) worked in Vienna under Wenckebach and became professor of clinical medicine at the New York Medical College from 1938. Special interests are cardiology and electrocardiography.

GROSSE-BROCKHOFF (FRANZ) *b.* 1907, and others

445 Spezielle Untersuchungsmethoden bei angeborenen und erworbenen Herzfehlern, von F. Grosse-Brockhoff, F. Loogen und A. Schaede.

Reprinted from *Handbuch der inneren Medizin*, 4e Aufl. Berlin, Göttingen, Heidelberg, Springer, 1960. Band 9, Teil 2, pp. 1242–87. Illus, diagrs, bibliog. 8vo, 25 cms.

Deals with cardiac catheterisation, haemodynamics, angiocardiography, aortography, etc. Bibliography of 6 pages.

446 Erworbene Herzklappenfehler, von F. Grosse-Brockhoff, K. Kaiser und F. Loogen.

Reprinted from *Handbuch der inneren Medizin*, 4e Aufl. Berlin, Göttingen, Heidelberg, Springer, 1960. Band 9, Teil 2, pp. 1288–1550. Illus, tables, diagrs, bibliog. 8vo, 25 cms. Bibliography of 35 pages.

The *Handbuch der inneren Medizin* was founded by Leo Mohr (1874–1918) and R. Staehelin in 1911. This fourth edition was published under the direction of G. von Bergmann, W. Frey and H. Schwiegk; Band 9 has the overall title *Herz und Kreislauf:* for a list of parts see copy of no. 448.

WOLLHEIM (Ernst) *b.* 1900 and MOELLER (Julius)

447 Hypertonie – Hypotonie. (*Handbuch der inneren Medizin.* 4e Aufl. Band 9, Teil 5.) *Berlin, Göttingen, Heidelberg, Springer, 1960.* xv, 943 pp. Illus, tables, diagrs, bibliog. 4to, 26 cms.

An encyclopaedic work on hypertension. Bibliography, 114 pages. Wollheim was professor at Wurzburg. (For series, see note under no. 446).

WOLLHEIM (Ernst) *b.* 1900 and ZISSLER (Josef)

448 Krankheiten der Gefässe. (*Handbuch der inneren Medizin,* 4e Aufl. Band 9, Teil 6). *Berlin, Göttingen, Heidelberg, Springer, 1960.* xvi, 895 pp. Illus, tables, diagrs, bibliog. 4to, 26 cms.

This book covers disease of arteries, veins, lymphatics, aneurysm, A-V fistula, etc. A vast bibliography of 277 pages. For series, see note under no. 446.

Italian

TESTA (Antonio Giuseppe) 1756–1814

449 Delle malattie del cuore loro cagioni specie, segni e cura. *Bologna, presso Giuseppe Lucchesini, 1810–1811.* 3 vols. Bibliog. (ftn. refs). 8vo, 24 cms.

Vol. 1 (civ, 215 pp.), libro 1: Cagioni; vol. 2 (cxxxii, 249 pp.), libro 2: Specie e segni, parte 1; Asimmetrie; and vol. 3 (473 pp.) (called vol. 2) parte 2, Infiammagioni. Despite the note on the title-page ("libri tre, volumi tre") there appears to be no libro 3. A fine uncut copy. Enclosed is correspondence with R. D. Gurney, antiquarian bookseller, about this book.

Testa was at the time of writing this book professor of clinical medicine at Bologna University. He was formerly professor of medicine and surgery in the Hospital at Ferrara. His book was one of the four major text-books on heart disease prior to Laennec's discovery of auscultation (nos. 455–9). He was familiar with angina pectoris and accepted Parry's coronary theory (no. 609) with some reservation. His book ran through several editions and a German translation. Of Testa himself and his works, Dezeimeris (no. 1101) remarks: "Il avait fait une longue étude des anciens, et l'amour qu'il avait pour cette littérature l'a entraîné dans des digressions bien diffuses et moins utiles que curieuses. Il passait pour un théoricien savant, mais pour un clinicien médiocre. Quoique diffus, ses ouvrages offrent de l'intérêt.'

Spanish

ARRILLAGA (Francisco C.) *b.* 1896

450 Insuficiencia cardiaca. *Buenos Aires, "El Ateneo", 1929.* 304 pp. Illus, diagrs (incl. tracings), bibliog. (ftn. refs). 8vo, 24 cms.

Presentation copy "à mon cher ami le Docteur F. Parkes Weber, avec l'espoir de vous visiter bientôt à Londres, tres sincèrement, votre devoué. . . ." From the library of Frederick Parkes Weber (1863–1962, M.D., F.R.C.P.).

DIAGNOSIS

Physical Diagnosis, Percussion, Auscultation and the Heart Sounds

The pioneers of physical diagnosis were Auenbrugger, Piorry, Corvisart and Laennec. Corvisart translated Auenbrugger's *Inventum* and introduced percussion in his clinic. Piorry first practised mediate percussion with a pleximeter, soon replaced by the physician's finger as used today.

Laennec, with his stethoscope, identified two sounds to each heart beat and described various kinds of murmur, thus making clinical signs audible as well as visible and palpable, and so paving the way for others to establish the signs of valvular disease. Despite many errors of interpretation Laennec opened up a new era in cardiac diagnosis.

AUENBRUGGER (LEOPOLD) 1722–1809

451 Inventum Novum. Faksimile nach der ersten Ausgabe begleitet von der französischen Übersetzung Corvisart's, der englischen von Forbes, der deutschen von Ungar. Herausgegeben und mit einter biographischen Skizze versehen von Dr. Max Neuburger. *Wien und Leipzig, Josef Šafár, 1922.* [311 pp. Various paging]. Ports, facsims, bibliog. 8vo, 24 cms.

No. 136 of limited edition. Has own overall title-page and frontispiece portrait of Auenbrugger. Individual pagination for each item.

Comprises the original treatise: *Inventum novum ex percussione thoracis humani ut signo abstrusos interni pectoris morbos detegendi.* (Vindobonae, typis Joannis Thomae Trattner, 1761. 95 pp.); French translation by J. N. Corvisart *Nouvelle méthode pour reconnaitre les maladies internes de la poitrine par la percussion de cette cavité.* ([Paris, de l'imprimerie de Migneret, 1824] 51 pp.); English translation by Sir John Forbes *On percussion of the chest* ([London, T. & G. Underwood, 1824] 36 pp.); German translation by S. Ungar *Neue Erfindung mittelst des Anschlagens an den Brustkorb, als eines Zeichens, verborgene Brustkrankheiten.* [Wien, J. B. Wallishausser, 1843] 55 pp.); and

NEUBURGER (Max) 1868–1955. *Leopold Auenbrugger und sein Inventum Novum: eine historische Skizze* [Wien und Leipzig, Josef Šafář, 1922]. 72 pp. Port., bibliog.

Auenbrugger was physician to the Spanish Hospital in Vienna and a successful practitioner there.

452 *The same.* On percussion of the chest: being a translation of Auenbrugger's original treatise entitled "*Inventum novum . . .*" by John Forbes M.D. [London, 1824]; introduction by Henry E. Sigerist. *Baltimore, Johns Hopkins Press, 1936.* [i], 31 pp. Port., facsim., bibliog. (ftn. refs). 4to, 27 cms.

Reprinted from *Bulletin of the Institute of the History of Medicine*, 1936, **4**, 373–403. Also published Camac (no. 1040), pp. 121–47, preceded by a biographical sketch pp. 117–19.

453 *The same.* Nouvelle méthode pour reconnaitre les maladies internes, de la poitrine par la percussion de cette cavité . . . Ouvrage traduit du latin et commenté par J. N. Corvisart. *Paris, de l'imprimerie de Migneret, 1808.* xxiv, 440, [1] pp. Bibliog. (ftn. refs). 8vo, 21 cms.

Last page errata. Text arranged in two columns for Latin original and French translation; French commentary covers the whole page width.

Autograph: Ex libris Bauer [?]. Corvisart introduced percussion into practice in his clinic in Paris.

AUENBRUGGER (LEOPOLD)

BISHOP (PATRICK JAMES) *b.* 1926

454 A bibliography of Auenbrugger's *Inventum novum* (1761).

Reprinted from *Tubercle*, 1961, **42,** 78–90. Port., facsims, bibliog. 8vo, 25 cms. Author's presentation copy.

LAENNEC (RÉNÉ THEOPHILE HYACINTHE) 1781–1826

455 De l'auscultation médiate ou Traité du diagnostic des maladies du poumon et du cœur, fondé principalement sur ce nouveau moyen d'exploration. *Paris, J. A. Brosson et J. S. Chaudé, 1819.* 2 tom. Illus (plates), bibliog. (ftn refs). 8vo, 21 cms.

Garrison and Morton 2673. Osler 1318. Tom. 1: xlviii [i.e. xlvi], 456, [8] pp.; tom. 2: xvi, 472 pp.

456 *The same.* Traité de l'auscultation médiate et des maladies des poumons et du cœur. *Paris, Masson, 1927.* 2 tom. Illus (plates), bibliog. (ftn. refs). 8vo, 24 cms.

Tom. 1: [xii], v–xxxvi, 728 pp.; tom. 2: [vii], 790 pp.

Facsimile reproduction of second edition 1826, published on the centenary of the death of Laennec. "La présente édition, publiée avec le concours du Comité du Centenaire de Laennec, reproduit en fac-simile le texte de la deuxième édition (1826). A titre documentaire, la préface de la première édition (1819) a été reproduite et placée en tête du volume, entre la titre et la préface de la deuxième édition."

457 *The same.* 4e éd., considérablement augmentée par M. Andral. *Paris, J. S. Chaudé, 1837.* 3 tom. Illus, bibliog. (ftn. refs). 8vo, 21 cms.

Preface by Andral and by Laennec with notes by Mériadec Laennec. Tom. 1: xxviii, 672 pp.; tom. 2: [iii], 704 pp. (page numbering 365–80 confused but text complete); tom. 3: [iii], 576 pp. (4 plates).

Provenance: presented by Brigadier William Kenneth Morrison, D.S.O., in Malta, 1943.

The first (1819) and second (1826) editions of *Traité de l'auscultation médiate* were published during Laennec's lifetime, the third edition (1831) was published by his cousin, Mériadec Laennec with his notes, and the fourth edition (1837) by Andral (1797–1876) with his notes. Forbes's translation of Laennec's *Traité* was first published in 1821, the second edition, 1827, third edition 1829 and fourth edition, 1834. An American edition of Forbes's translation was published in Philadelphia, 1823, and a second American edition (of the third English edition) in New York, 1830 and a third in 1835 (fourth English edition). The first German edition was published in Weimar, 1822.

Laennec's contribution to diseases of the lungs was of more importance than that to heart disease, for the cause of the heart sounds was unknown in 1819. He made a fundamental error in attributing the second sound to atrial systole. In his first edition (1819), he regarded the bellows murmur as evidence of valvular obstruction; in the second edition (1826) he revised his opinion and regarded the murmur as due to spasm of the heart, a muscular sound. He also discarded the new laether sound described by Collin (no. 465), his chef de clinique, as due to pericarditis, and attributed it to cardio-pulmonary bruit. So in the second edition he fell into worse error than in the first.

458 *The same.* A Treatise on the diseases of the chest and on mediate auscultation . . . trans. from the latest French edition, with copious notes and a sketch of the author's life by John Forbes . . . 4th ed., considerably enlarged and improved with many additional notes and an extensive bilbiography of the different diseases. *London, Longman, Rees, Orme, Brown, Green & Longman; Whittaker; Simpkin and Marshall; J. Chidley; E.*

Portwine: and Henry Renshaw, 1834. xliv, 676 pp. Illus (plates), bibliog. (sections, ftn. refs). 8vo, 24 cms.

Book-stamp: Medical Officers Library, Cambridge Hospital, Aldershot. Signatures: Neale (possibly William Michael Neale, 1813–1877, of Worksop, Notts.) and W. Finlay (several of this name, perhaps W. Finlay, *b.* 1845, of Army Medical Department).

This edition contains Forbes's extensive bibliography of early works on the heart. He published an alphabetical *Manual of select medical bibliography* . . . (London, Sherwood, Gilbert and Piper, 1835) covering all diseases.

459 *The same.* A Treatise on the diseases of the chest, with plates, trans. from the French of R. T. H. Laennec M.D., with a preface and notes by John Forbes, M.D. (New York. Academy of Medicine Library. History of Medicine Series no. 17). *New York, Hafner, 1962.* [vi], xliii, 437 pp. Illus (plates), bibliog. (ftn. refs). 8vo, 21 cms.

Facsimile reprint of 1821 edition. This translation is also published in Camac (no. 1040), pp. 157–204, and is preceded by a biographical sketch of Laennec, pp. 151–6.

460 Proposition sur la doctrine d'Hippocrate, relativement à la médecine-pratique. [*Thesis*]. (*n.p., n.d., 1926?*) 39, [5] pp., 3 inserted leaves. 4to, 26 cms.

Facsimile reproduction of Laennec's M.D. thesis (*Paris, Didot jeune*, 1804) which contains Laennec's notes written in the margins and inserted at the end.

461 Laennec, 1781–1826 (Documents inédits). *Paris, Masson, 1926.* 42 pp. Facsims. 8vo, 25 cms.

Cover title reads: *Laennec. Documents inédits publiés a l'occasion de son centenaire.* No. 765 of 1000 copies distributed by the Centenary Committee. Contains notes and documents from the library of the Faculty of Medicine, Paris, and the Laennec Museum of Nantes Medical School.

SAINTIGNON (HENRI)

462 Laennec, sa vie et son œuvre. *Paris, J. B. Baillière, 1904.* 488 pp. Ports, bibliog. 8vo, 20 cms.

Presentation copy to a M. Labarre. A standard life of Laennec.

WEBB (GERALD BERTRAM) 1871–1948

463 René Théophile Hyacinthe Laennec; a memoir. *New York, Paul B. Hoeber, 1928.* xix, 146 pp. Illus, ports, facsims. 12mo, 20 cms.

LE JUMEAU DE KERGARADEC (JEAN ALEXANDRE) 1787–1877

PINKERTON (JOHN HENRY MCKNIGHT) *b.* 1920

464 Kergaradec, friend of Laennec and pioneer of foetal auscultation.

Reprinted from *Proceedings of the Royal Society of Medicine*, 1969, **62**, 477–483 (Section of the History of Medicine, pp. 15–21), Illus, port.

A copy of DEB's letter to Professor Pinkerton at the Department of Gynaecology, Queen's University, Belfast, with dates of the general use of auscultation and the author's reply are enclosed. Le Jumeau's *Mémoire* (RCP; Garrison and Morton 6171) was published in 1822.

COLLIN (VICTOR)

465 A Treatise on the different methods of investigating the diseases of the chest, particularly percussion, and the use of the stethoscope; trans. from the French of M. Collin, with an additional preface, by W. N. Ryland, M.D. *London, Burgess & Hill, 1825.* xii, [i], 67 pp. Illus. (plate, frontispiece of stethoscope). 12mo, 16 cms.

Book-stamp: Norwich and Norfolk United Medical Book Society.

First French edition, 1824, second 1831. American edition, 1829, German edition, 1832. Forbes gave a synopsis of Collin's treatise in the appendix to this *Original cases*, 1824 (see no. 466). Collin gave the first description of pericardial friction "creaking of new leather". One of the classics of auscultation. The title of Collin's M.D. thesis *Des diverses méthodes d'exploration de la poitrine* (Paris, 1823) shows an early interest in the subject.

FORBES (Sir JOHN) 1787–1861

466 Original cases with dissections and observations illustrating the use of the stethoscope and percussion in the diagnosis of diseases of the chest; also commentaries on the same subjects selected and translated from Auenbrugger, Corvisart, Laennec and others. *London, T. and G. Underwood, 1824.* xxxvi, 304 pp. Illus (plates). 8vo, 23 cms.

Auenbrugger's treatise on percussion of the chest, pp. 1–64; On mediate auscultation (a brief outline of Laennec), pp. 65–82; "Cases, with dissections and remarks; illustrating the application of the stethoscope and percussion to the diagnosis of diseases of the chest", pp. 83–276; "Apendix: outline of an essay on the physical diagnosis of diseases of the chest; translated and abridged (with some additions) from a work by Dr. Collin, entitled "Des diverses méthodes d'exploration de la poitrine, et leur application au diagnostic de ses maladies"; published at Paris in 1824, pp. 277–302.

The earliest English work on the stethoscope. Forbes translated Laennec's book in 1821 (no. 459), since when he used auscultation and percussion regularly at the Chichester Dispensary. Collin's treatise is summarised in the appendix.

Forbes's translation of Auenbrugger was reproduced in Neuburger's collection (no. 451) and in 1936 separately by Johns Hopkins Press (no. 452).

467 Two lectures on some of the physical signs of diseases of the chest delivered before the members of the Portsmouth Philosophical Society in January 1829. *Winchester, [printed by] Robbins and Wheeler, 1830.* [ii], 26 pp. Bibliog. (ftn. refs). 8vo, 21 cms.

"Extracted from the *Provincial medical Gazette*, published at Winchester": the journal is untraced and Callisen (Bd. 6, item 2324, and Bd. 33, item 4469) can give no details. The text is in double columns. Lecture 1, On percussion, pp. 1–12; 2, On the stethoscope, pp. 12–26.

BISHOP (PATRICK JAMES) *b.* 1926

468 The Life and writings of Sir John Forbes (1787–1861).

Extracted from *Tubercle*, 1961, **42**, 255–61. Port., bibliog.

PARKES (EDMUND ALEXANDER) 1819–1876

469 Memoir of Sir John Forbes, Kt., M.D., D.C.L., F.R.S., etc. *London, printed [for private circulation] by Savill & Edwards, 1862.* vi, 7–70 pp. Port. (frontispiece). 8vo, 21 cms.

Reprinted from *British and foreign medico-chirurgical Review*, 1862, **29**, 271–82.

The author of the memoir is E. A. Parkes, not Alexander C. Forbes, son of Sir John, as in the British Museum *Catalogue of printed books*. As Forbes acknowledges in the preface, "By the kindness and courtesy of Mr. Churchill"—the publisher of *British and foreign medico-chirurgical Review* "and Dr. Parkes"—author of the original article—"I am permitted to reprint in a separate form the accompanying memoir of my late father, Sir John Forbes."

STOKES (WILLIAM) 1804–1878

470 An Introduction to the use of the stethoscope. *Edinburgh, Maclachlan & Stewart; London, Baldwin, Cradock and Joy; Dublin, Hodges and M'Arthur, 1825.* xiv, 226 pp. Bibliog. (ftn. refs). 8vo, 19 cms.

Our copy has pp. 225–6 (index) after p. xiv, possibly as substitute for a list of contents. Autographs: Henry J. Smith, Newpark; S. B. Sachs, M.B., 1936. Acquired 1940.

The first systematic English treatise on the stethoscope. According to his son's biography (no. 283, p. 33), Stokes "before he obtained any medical qualification, prepared and published in Edinburgh in 1825 a small treatise on the use of the stethoscope, for which work he received the sum of £70". Nevertheless Stokes took his degree in 1825 (thesis *De ascite*, which is not listed in the bibliography of no. 283), and our copy gives M.D. after his name. Cullen, to whom the work is dedicated, had already published cases on the practical uses of the stethoscope in diagnosing thoracic diseases, as had Forbes, whose *Original cases* (no. 466) showed that he was using the stethoscope at his Chichester Dispensary as early as 1822. The work itself shows a knowledge of Bayle, Laennec, Andral and Forbes in addition to practical pathological and clinical work.

PIORRY (PIERRE ADOLPHE) 1794–1879

471 De la percussion médiate et des signes obtenus à l'aide de ce nouveau moyen d'exploration dans les maladies des organes thoraciques et abdominaux. *Paris, J. S. Chaudé, J. B. Baillière, 1828.* x, 336 pp. Illus (plates). 8vo, 22 cms.

Piorry invented the pleximeter and modified Laennec's stethoscope. A classic on percussion in its day.

472 Atlas de plessimétrisme . . . suivi d'un dictionnaire des termes . . . *Paris, J. B. Baillière, 1851.* [iv], 108 pp. Illus ("42 planches"), table. 8vo, 23 cms.

Comprises diagrams of percussion with the pleximeter—he carried mensuration by percussion to an almost ludicrous stage. This volume also has *Table alphabétique des matières* [du Traité] par MM. A. Chevallier fils et [L.] Baillard. (Paris, J. B. Baillière, 1852, iv, 5–55 pp.).

Both these form part of Piorry's work originally entitled *Traite de pathologie iatrique ou médicale, et médecine pratique, professée à la Faculté de Médecine de Paris*, (Paris, Pourchet & J. B. Baillière, 1841–51. 8 tom.). "Tom 1 contains "Généralités" and is without numeration. Tom. 2–8 comprise "Monographies ou spécialités" in 7 volumes, the title of the work being altered to "Traité de médecine pratique," etc. The "Atlas" and "Table" have each a distinct title-page and pagination" (note in British Museum *General Catalogue of printed books*, vol. 190, column 462), and were issued separately.

WILLIAMS (CHARLES JAMES BLASIUS) 1805–1889

473 The Pathology and diagnosis of diseases of the chest, comprising a rational exposition of their physical signs. 4th ed. With an appendix; containing various opinions and experiments on the motions and sounds of the heart, and on the bronchi. *London, John Churchill, 1840.* xii, 331 pp. Illus. 8vo, 23 cms.

Publisher's catalogue (16 pp.) bound in at front.

Book-stamp: Staffordshire General Infirmary.

First published as *A Rational exposition of the physical signs of the diseases of the lungs and pleura* (London, T. & G. Underwood, 1828; 2nd ed. 1834); third edition, entitled *The Pathology and diagnosis* . . . was published 1835. American editions were published in Philadelphia in 1830 (1st ed., Carey & Lea), 1834 (2nd ed., Carey, Lea & Blanchard), 1837, 1851 (Blanchard & Lea, revised 1853).

A German translation was made from the third edition by Hermann Velton (Bonn 1835; 2nd ed., 1838), an Italian by Carlo de Vecchi (Milano, 1839) and a Swedish by J. Lewertin (Stockholm, 1839).

Williams studied in Paris under Laennec at the Charité Hospital and investigated the heart sounds with James Hope with whom a dispute as to priority arose. He became a leading authority on auscultation, percussion and heart sounds and coined the onomatopœia "lub-dup".

474 Authentic narrative of the case of the late Earl St. Maur . . . with the short-hand notes of the retraction and apology. *London, Longmans Green, 1870.* 44 pp. 8vo, 21 cms.

Autograph presentation letter of March 19, 1870, from author to Dr. (later Sir George) Johnson.

Second edition, also 1870. Williams had been physician to the Earl St. Maur, son of the Duke and Duchess of Somerset, during his final illness (probably aneurysm of the arch of the aorta pressing against the trachea and its nerves). The distraught Duchess, who was the daughter of the playwright Sheridan, libelled Williams in the press for misconduct and incompetence, but withdrew the allegations at the ensuing trial before Williams's defence was given. The pamphlet is Williams's defence.

475 Memoirs of life and work. *London, Smith Elder, 1884.* xxiv, 522 pp. Ports, bibliog. (ftn. refs). 8vo, 23 cms.

Publisher's catalogue (2 pp.) bound in at end.

Autographs: Chevalier D'Eon (? a descendant or relation of Charles Geneviève Louis Auguste André Timothée de Beaumont d'Eon, 1728–1810, a secret agent of Louis XV especially in Russia and London, known as la Chevalière d'Eon on account of his often assuming a female disguise). W. B. Phillimore, 1884. Acquired 1941.

BISHOP (PATRICK JAMES) *b.* 1926

476 Life and work of C. J. B. Williams (1805–1889), an eminent pupil of Laennec.

Reprinted from *Tubercule*, 1960, **41**, 383–95. Ports.

SHARPE (JAMES BIRCH) *d. c.* 1842?

477 A manual of auscultation and percussion. 2nd ed. *London, Samuel Highley, 1838.* xxiv, 118 pp. Illus. 12mo, 16 cms.

Publisher's catalogue (2 pp.) bound in at end.

Provenance (stamp): J [?] Beynton [?].

First edition, 1832. Largely abstracts from Mériadec Laennec's edition of Laennec's book on mediate auscultation (see no. 455). Sharpe became M.R.C.S. in 1811, lived at Windsor, and was included in the lists of the Royal College of Surgeons until 1842. The 1843 and subsequent lists were compiled from circulars of members and no reply from Sharpe was received. (The 1845 *Medical Directory* has the briefest mention of him, but is not always correct). From the preface he was certainly alive in November 1838.

KENNEDY (EVORY) 1808–1886

478 Observations on obstetric auscultation with an analysis of the evidences of pregnancy, and an inquiry into the proofs of the life and death of the foetus in utero. With an appendix containing legal notes, by John Smith Esq., Barrister-at-law. *Dublin, Hodges & Smith, 1833.* viii, 288 pp. Illus. (4 engraved plates,) bibliog. (ftn refs). 12mo, 19 cms.

Appendix pp. 261–88. This copy lacks p. vii (Dedication to Joseph Clarke M.D., F.R.C.P.I.) and p. viii (errata).

Provenance: sold at Sotheby's 16 July 1969 in lot 720 to Elliott, and purchased from him, £22 10 shillings. Originally in the Edinburgh Medical Society Library (book-stamp: Ex libris Medicae Societatis Edinensis).

An important early work on foetal auscultation cited by Barth and Roger, (no. 480, p. 562; Newbigging's translation (no. 481, p. 315) has "*Dublin Hosp. Reports*, vol. 5" which refers to a paper in 1830 (see Callisen, Bd. 10 item 797), Bowditch (no. 483, pp. vi, 179) and by Pinkerton (no. 464). American edition "with notes and additional illustration, by Isaac E. Taylor, New York, J. & H. G. Langley, 1843.

ŠKODA (JOSEF) 1805–1881

479 Abhandlung über Perkussion und Auskultation. 5e Aufl. *Wien, L. W. Seidel, 1854.* xiii, 338 pp. Bibliog. (ftn. refs). 8vo, 23 cms.

This edition contained important additions and revisions. The book went through several editions (first, 1839; second, 1842; third, 1844; fourth, 1850; sixth, 1864; editions 1–3, Braumüller und Seidel) and translations from the fourth edition into English (by W. O. Markham, London, Highly, 1853; American edition, Philadelphia, Blakiston & Lindsay, 1854) and French (Dr. F. A. Aran (no. 382), Paris, Labé, 1854). Škoda and Rokitansky (nos. 799, 905) made Vienna a famous teaching centre after Paris, and Škoda put physical signs on a scientific basis and created cardiology as a specialty.

BARTH (JEAN BAPTISTE PHILIPPE) 1806–1877 and ROGER (HENRI LOUIS) 1809–1891

480 Traité pratique d'auscultation ou exposé méthodique des diverses applications de ce mode d'examen à l'état physiologique et morbide de l'économie, suivi d'un précis de percussion. 4e éd. *Paris, Labé, 1854.* xviii, 719 pp. Bibliog. (ftn. refs). 12mo, 14 cms.

Barth's presentation copy to Dr. Baillarger (Jules Gabriel François Baillarger 1809–1890, mental specialist, president of the Académie de Médecine, Paris for 1878). Copy also signed by both authors; unsigned copies are counterfeit.

A classic for 50 years and the best contemporary account of the heart sounds. First published in 1841, it went through many editions, (2nd 1844, 3rd 1850, 6th 1865, 8th 1874, 12th 1895, 13th 1898 cited by Edens, no. 441, p. 768) and was translated into English. Separate American editions appeared in 1845, 1847 and 1849. There were translations also into German, 1842, and Italian, 1844.

481 *The same.* A Practical treatise on auscultation. Trans., with notes by Patrick [Small Keir] Newbigging. *Edinburgh, Maclachlan, Stewart; London, Whittaker, 1842.* xxii, 398 pp. Tables. 8vo, 20 cms.

Translation of first French edition of 1841, with references in the text. The translator (*c.* 1814–1864) was President of the Royal College of Surgeons of Edinburgh, 1861–1863, and physician to the Sick Children's Hospital.

HUGHES (HENRY MARSHALL) 1805–1858

482 A Clinical introduction to the practice of auscultation and other modes of physical diagnosis: intended to simplify the study of the diseases of the lungs and heart. *London, Longman, Brown, Green & Longmans, 1845.* xxiii, 246, [2] pp. Illus. 8vo, 20 cms.

Autograph: E. J. Galton, Brixton (Edmund John Galton, L.S.A., *d.* 1879?). Acquired 1942.

This book, cited in contemporary works, reached a second edition, 1854. Hughes was assistant physician to Guy's Hospital and sought to simplify terminology for students.

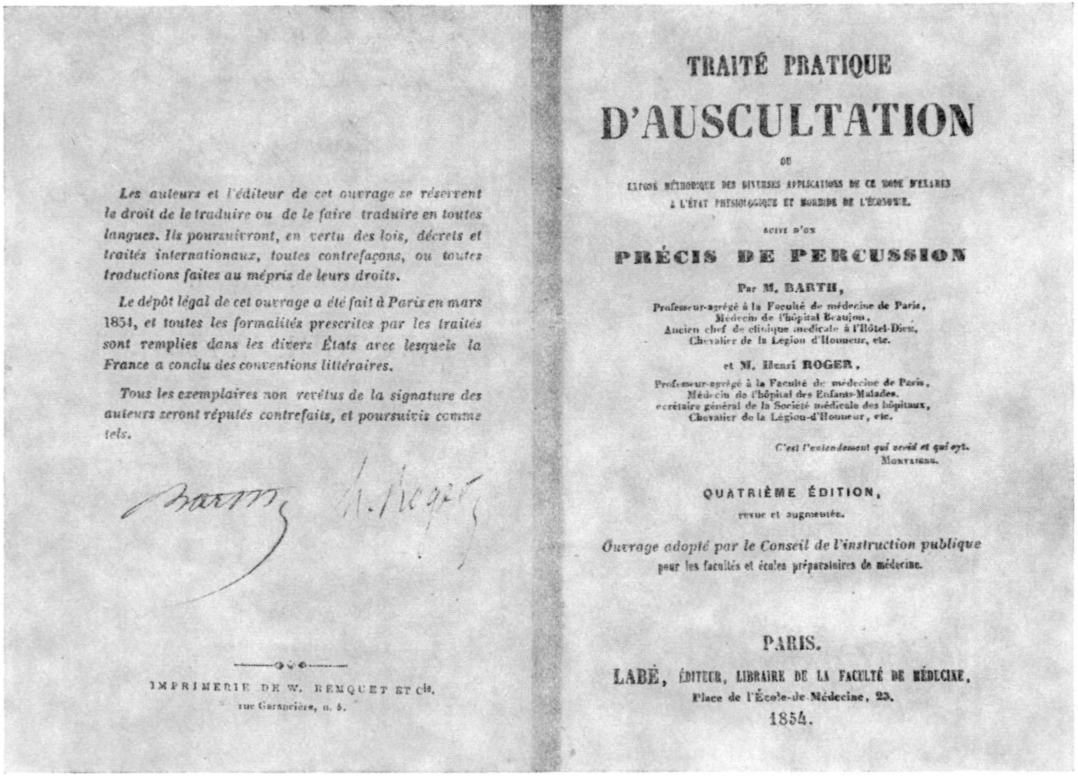
Les auteurs et l'éditeur de cet ouvrage se réservent le droit de le traduire ou de le faire traduire en toutes langues. Ils poursuivront, en vertu des lois, décrets et traités internationaux, toutes contrefaçons, ou toutes traductions faites au mépris de leurs droits.

Le dépôt légal de cet ouvrage a été fait à Paris en mars 1854, et toutes les formalités prescrites par les traités sont remplies dans les divers États avec lesquels la France a conclu des conventions littéraires.

Tous les exemplaires non revêtus de la signature des auteurs seront réputés contrefaits, et poursuivis comme tels.

IMPRIMERIE DE W. REMQUET ET Cie,
rue Garancière, n. 5.

TRAITÉ PRATIQUE

D'AUSCULTATION

OU

EXPOSÉ MÉTHODIQUE DES DIVERSES APPLICATIONS DE CE MODE D'EXAMEN
A L'ÉTAT PHYSIOLOGIQUE ET MORBIDE DE L'ÉCONOMIE.

SUIVI D'UN

PRÉCIS DE PERCUSSION

Par M. BARTH,
Professeur-agrégé à la Faculté de médecine de Paris,
Médecin de l'hôpital Beaujon,
Ancien chef de clinique médicale à l'Hôtel-Dieu,
Chevalier de la Légion d'Honneur, etc.

et M. Henri ROGER,
Professeur-agrégé à la Faculté de médecine de Paris,
Médecin de l'hôpital des Enfants-Malades,
secrétaire général de la Société médicale des hôpitaux,
Chevalier de la Légion-d'Honneur, etc.

C'est l'entendement qui void et qui oyt.
MONTAIGNE.

QUATRIÈME ÉDITION,
revue et augmentée.

Ouvrage adopté par le Conseil de l'instruction publique
pour les facultés et écoles préparatoires de médecine.

PARIS.
LABÉ, ÉDITEUR, LIBRAIRE DE LA FACULTÉ DE MÉDECINE,
Place de l'École-de-Médecine, 23.
1854.

No. 480. Unsigned copies of this book are counterfeit

BOWDITCH (Henry Ingersoll) 1808–1893

483 The Young stethoscopist . . . with an introduction by Saul Jarcho. (New York Academy of Medicine Library. History of Medicine Series no. 20). *New York, London, Hafner, 1964.* ix, vii, 278 pp. Illus, diagrs. 8vo, 21 cms.

Facsimile reprint of the original edition (New York, J. & H. G. Langley; Boston, William D. Ticknor 1846).

This book is reputed to have marked the formal acceptance of physical diagnosis in U.S.A. and includes a chapter on obstetric auscultation.

BILLING (Archibald) 1791–1881

484 Practical observations on diseases of the lungs and heart. *London, S. Highley, 1852.* [iii], 138 pp. Bibliog. (ftn. refs). 8vo, 23 cms.

Billing was physician to the London Hospital and one of the last to visit his patients on horseback. He supported the view that the heart sounds were valvular in origin rather than muscular. He was an expert on jewels and precious stones.

VERNEUIL (Aristide Auguste Stanislas) 1823–1895

485 Recherches sur la locomotion du cœur: thèse pour le doctorat en médecine. (Faculté de Médecine de Paris). *Paris, Rignoux, 1852.* 57 pp. Diagrs, bibliog. 4to, 26 cms.

Autograph: "A Mr Martin, bon souvenir de l'école pratique Verneuil."

A Paris thesis concerned with the apex beat which cites the work of Carson of Liverpool. He wrongly concluded that the apex beat was due to diastole.

HÉRARD (Hippolyte Victor) 1819–1913

486 Des signes stéthoscopiques du rétrécissement de l'orifice auriculo-ventriculaire gauche du cœur, et spécialement du souffle au second temps. *Paris, Rignoux, 1853.* 52 pp. Bibliog. (refs in text). 8vo, 21 cms.

Reprinted from *Archives générales de Médicine*, 1853, 5e série, **2** (vol. 2) 543–63; 1854, **3** (vol. 1) 165–94.

Autograph: "donné par M. Hérard à J. [?] Dourlens [?] son interne, l'hopital St. Antoine avril 1854."

An important early work on the murmurs of mitral stenosis; he states that mitral stenosis may produce a systolic, presystolic or diastolic murmur, or no murmur, and notes the bruit de rappel of Bouillaud. A very modern view on the subject.

HALORD (George Britton) 1824–1920

487 The action and sounds of the heart: a physiological essay. *London, John Churchill, 1860.* 47 pp. Illus, table, diagrs. 8vo, 22 cms.

Author's presentation copy to Dr. (later Sir George) Johnson (1818–1896), whose manuscript notes are on the fly-leaf.

488 On the time and manner of closure of the auriculo-ventricular valves. *London, John Churchill, 1861.* 8 pp. Illus, diagrs. 8vo, 22 cms.

Author's presentation copy to Dr. G. (later Sir George) Johnson whose manuscript notes are on the fly-leaf.

Halford's experiments on the heart sounds were widely cited in contemporary works.

ROGER (Henri Louis) 1809–1891

489 Clinical researches on auscultation of the head; trans. from the French by Alfred Meadows. *London, Henry Henshaw, 1863.* ii, 47 pp. 8vo, 21 cms.

Translation of Roger's "Recherches cliniques sur l'auscultation de la tête" in *Mémoires de l'Académie Impériale de Médecine*, 1860, **24,** 39–96.

Translator's presentation copy to George Johnson, later Sir George Johnson (1818–1896).

Roger was physician to the Hôpital des Enfants Malades in Paris and first described the murmur of ventricular septal defect (Maladie de Roger). Both Roger's disease and associated murmur are described in his "Recherches cliniques sur la communication congénitale des deux cœurs, par inocclusion du septum interventriculaire" in *Bulletin de l'Académie médicale*, Paris, 1879, **8,** 1074–94, 1189–91).

COCKLE (John) 1813?–1900

490 On Insufficiency of the aortic valves in connection with sudden death; with notes historical and critical. *London, J. W. Davies, 1861.* 30 pp. Bibliog. (ftn. refs). 8vo, 21 cms.

Second edition, 1880. A valuable history of aortic incompetence, with appendix describing a Gibson murmur.

[*and*] On the second sound and murmur of the heart and great vessels in their relation to diagnosis. *London, printed by T. Richards [for the British Medical Association], 1857.* 20 pp. 12mo, 18 cms.

Reprinted from *British medical Journal*, 1857, 337–8, 361–3.

Presentation copy to Dr. (later Sir) George Johnson (1818–1896).

LEARED (Arthur) 1822–1879

491 On the sounds caused by the circulation of the blood; being a thesis read in the University of Dublin for the degree of M.D., at the winter commencement, 1860. *London, John Churchill, 1861.* 22 pp. Bibliog. (ftn. refs). 8vo, 22 cms.

Leared made experiments with a primitive artificial circulation, and his contribution was widely quoted in the literature of the heart sounds.

GERHARDT (Carl Adolf Christian Jacob) 1833–1902

492 Lehrbuch der Auscultation und Percussion, mit besonderer Berücksichtigung der Besichtigung, Betastung und Messung der Brust und des Unterleibes zu diagnostischen Zwecken. 5e Aufl. *Tübingen, H. Laupp, 1890.* viii, 363 pp. Illus, diagrs (tracings). 8vo, 24 cms.

First edition with same publisher 1866. An important early work on physical diagnosis much cited in contemporary literature.

POTAIN (Pierre Carl Édouard) 1825–1901

493 Du rhythme cardiaque appelé bruit de galop, de son mécanisme et de sa valeur séméiologique. [*Paris, J. B. Baillière, 1876*] 32 pp. Diagrs (tracings), bibliog. (ftn. refs).

Reprinted from *Union médicale*, 1875, 3e série **20,** 706–11, 745–6; 1876, **21,** 22–6, 141–7, 322–6, 396–400.

Author's presentation copy, with autographed letter, to George (later Sir George) Johnson (1818–1896).

[*and*] EXCHAQUET (THÉODORE)
D'un phénomène stéthoscopique propre à certaines formes d'hypertrophie simple du cœur. *Paris, Adrien Delahaye, 1875.* 94 pp. Diagrs (tracings).

[*and*] POTAIN (PIERRE CARL ÉDOUARD) 1825–1901
Note sur les dédoublements normaux des bruits du cœur. *Paris, typographie Felix Malteste, 1866.* 36 pp. Diagrs (tracings), bibliog. (ftn. refs).

Reprinted from *Union médicale* (nouvelle série, [2e] série) 1866, **31**, 307–11, 357–64, 438–47, 595–99, 610–17.

[*and*] POTAIN (PIERRE CARL ÉDOUARD) 1825–1901
Des mouvements et des bruits qui se passent dans les veines jugulaires. *Paris, J. B. Baillière, 1868.* 31 pp. Diagrs (tracings).

Reprinted from *Mémoires de la Société médicale des Hôpitaux de Paris*, 1867, 2e série **4**, 3–27.
Four papers bound together. Spine title: Bruit de galop.

GEE (SAMUEL JONES) 1839–1911

494 Auscultation and percussion: together with the other methods of physical examination of the chest. 2nd ed. *London, Smith, Elder, 1877.* xvi, 324 pp. Illus, diagrs, bibliog. (ftn. refs). 8vo, 18 cms.

Publisher's catalogue (12 pp.) bound in at end. Autograph: Rowland H. Coombs (Rowland Hill Coombs, *d.* 1929, J.P. of Bedford, physician of Bedford County Hospital).
First edition, 1870; third, 1883 (RCP); fourth, 1893; fifth, 1906 (Oxford Medical Publications, Henry Frowde, Hodder & Stoughton, 1907) (RCP).

PATON (GEORGE) *d. c.* 1882?

495 Researches on the action and sounds of the heart. *London, J. & A. Churchill, 1873.* 64 pp. Bibliog. (ftn. refs). 8vo, 23 cms.

Publisher's catalogue, Oct. 1872 (24 pp.) bound in. Acquired (H. K. Lewis), 1942. Second edition also 1873 (93 pp., pp. 1–64 duplicate of our edition).
Comprises a revised version of two papers from *British medical Journal* and *Dublin quarterly Journal of medical Science* (see *Preface*). From experiments on turtles, Paton concludes that the second sound is due to atrial contraction.
Paton, who graduated M.D. at Jena in 1840, lived in Ontario; he is last recorded in the *Medical Directory* for 1882.

FLINT (AUSTIN) 1812–1886

496 A Manual of percussion and auscultation; of the physical diagnosis of diseases of the lungs and heart, and of thoracic aneurism. *London, J. & A. Churchill, 1876.* viii, 13–255 pp. 8vo, 21 cms.

The only other copy located in Britain at Glasgow University has the same peculiar pagination. The pagination of the American edition is given in the *Index-catalogue of the library of the Surgeon General's Office*, 4th series, as viii, 255 pp., suspiciously like our copy. Moreover, the pagination of the second and third editions, given less precisely in this series as 240 pp. and 242 pp., is shown in the first series as viii, 13–240 pp. and xii, 13–242 pp. respectively. Gatherings are in twelves in our copy and the preliminary leaves (printed last) were probably expected to occupy the whole of the first gathering. Our copy is therefore almost certainly complete.
The author is often catalogued as "senior" or "the elder" to distinguish him from his son, Austin Flint 1836–1915.

SANSOM (Arthur Ernest) 1838–1907

497 Manual of the physical diagnosis of the heart, including the use of the sphygmograph and cardiograph. 3rd ed. *London, J. & A. Churchill, 1881.* xii, 300 pp. Diagrs (tracings), bibliog. (ftn. refs). 8vo, 18 cms.

Publisher's catalogue October 1880, (16 pp.) bound in at end. Book-stamp: Royal Army Medical College Library.

First edition (London, Churchill, 1876) and second (also 1876) called *Lectures on the physical diagnosis....* Sansom was physician to the London Hospital, and designed a binaural stethoscope and first explained the opening snap of mitral stenosis.

BARR (Sir James) 1849–1938

498 On reduplication of cardiac sounds; read before the Liverpool Medical Society. *London, printed by Pardon & Son, 1877.* 30 pp. Diagrs (tracings). 12mo, 17 cms.

Reprinted from *Medical Times and Gazette*, 1877, **54,** 31–4, 60–1, 88–9.

Author's presentation copy.

Barr wrongly concluded that P2 (pulmonary second sound) preceded A2 (second sound in the aortic region) in split second sound. He was criticised by George Johnson (later Sir George Johnson, 1818–1896) in the same journal (pp. 140–1) and again (p. 229) to Barr's rejoinder (pp. 194–5).

WEIL (Adolf) 1848–1916

499 Handbuch und Atlas der topographischen Percussion. *Leipzig, F. C. W. Vogel, 1877.* x, 183 pp. Illus (26 plates), bibliog. (beginning of sections). 8vo, 23 cms.

A much cited early work on percussion of thorax and abdomen. (Second edition, 1880).

STEELL (Graham) 1851–1942

500 The Physical signs of cardiac disease. *Edinburgh, Maclachlan and Stewart; London, Simpkin, Marshall; Manchester, J. E. Cornish, 1881.* [vii], 63 pp. Illus, diagrs (tracings), bibliog. (ftn. refs). 8vo, 19 cms.

This booklet contains the first account of Graham Steell's murmur of relative pulmonary incompetence prior to his paper of 1888 (*Medical Chronicle* (Manchester), 1888–9, **9,** 182–8. Garrison and Morton 2794. See also no. 1009, pp. 680–5).

RUSSELL (William) 1852–1940

501 The Murmurs of debility in the pulmonary and tricuspid areas.

Reprinted from *Edinburgh medical Journal*, 1882–1883, **28,** 130–6. Bibliog. (ftn. refs).

Russell graduated from Edinburgh in 1876 (M.D. 1884) and after some time in Wolverhampton, went to the Royal Infirmary in Edinburgh, 1891. He became professor of medicine at the University in 1913. Besides study of the cancer cell, his interest was circulatory disorders and later problems of blood pressure and gastro-intestinal disorders. A considerable man of affairs, he was President of the Royal College of Physicians of Edinburgh and of the Medico-Chirurgical Society of Edinburgh. First editor of the *Scottish medical and surgical Journal* he wrote many papers. With George Alexander Gibson (author of nos. 312, 313, 630) he published *Physical diagnosis* (Edinburgh, Pentland, 1890; 2nd ed., 1893; 3rd ed., 1902).

WEST (Samuel Hatch) 1848–1920

502 How to examine the chest: a practical guide for the use of students. 3rd ed. *London, J. & A. Churchill, 1900.* xvi, 206 pp. 8vo, 17 cms.

Publisher's catalogue (no. 1, 1901) (32 pp.) bound in at end. Autograph: Glen Davison, 26 Belgrave Terrace, Newcastle-on-Tyne, May 13, 1904. (Not in the *Medical Registers* of the period).

First edition, 1883; second 1890 (same publisher). A popular handbook, clearly written, on examination of the heart and lungs and pulse by West, physician to St. Bartholomew's Hospital.

FOWLER (Sir James Kingston) 1852–1934

503 On the origin of anaemic murmurs. *London, J. & A. Churchill, 1884.* 45 pp. Tables, bibliog. (ftn. refs). 8vo, 23 cms.

Author's presentation copy to Middlesex Hospital Library; book-stamp: Middlesex Hospital Library.

Fowler's inaugural M.D. thesis. He notes that the conus arteriosus occupies the second interspace, and that the pulmonary systolic murmur in anaemia precedes the mitral murmur.

NIXON (Sir Christopher John) 1849–1914

504 The Cardiac murmurs of the mitral area. *Dublin, printed for the author by John Falconer, 1886.* 20 pp. Illus. (4 plates). 8vo, 21 cms.

Reprinted from *Dublin Journal of medical Sciences*, 3rd series, **81**, 473–90 (RCP). Our copy has only pp. 19–20 (covering Mitral bruit de scie), one plate and title-page signed "with the writer's compliments [?]".

BALFOUR (George William) 1823–1903

505 On the evolution of cardiac diagnosis from Harvey's days till now. (Harveian Discourse for 1887). *Edinburgh, printed by Oliver & Boyd, 1887.* 19 pp. Bibliog. (ftn. refs). 8vo, 21 cms.

Reprinted from *Edinburgh medical Journal*, 1887, **32**, 1065–81.

One of the best general reviews of contemporary knowledge of the heart sounds and murmurs, with full references.

BARIÉ (Ernest) 1845–1931

506 Bruits de souffle et bruits galop (Bibliothèque Médicale). *Paris, Rueff, [1894?].* [iii], 214 pp. Tables, diagrs (incl. tracings). 8vo, 18 cms.

Bulletin des annonces (8 pp.) bound in at end.

A good historical account of murmurs and gallop rhythm.

GILLET (Henri) 1858–?

507 Rythmes des bruits du cœur. (Bibliothèque Médicale). *Paris, Rueff, 1894.* [vi], 218 pp. Tables, diagrs (incl. tracings), bibliog. (ftn. refs). 8vo, 19 cms.

Pp. [217-8] "Du même auteur." "Bulletin des annonces" (8 pp.) bound in at end.

Deals with heart sounds, murmurs, and gallop rhythm, etc.

MERKLEN (MARIE JOSEPH FÉLIX PIERRE) 1852–1906 and HEITZ (JEAN) 1876–1930

508 Examen et sémiotique du cœur: techniques classiques, radioscopie, électrocardiographie. 5e éd., (Encyclopédie Scientifique des Aide-mémoire). *Paris, Masson, Gauthier-Villars, [1914].* 203 pp. Illus, tables, diagrs (tracings). 8vo, 19 cms.

Publisher's catalogue (16 pp.) bound in at end.

First edition, 1894? A very popular work on the clinical signs of heart diseases by Merklen, a renowned French teacher.

MEYER (JEAN DE) 1878–1934

509 Les Méthodes modernes d'examen du cœur et des vaisseaux: méthodes, techniques, documents graphiques. Préface de M. le Dr. Vaquez. *Paris, J. B. Baillière, 1914.* 538 pp. Illus, tables, diagrs (tracings), bibliog. 8vo, 24 cms.

Provenance: This copy was obtained by Prof. P. Rijlant of Brussels in 1949.

This work, by a Belgian physiologist, is a veritable encyclopaedia of the early instruments used to investigate the heart and circulation such as sphygmomanometers, polygraphs, phoncardiographs, and early electrocardiographs, with a comprehensive bibliography (501 references) which makes it of much historical interest.

GROEDEL (FRANZ MAXIMILIAN) 1881–1951

510 Die diagnostiche Bedeutung der graphischen Darstellung des Herztöne. *Leipzig, Georg Thieme, 1930.* 41 pp. Diagrs (tracings). 8vo, 25 cms.

Reprinted from *Fortbildungs—Lehrgang in Bad Nauheim, 6e, 1929. Pathologie und Therapie der Zirkulationsstörungen.* [Leipzig, Georg Thieme, 1930]. Acquired 1944.

DRESSLER (WILHELM) *b.* 1890

511 Die Brustwandpulsationen als Symptome von Herz- und Gefässkrankheiten. *Wien, Wilhelm Maudrich, 1933.* vii, 181 pp. Illus, diagrs (tracings), bibliog. 8vo, 25 cms.

Publisher's catalogue (3 pp.) bound in at end.

Presentation copy to DEB from the author, 1934.

An important work on diagnosis by palpation.

512 *The same.* Pulsations of the wall of the chest.

Reprinted from *Archives of internal Medicine*, 1957, **60**, 225–39, 437–40, 441–8, 654–62, 663–7.

An important work covering pulsation in valvular disease, adhesive pericarditis and aneurysmal dilatation of left atrium. The author was assistant at the "Herzstation" in Vienna; the translator, Hugo Roesler, also worked there. Later, when Dressler also went to the U.S.A., they collaborated on *An Atlas of electrocardiography* (Springfield, Ill., Thomas, 1949).

COSSIO (PEDRO) *b.* 1900

513 Temas de fonocardiografía. *Buenos Aires, El Ateneo, [1936?].* 193 pp. Diagrs, bibliog. (chapters). 8vo, 23 cms.

Written in collaboration with O. Orias, E. Braun Menéndez, M. Lascalea and E. Fongi. Preface dated December 1935.

Author's presentation copy to DEB January 25, 1937.

Deals with first sound, gallop rhythm, duplication of sounds, sounds in complete heart block, atrial sound and opening snap. Summary in French, English and German. Bibliography of all classical accounts of heart sounds.

514 Comentarios sobre los fenómenos acústicos de la estrechez mitral y de algunos ruidos de soplo, según el registro grafico de los mismos. *Buenos Aires*, [*Proventas*], *1938*. 60 pp. Diagrs (tracings), bibliog. 8vo, 23 cms.

Author's presentation copy to DEB May 28, 1938.

Deals with heart sounds and murmurs of mitral stenosis with phono-cardiograms. Summary in English. An important early comprehensive account.

ORÍAS (OSCAR) and BRAUN-MENÉNDEZ (EDUARDO) *b.* 1903

515 Los Ruidos cardíacos en condiciones normales y patólogicas. *Buenos Aires, El Ateneo, 1937*. xvii, 279 pp. Ports, diagrs (tracings), bibliog. 8vo, 23 cms.

Presentation copy to DEB from the authors. The standard work on phonocardiography and the heart sounds in its day, with an important bibliography of 23 pages.

516 *The same*. The Heart sounds in normal and pathological conditions. (Oxford Medical Publications). *London, New York, Toronto, Oxford University Press, 1939*. xx, 258 pp. Illus, diagrs (tracings), bibliog. 8vo, 23 cms.

Translated from the Spanish by R. A. Gregory. Acquired July 1941.

LIAN (CAMILLE CONSTANT) 1882–1969, and others

517 Phonocardiographie: auscultation collective (acoustique—technique—clinique) [par] C[amille] Lian, G[eorges] Minot et J[ean] J[acques] Welti. *Paris, Masson, 1941*. vi, 256 pp. Ilus, diagrs (tracings), bibliog. 8vo, 25 cms.

Lian was a pioneer worker at phonocardiography at the Tenon Hospital, Paris, and his treatise summarises 15 years of investigation of the heart sounds and murmurs. With Georges Minot he invented the Lian-Minot electrokymographe (*Archives des Maladies du Cœur et des Vaisseaux*, 1939, **32**, 497–505). Inserted is an obituary of Camille Lian by Jean Lenègre (1904–1972) reprinted from *Bulletin de l'Académie Nationale de Médecine*, 1970, **154**, 102–8. Port., bibliog.

LEVINE (SAMUEL ALBERT) 1891–1966 and HARVEY (WATKINS PROCTOR) *b.* 1918

518 Clinical auscultation of the heart. *Philadelphia, London, W. B. Saunders, 1949*. viii, 327 pp. Diagrs (tracings). 8vo, 24 cms.

Deals with clinical auscultation in various forms of heart disease, illustrated by phonocardiograms, by a great American teacher and his assistant.

SOULIÉ (PIERRE LOUIS JEAN) 1903–1970, and others

519 Le Cathétérisme du cœur au micromanomètre. "Le son intracardiaque". *Paris, J. B. Baillière,* [*1961*]. viii, 155 pp. Diagrs (tracings). 8vo, 24 cms.

Note on first page of text only: *Archives des Maladies du Cœur*, 54e année, supplement I, 1961. Author's presentation copy to DEB.

History and Bibliography

KEELE (KENNETH DAVID) *b.* 1909

520 The Evolution of clinical methods in medicine. (FitzPatrick Lectures, 1960–1961). *London, Pitman Medical, 1963*. xi, 115 pp. Illus, ports, facsims, table, diagrs, bibliog. 8vo, 24 cms.

Garrison and Morton 2243.2. Also published in Springfield, Ill., C. C. Thomas, 1963.

Covers auscultation, percussion and early instrumental investigation of the heart.

RAVIN (ABE) *b.* 1908 and FRAME (FLORENCE K.)

521 International bibliography of cardiovascular auscultation and phonocardiography. Journal articles 1820–1966. Books, theses, dissertations, phonodiscs 1819–1968. (American Heart Association Monograph, no. 31). *New York, American Heart Association, 1971.* x, 318 pp. 4to, 27 cms.

Journal articles (inverse chronological arrangement) pp. 1–190; books, theses, etc. (same arrangement) pp. 191–9; author and subject indexes.

Graphic Methods, Electrocardiography and Arrhythmias

Mackenzie and Wenckebach investigated cardiac irregularities with the sphygmograph and polygraph, and later Lewis and others employed the electrocardiograph for this purpose. Eventually three common types of irregularity were identified, namely, sinus arrhythmia, extra systole, and atrial fibrillation; heart block and paroxysmal tachycardia were less common disturbances of rhythm.

HOFFMANN (AUGUST) 1862–1929

522 Die Paroxysmale Tachycardie. (Anfälle von Herzjagen). *Wiesbaden, J. F. Bergmann, 1900.* 215 pp. Diagrs (tracings), bibliog. 8vo, 25 cms.

Gives a good bibliography (336 references) of early papers prior to graphic methods, arranged alphabetically under I, Klinische Literatur, II, Anatomische und physiologische Literatur. Publisher's catalogue on additional first [4] and last [16] pp. and original covers.

Presentation copy to Dr. E. von Leyden (Ernst von Leyden, 1832–1910, professor of clinical medicine and director of the First Medical Clinic of the University of Berlin. His work included neurology, tuberculosis and cancer. He was assistant and then successor to Ludwig Traube).

WENCKEBACH (KAREL FREDERICK) 1864–1940

523 Arhythmia (*sic*) of the heart: a physiological and clinical study; trans [from the German] by Thos. Snowball. *Edinburgh and London, William Green,* 1904. ix, 198 pp. Illus (7 folding plates of tracings), bibliog. 4to, 26 cms.

Translation of *Die Arythmie als Ausdruck bestimmter Funktionsstörungen des Herzens*; eine physiologisch-klinische Studie (Leipzig, W. Engelmann, 1903).

Wenckebach, a Dutch physician, was a friend of Einthoven and of Mackenzie, and his pioneer work on the arrhythmias was done like Mackenzie's with the polygraph before the advent of the clinical electrocardiograph. He was the first to recognise extrasystoles in man and "Wenckebach's periods" in partial heart-block. He was professor of medicine at Groningen, later at Strasbourg and finally at Vienna.

HAY (JOHN) 1873–1959

524 Graphic methods in heart disease; with an introduction by James Mackenzie. (Oxford Medical Publications). *London, H. Frowde; Hodder & Stoughton, 1909.* xvii, 184 pp. Illus, diagrs (tracings). 8vo, 20 cms.

An early work on polygraphic records.

KRAUS (FRIEDRICH) 1858–1936 and NICOLAI (GEORG FREDRICK) *b.* 1872

525 Das Elektrokardiogramm des gesunden und kranken Menschen. *Leipzig, Veit, 1910.* xxii, 322 pp. Illus, tables, diagrs (tracings), bibliog. 8vo, 23 cms.

Alphabetical bibliography of cited references pp. xi–xxii.

Kraus graduated at Prague and in 1902 became professor of medicine at the Charité Hospital, Berlin. He worked with the early string electrocardiograph of Edelmann and Sons of Munich (see no. 571) and this book represents the first clinical application of the electrocardiograph outside Leyden.

LEWIS (Sir THOMAS) 1881–1945

526 The Mechanism and graphic registration of the heart beat. 3rd ed. *London, Shaw, 1925.* xix, 529 pp. Illus, tables, diagrs (incl. tracings), bibliog. 8vo, 25 cms.

Well illustrated. Alphabetical bibliography (pp. 449–516) of 1003 references (full referencing and cross-indexing). First published as *The Mechanism of the heart beat with especial reference to its clinical pathology* (London, Shaw, 1911) (RCP); [second] (RCP) under our title published by Shaw (1920). This book remained for long the most authoritative work on electrocardiography.

527 Clinical disorders of the heart beat: a handbook for practitioners and students. *London, Shaw, 1912.* xii, 104 pp. Illus, tables, diagrs (incl. tracings). 8vo, 22 cms.

528 *The same.* 2nd ed. *London, Shaw, 1913.* xii, 116 pp. Illus, tables, diagrs (incl. tracings). 8vo, 22 cms.

Provenance (autograph): F. Silva Jones 1915. (Frank Silva Jones, *d.* 1916, M.B., B.S.).

"The chief alteration is the addition of a chapter upon *Auricular Flutter.*" (*Preface*, p. viii.)

529 *The same.* 6th ed. *London, Shaw, 1925.* xii, 131 pp. Illus, tables, diagrs (incl. tracings). 8vo, 22 cms.

The third, fourth, fifth and seventh editions appeared from the same publishers in 1915, 1918, 1920 and 1933 respectively. A classic of cardiology.

530 Clinical electrocardiography, 2nd ed. *London, Shaw, 1918.* viii, 120 pp. Illus, diagrs (incl. tracings). 8vo, 22 cms.

531 *The same.* 4th ed. *London, Shaw, 1928.* viii, 128 pp. Illus, tables, diagrs (incl. tracings). 8vo, 22 cms.

The first edition was published in 1913 (RCP). Subsequent editions appeared in 1918 (3rd) (RCP), 1931 (5th) and 1937 (6th).

532 Electrocardiography and clinical disorders of the heart beat: a handbook for practitioners and students. *London, Shaw, 1949.* xiv, 285 pp. Illus, tables, diagrs (incl. tracings). 8vo, 22 cms.

A combination of his *Clinical electrocardiography* and *Clinical disorders of the heart beat.* Sir Thomas completed the work just before his death (*Publisher's note*).

VAQUEZ (Louis Henri) 1860–1936

533 Les Arythmies. Leçons recueillies par le Dr. Ch. Esmein. *Paris, J. B. Baillière, 1911.* [iii], x, 437 pp. Illus, diagrs (tracings). 8vo, 25 cms.

An important early work on the arrhythmias. Vaquez was using the electrocardiograph in his clinic at this date.

RITCHIE (William Thomas) 1873–1945

534 Auricular flutter. *Edinburgh and London, W. Green & Son, 1914.* xii, 144 pp. Illus, tables, diagrs (tracings), bibiliog. (ftn. refs). 4to, 26 cms.

In addition to footnote references, an index of authors cited leads to relevant reference.

A pioneer work on auricular flutter based on 11 personal cases and 42 recorded by others. William Adam Jolly (1873–1939) and Ritchie first named this arrhythmia; ("Auricular flutter and fibrillation", *Heart,* 1910, **2,** 177–81. Garrison and Morton 2833) and Ritchie first recognised it in man ("Complete heart-block, with dissociation of the auricles and ventricles." *Proceedings of the Royal Society of Edinburgh,* 1905–1906, **25,** 1085–91. Garrison and Morton 2821). Ritchie later became professor of medicine at Edinburgh.

LUTEMBACHER (René) *b.* 1884

535 Les Nouvelles méthodes d'examen du cœur en clinique. *Paris, Masson, 1921.* vii, 186 pp. Illus, diagrs (incl. tracings). 8vo, 22 cms.

Includes a reference to Lutembacher's syndrome (interatrial septal defect with mitral stenosis and dilatation of the pulmonary artery) (p. 168). It was first described by Lewis Martineau (*d.* 1888) in 1865; the subject was subsequently reviewed by Lutembacher in *Archives des Maladies du Cœur,* 1916, **9,** 237–60, "De la sténose mitrale avec communication interauriculaire".

WALLER (Augustus Désiré) 1856–1922

536 The Electrical action of the human heart. *London, University of London Press, 1922.* ix, 103 pp. Illus (4 plates of tracings), diagrs, bibliog. 8vo, 22 cms.

The lectures forming the basis of this book delivered in 1913 but publication delayed by the war. (See *Preface*).

Waller was born in Paris, trained in Geneva, qualified in Edinburgh in 1881, and became director of the physiological laboratory of London University. He was the first to record the electrical activity of the human heart by leads from the body surface and so was the founder of clinical electrocardiography. He was elected physician to the National Heart Hospital in 1912.

WEBSTER (Alfred) *d.* 1950

537 Cardiac arrhythmia and the neocardiology. *London, Watts, 1922.* vii, 195 pp. Diagrs (tracings), bibliog. (occasional ftn refs). Oblong folio, 23 × 30 cms.

Provenance: Presented to DEB by John Hay (author of 524). A review copy with Dr. Hay's annotations and his very critical review in *British medical Journal,* 1922, **1,** 921–2.

Webster was the first to record atrial waves in the radial pulse in complete heart-block. "Webster's case" was reproduced in Mackenzie's textbook (e.g. 325, p. 178). Webster's best-known writing is "Cardiac arrhythmia in relation to cerebral anaemia and epileptiform crises" in *Glasgow Hospital Reports,* 1900/1901, **3,** 413–61, mentioned both in Hay's review with approval and the bibliography of Mackenzie (*ibid.*, p. 359).

GAILLARD (Ch.)

538 Le Syndrome de Stokes-Adams et les troubles de la conductibilité d'après 54 observations. [Thesis for the Faculté de Médecine, Université de Lyon?] *Lyon, Bosc frères et Riou, [n.d., c. 1923?].* 223 pp. Diagrs (tracings), bibliog. 8vo, 25 cms.

EMANUEL (JOSEPH GEORGE) 1871–1958

539 Auricular fibrillation. (The Ingleby Lectures, delivered at the University of Birmingham May 6th and May 13th, 1925.) *Birmingham, Cornish Bros., 1926.* 31 pp. (+16 plates). Diagrs (tracings), tables. 8vo, 25 cms.

Acquired, 1926.

PARKINSON (Sir JOHN) 1885–1976 and BEDFORD (DAVIS EVAN) *b.* 1898

540 Successive changes in the electrocardiogram after cardiac infarction (coronary thrombosis).

Reprinted from *Heart*, 1928, **14**, 196–239. Diagrs, (tracings, incl. plates pp. 213–39), bibliog.

LEVY (ROBERT JEAN) *b.* 1895

541 Les anomalies du complexe ventriculaire électrique; leur importance en clinique (essai d'électro-cardio-pronostic). Préface du Dr. [A] Clerc. *Paris, Masson, 1929.* [vii], iii, 202 pp. Diagrs (tracings), bibliog. 4to, 26 cms.

Bibliography, 417 references (pp. 179–99). Du même auteur pp. [vi–vii]. Publisher's catalogue (48 pp.) bound in at end.

Contains one of the early accounts of cardiac infarction.

CRAIB (WILLIAM HOFMEYR) *b.* 1895

542 The Electrocardiogram. (Medical Research Council. Special Report Series, No. 147). *London, His Majesty's Stationery Office, 1930.* 57 pp. Illus (4 plates), diagrs, bibliog. 8vo, 25 cms.

List of M.R.C. publications (8 pp.) bound in at end.

One of the classics of electrocardiography. Craib introduced the dipole theory while working in the clinic of Sir Thomas Lewis.

DRESSLER (WILHELM) *b.* 1890

543 Klinische Elektrokardiographie, mit einem Grundriss der Arrhythmien, . . . mit einer Geleitwort von Prof. Dr. C. J. Rothberger. 4e Aufl. *Berlin und Wien, Urban & Schwarzenberg, 1937.* viii, 180 pp. Illus, tables, diagrs (tracings). 4to, 26 cms.

Author's presentation copy to DEB. First edition (same publishers) 1930; second edition, 1932.

An important popular work on clinical electrocardiography.

WOLFF (LOUIS) *b.* 1898

544 Bundle-branch block with short P-R interval in healthy young people prone to paroxysmal tachycardia; by Louis Wolff, [Sir] John Parkinson and Paul D[udley] White. *[St. Louis, American Heart Journal, 1930].* 20 pp. Diagrs (tracings), bibliog. 4to, 26 cms.

Reprinted from *American Heart Journal*, 1930, **5**, 685–704. Presentation copy from J[ohn] P[arkinson]. The original account of the Wolff-Parkinson-White syndrome. Garrison and Morton 2860.

WOLFF (Louis)

545 Electrocardiography, fundamentals and clinical application. *Philadelphia and London, Saunders, 1950.* viii, 187 pp. Illus, diagrs (tracings). 8vo, 25 cms.

Second edition (same publishers) 1956; third edition, 1962. A most useful teaching book in its day.

FROMENT (Roger) *b.* 1907

546 Les Tachycardies paroxystiques ventriculaires. Préface du Docteur L. Gallavardin. *Paris, Masson, 1932.* 541 pp. (+errata leaf). Diagrs (tracings), bibliog. 8vo, 24 cms.

Extensive alphabetical bibliography, pp. 503–36. Author's presentation copy to DEB, May 1932.

An important monograph from Gallavardin's clinic on ventricular tachycardia in which he was a pioneer worker.

ROUTIER (Daniel) 1887–1963 and THIROLOIX (Paul Louis Jules) *b.* 1901

547 L'Arythmie complète. Préface du Docteur Ch. Laubry. (La Practique Médicale Illustrée). *Paris, G. Doin, 1934.* [iii], 46 pp. Illus, diagrs (tracings). 4to, 27 cms.

Presentation copy to DEB from Routier.

TAQUINI (Alberto C.) *b.* 1905

548 Exploración del corazón por vía esofágica. (Universidad Nacional de Buenos Aires, Facultad de Ciencias medicas. Tesis de doctorado. Año 1936, num. 4895). *Buenos Aires, El Ateneo, 1936.* xvi (i.e. x), 231, [i] pp. Illus, diagrs (tracings), bibliog. 8vo, 23 cms.

Author's presentation copy to DEB, 1937.

Gives history of recording oesophageal pulsations, phonocardiograms and radiological exploration of oesophagus. Good bbliography (pp. 207–19).

BATTRO (Antonio) 1901–1948

549 Las Arritmias en clinica (diagnóstico, prognóstico y tratamiento). *Buenos Aires, El Ateneo, 1937.* 476 pp. Illus, diagrs (tracings), bibliog. 8vo, 23 cms.

Author's presentation copy to DEB, November 1937.

The classified bibliography (pp. 407–56) and indexes (pp. 457–76) are extensive. A new edition appeared in 1948.

SCHERF (David) *b.* 1899 and BOYD (Linn John) *b.* 1895

550 Clinical electrocardiography. 2nd rev. ed. *London, William Heinemann, 1945.* xiii, 403 pp. Illus, diagrs (tracings), bibliog. 8vo, 23 cms.

First edition, St. Louis, Mosby, 1940 (2nd impression 1941); second edition, Philadelphia, Lippincott, 1946. Portuguese edition 1941; Spanish edition 1942; French edition 1943.

This popular treatise was the best available in its time on clinical electrocardiography. Scherf worked in Wenckebach's clinic in Vienna for many years.

SCHERF (David) *b.* 1899 and SCHOTT (Ernst Adolf)

551 Extrasystoles and allied arrhythmias. *Melbourne, London [etc], William Heinemann, 1953.* xv, 531 pp. Facsims, tables, diagrs (tracings), bibliog. 4to, 26 cms.

Presentation copy to DEB from the authors, 1953. Contains an excellent historical account of the pulse (pp. 1–26, facsims, bibliog.) and cardiac irregularities.

WILSON (Frank Norman) 1890–1952, and others

552 The Precordial electrocardiogram, by Frank N. Wilson, M.D., in collaboration with Drs. Franklin D. Johnston, Francis F. Rosenbaum, Herman Erlanger, Hans Hecht, Nelson Cotrim, Paul S. Barker, Roberto Scarsi and Roberto Menezes de Oliveira. Read at the Assoc. of Life Insurance Medical Directors of America, Oct. 21–22, 1942. *New York, Press of the Recording and Statistical Corporation for the Association of Life Insurance Medical Directors of America, 1943.* 100 pp. Diagrs (tracings), bibliog. 8vo, 23 cms.

Wilson worked with the electrocardiograph on arrhythmias, and from 1920 onwards he investigated the ventricular complex using chest leads which he standardised, and identified pathological Q waves of myocardial infarction.

OHNELL (Richard Fredrik) *b.* 1913

553 Pre-excitation, a cardiac abnormality: patho-physiological, patho-anatomical and clinical studies of an excitatory spread phenomenon bearing on the problem of the WPW (Wolff, Parkinson and White) electrocardiogram and paroxysmal tachycardia; [trans. by Ulla Schött.] *London, Kimpton, 1944.* 167 pp. Illus, tables, diagrs (tracings), bibliog. 8vo, 23 cms.

A full bibliography of the Wolff-Parkinson-White syndrome. Also published in Stockholm, [Norstedt], 1944.

SODI PALLARES (Demetrio)

554 Nuevas bases de la electrocardiografia. 3 ed., corregida y aumentada. Prólogo de Dr. Ignacio Chavez. *Mexico, Instituto Nacional de Cardiologia, la Prensa Medica Mexicana, 1951.* xv, 625 pp. Illus, tables, diagrs (incl. tracings), bibliog. 8vo, 24 cms.

Presentation copy to DEB by author. First edition, 1945. English translation, St. Louis, Mosby, 1956.

Deals with original work of the Mexican school on electrocardiograpy. Alphabetical bibliography, pp. 587–611.

GALLAVARDIN (Léon)

555 L'Extrasystolie auriculaire: extrasystoles isoleés; extrasystolie en salves. *Paris, G. Doin, 1946.* [iii], 208 pp. Diagrs (tracings), bibliog. 8vo, 24 cms.

Author's presentation copy to DEB, 1946.

CORDEIRO (Arsénio)

556 Contribuição de para o estudo do sindroma de Wolff-Parkinson-White. (Dissertação de doutoramento apresentada à Faculdade de Medicina, [Universidade] de Lisboa). *Lisboa, [Universidade de Lisboa], 1947.* xv, 154 pp. Diagrs (tracings), bibliog. 8vo, 22 cms.

Author's presentation copy to DEB.

SCHOTT (Ernst Adolf)

557 Wolff-Parkinson-White syndrome (short P-R intervals associated with disturbances of intraventricular conduction) with attacks of paroxysmal tachycardia in an infant aged 8

months suffering from probable congenital heart disease [by] A. Schott. [*London, Royal Society of Medicine, 1947*]. 4 pp. Illus, diagrs (tracings), bibliog. 8vo, 25 cms.

Reprinted from *Proceedings of the Royal Society of Medicine*, 1947, **40**, 472–5 (Clinical Section, pp. 20–3).

The case mentioned was seen by DEB 12 February, 1953.

CABRERA COSÍO (ENRIQUE)

558 Bases électrophysiologiques de l'électrocardiographie: ses applications cliniques. Préface du Dr. Daniel Routier. *Paris, Masson, 1948.* [vii], 209 pp. Illus, tables, diagrs, bibliog. 8vo, 25 cms.

An important early account of the Mexican work on electrocardiography.

EVANS (WILLIAM) *b.* 1895

559 Cardiography. (Butterworths Medical Publications). *London, Butterworth, 1948.* ix, 132, 8 pp. Tables, diagrs (tracings). 8vo, 25 cms.

Series title on cover only. Deals with electrocardiography (part I, pp. 1–95) and phono-cardiography (part II, pp. 97–132).

DUCHOSAL (PIERRE W.) and SULZER (ROBERT)

560 La Vectocardiographie; méthode d'exploration du champ électrique créé dans le corps humain par les courants d'action du cœur dans les conditions normales et pathologiques. (Bibliotheca Cardiologica, fasc. 3). *Bâle (Suisse); New York, S. Karger, 1949.* 172 pp. Illus, diagrs, bibliog. 8vo, 25 cms.

A pioneer work on vectorcardiography.

HECHT (HANS H.) *b.* 1913

561 Basic principles of clinical electrocardiography. (American Lecture Series, no. 87. American Lectures in Circulation). *Springfield, Illinois, Charles C. Thomas, 1950.* ix, 88, [1] pp. Illus, tables, diagrs (tracings), bibliog. 8vo, 22 cms.

Acquired 1951.

REINDELL (HERBERT) *b.* 1908 and KLEPZIG (HELMUT) *b.* 1916

562 Die neuzeitlichen Brustwand- und Extremitaten-Ableitungen in der Praxis; mit einen Vorwort von Prof. Dr. Ludwig Heilmeyer. *Stuttgart, Georg Thieme, 1951.* vii, 179 pp. Illus, tables, diagrs (tracings), bibliog. 8vo, 25 cms.

Second edition, 1953. One of the first post-war German works on electrocardiography describing the new knowledge on chest leads developed in U.S.A. and England during the war. A letter, dated 8th November 1951, from Dr. Gerhart Schoenewald (then living in Wimpole Street) giving the German viewpoint on this book is enclosed.

ACCELERATED CONDUCTION

563 Accelerated conduction: the Wolff-Parkinson-White syndrome and related conditions; by Myron Prinzmetal [and others]. (Modern Medical Monographs, 3). *New York,*

Grune & Stratton, 1952. viii, [ii], 110 pp. Illus, diagrs (tracings), bibliog. (66 refs). 8vo, 22 cms.

Other contributors: Rexford Kennamer, Eliot Corday, John A. Osbourne, Joshua Fields, L. Allen Smith (all from the University of California Medical School, Los Angeles, California).

Presentation copy to DEB from Prinzmetal.

AURICULAR ARRHYTHMIAS

564 The Auricular arrhythmias, by Myron Prinzmetal [and others]. *Springfield, Ill., Charles C. Thomas, 1952.* xix, 387, [1] pp. Illus, diagrs (incl. tracings), bibliog. 4to, 29 cms.

Other authors: Eliot Corday, Isidor C. Brill, Robert W. Oblath, H. E. Kruger.

Associate authors: Joshua Fields, Walter Flieg, Alfred Goldman, Harold Karpman, S. Rexford Kennamer, John A. Osbourne, Alvin L. Sellers, L. Allen Smith.

Author's presentation copy to DEB from Myron Prinzmental, March 1952.

The high-speed cinematograph was used to investigate atrial arrhythmias; the circus movement theory (for a historical outline see pp. 53–4) was not confirmed.

The bibliography (pp. 359–79) has 686 references.

LENÈGRE (JEAN) 1904–1972

565 Électrocardiographie clinique, par J. Lenègre, G. Carouso et H. Chevalier. Préface du Pr. Ch. Laubry. *Paris, Masson, 1954.* [viii], ii, 810 pp. Illus, tables, diagrs (tracings), bibliog. 8vo, 25 cms.

Presentation copy to DEB by Lenègre.

Well illustrated. Alphabetical bibliography (pp. 769–98) of 648 references. Detailed index and list of contents. One of the best books on electrocardiography with clinical and necropsy findings correlated.

566 Contribution a l'étude des blocs de branche comportant notamment les confrontations éléctriques et histologiques. *Paris, Baillière, 1958* (i.e. 1957). [iii], 343 pp. Illus, tables, diagrs (tracings). 8vo, 24 cms.

Author's presentation copy to DEB, 6 November, 1957.

The most important clinico-pathological work on bundle-branch block since Mahaim's monograph of 1931 (no. 874).

GRANT (ROBERT PURVES) *b.* 1921

567 Clinical electrocardiography: the spatial vector approach. *New York, Blakiston Division, McGraw Hill, 1957.* ix, 225 pp. Illus, diagrs, bibliog. 8vo, 22 cms.

Interprets the scalar electrocardiogram in terms of vectorcardiography quite simply.

POZZI (LUCIANO)

568 Basic principles in vector electrocardiography; with a foreword by Professor P. Rijlant. *London, Henry Kimpton, 1961.* xii, 292 pp. Illus (incl. plates), diagrs, bibliog. 8vo, 25 cms.

Acquired Mexico, 1962—author's presentation.

The original Italian text, *Introduzione alla eletrocardiografia vettoriale* (Firenze, Malesci, 1960) modified by various contributors for the English edition. Classified bibliography (pp. 251–75).

COSSIO (PEDRO) *b.* 1900 and PECORINI (VICTORIO)

569 Electrovectorcardiographía clínica. *Buenos Aires, Fundación Cossio, 1962.* xii, 402 pp. Illus, ports, diagrs (tracings), bibliog. 8vo, 24 cms.

Transparent flimsy to put over drawings of standard size. Fully illustrated. Extensive alphabetical bibliography pp. 355–94. Presentation copy to DEB from Cossio.

STOCK (JOHN PETER PENDERELL) 1910–1973

570 Diagnosis and treatment of cardiac arrhythmias. *London, Butterworth, 1969.* x, 234 pp. Illus, diagrs (tracings), bibliog. 4to, 26 cms.

Also published New York, Appleton-Century-Crofts, 1969. A comprehensive account, theoretical and practical, of the arrhythmias.

History

BURCH (GEORGE EDWARD) *b.* 1910 and DE PASQUALE (NICHOLAS P.) *b.* 1927

571 A History of electrocardiography. *Chicago, Year Book Medical Publishers, 1964.* 309 pp. Illus, ports, diagrs, bibliog. 8vo, 22 cms.

Garrison and Morton 3161.1. The following are enclosed: a review of Burch and Pasquale's inclusion of W. H. Craib from *Sciendaba*, the internal newspaper of C.S.I.R. (South Africa) 1965, Vol. 1 no. 6 (Tribute to Dr. Craib for his research in the wake of Einthoven), and American Heart Association. *Standardization of precordial leads.* New York, American Heart Association, [1938]. [8] pp. 8vo, 22 cms.

Part 3, Great Men of Electrocardiography, includes Willem Einthoven (1860–1927), Aloysio Luigi Galvani (1737–1798), Carlo Matteucci (1811–1868), Emil DuBois-Reymond (1818–1896), Hermann Ludwig Ferdinand von Helmholtz (1821–1894), Sir John Scott Burdon-Sanderson (1828–1905), Julius Bernstein (1839–1917), Gabriel Lippmann (1845–1921), Walter Holbrook Gaskell (1847–1914), Sir James Mackenzie (1853–1925), Augustus Désiré Waller (1856–1922), Frederick Kraus (1858–1936), Sir William Maddock Bayliss (1860–1924), James Bryan Herrick (1861–1954), Augustus Hoffmann (1862–1929), Karel Frederik Wenckebach (1864–1940), Heinrich Ewald Hering (1866–?), Horatio Burt Williams (1877–1955), Alfred Einstein Cohn (1879–1957), Sir Thomas Lewis (1881–1945), George Edmeston Fahr (*b.* 1882), Harold Ensign Bennet Pardee (*b.* 1886), Frank Norman Wilson (1890–1952), Fritz Schellong (1891–1953), Hubert Mann (*b.* 1891), and W. H. Craib (*b.* 1895).

A fascinating account of the early work on electrocardiography and the first instruments used, together with a few of the earliest records taken by Einthoven, and in U.S.A.

Cardiac Radiology

Williams, of Boston, U.S.A., was the first to x-ray the heart (1896) after which cardiac radiology was developed mainly in Europe, in advance of England and the U.S.A.

The pioneers were Holzknecht, Schwarz, Rœsler and Zdansky in Vienna, Moritz, Groedel, Dietlen and Assmann in Germany, Béclère, Vaquez, Bordet, Laubry and Chaperon in Paris, and Schinz in Zurich. Mensuration of the heart by orthodiagraphy occupied the attention of the early radiologists and elaborate tables of normal heart size in relation to weight and height were constructed, and the prediction tables of Hodges and Eyster were much employed. Three dimensional models of the heart constructed by orthodiagraphic methods or from films by Palmieri's method and Röher's formula for calculating heart volume (*Fortschritte auf dem Gebiete der Röntgenstrahlen*, 1916–17, **24**, 285) also came into use for a time.

More recently radiological anatomy has been perfected by angiocardiography.

HOLZKNECHT (GUIDO) 1872–1931

572 Die Röntgenologische Diagnostik der Erkrankungen der Brusteingeweide. (Archiv und Atlas der normalen und pathologischen Anatomie in typischen Röntgenbildern. Fortschritte auf dem Gebiete der Röntgenstrahlen, Ergänzungsheft 6). *Hamburg, Lucas Gräfe & Sillem, 1901.* ix, 229 pp. Illus (incl. 50 x-rays on 8 plates), diagrs, bibliog. (occasional ftn. refs). 4to, 30 cms.

Autograph: John Parkinson, 1936 (Sir John Parkinson, 1885–1976).

Holzknecht was a pioneer radiologist of the heart and chest and is known for his description of "Holzknecht's Space" behind the heart.

SCHWARZ (GOTTWALD) 1880–1959

573 Die Röntgenuntersuchung des Herzens und der grossen Gefässe: 5 vorträge. *Leipzig und Wien, Franz Deuticke, 1911.* [v], 61 pp. Illus (plates), diagrs, bibliog. (ftn. refs). 4to, 26 cms.

One of the earliest treatises on cardiac radiology prior to Dietlen, Assmann and Vaquez and Bordet. Schwarz introduced orthodiagraphy in the upright posture with a fixed screen and movable tube. This German roentgenologist is remembered for Schwarz's sign—x-ray shadow of fat at apex of the heart, often confused with cardiac enlargement: Ueber einen typischen Röntgenbefund am Herzen Fettliebiger und dessen anatomischer Grundlage (*Wiener klinische Wochenschrift*, 1910, **23**, 1850–2)—and Schwarz's test (also called the fibroderm bismuth capsule test) for anacidity of the stomach.

GROEDEL (FRANZ MAXIMILIAN) 1881–1951

574 Die Röntgendiagnostik der Herz- und Gefässerkrankungen. (Bibliothek der physikalisch-medizinischen Techniken, Band 2). *Berlin, Hermann Meusser, 1912.* vii, 188 pp. Illus (incl. plates), diagrs (orthodiagrams), bibliog. 8vo, 23 cms.

Additional [3] pp. publisher's advertisements, followed by 12 plates.

A pioneer work on cardiac radiology. Groedel, a pioneer in cardiac radiology, designed one of the earliest orthodiagraphs for use in the sitting posture. The orthogonal projection was marked on paper by a pneumatic marker. The Groedel orthodiagraph was used at the National Heart Hospital up to about 1927.

VAQUEZ (LOUIS HENRI) 1860–1936 and BORDET (ÉMILE) *b.* 1871

575 Radiologie du cœur et des vaisseaux de la base. 4me éd. *Paris, J. B. Baillière, 1928.* [v], 499 pp. Illus, tables, diagrs (orthodiagrams), bibliog. (occasional ftn. refs). 4to, 26 cms.

This radiological classic, first published in 1913, and based on orthodiagraphy, was translated into German (1916) and an American edition was published in 1920.

576 Radiologie des vaisseaux de la base du cœur. *Paris, J. B. Baillière, 1920.* 252 pp. Illus, diagrs. 8vo, 25 cms.

Half-title page p. [3]; pp. [1]–[2] blank.

This volume was intended to complete their original work on cardiac radiology, *Le Cœur et l'aorte* (3me éd. Paris, Baillière, 1920).

DIETLEN (HANS) 1879–1955

577 Herz und Gefässe im Röntgenbild: ein Lehrbuch . . . mit einem Beitrag über Röntgenbefunde bei den Arhythmien des Herzens von Prof. Dr. Arthur Weber. *Leipzig, Johann Ambrosius Barth, 1923.* xii, 455 pp. Illus, tables, diagrs (orthodiagrams), bibliog. 8vo, 25 cms.

A classic of cardiac radiology based on the orthodiagraph with extensive bibliography of earlier work (472 references).

MORISON (JOHN MILLER WOODBURN) 1875–1951

578 Elevation of the diaphragm; unilateral phrenic analysis: a radiological study, with special reference to the differential diagnosis. *London, William Heinemann, 1923.* [v], 30 pp. Illus, diagrs, bibliog. 4to, 28 cms.

Reprinted from *Archives of Radiology and Electrotherapy*, 1922–1923, **27,** 353–64; 1923–1924, **28,** 72–85, 111–23.

Autograph: Charlton Briscoe (Sir Charlton Briscoe, 1874–1960, M.D., F.R.C.P.).

BORDET (ÉMILE) *b.* 1871

579 La Dilatation du cœur: étude radioscopique. Préface du Pr. H. Vaquez. *Paris, J. B. Baillière, 1926.* 153 pp. Illus, diagrs (orthodiagrams). 8vo, 23 cms.

PEZZI (CESARE) 1874–1945

580 Radiologia clinica del cuore e dei grossi vasi. *Milan, Cooperativa Farmaceutica, 1928.* 335 pp. Illus, diagrs (orthodiagrams), bibliog. 8vo, 23 cms.

Author's presentation copy to DEB, March 1928.

Pezzi worked in Paris with Laubry and first described the "hilar dance" in pulmonary incompetence, later noted in atrial septal defect.

SCHINZ (HANS RUDOLF) *b.* 1891, and others

581 Lehrbuch der Röntgendiagnostik. 3 Aufl. *Leipzig, Georg Thieme, 1932.* 2 Bande. Illus, diagrs, tables, bibliog. 4to, 28 cms.

Band 1: wanting; Band 2: Innere Organe (pp. 705–1623).

The heart section by Max Holtzmann (*b.* 1891)—Erkrangungen des Herzens und der Gefässe (pp. 983–1128)—is profusely illustrated with x-ray plates and orthodiagrams and has an ample bibliography. Schinz's work was one of the most important on radiology at this period especially for the heart and chest. First published in 1928 (?), a fourth edition was published in 1939, and a fifth in 1950; an English translation appeared in 1951–1954.

KIRSCH (OSKAR)

582 Grundlagen der orthodiagraphischen Herzgrössen- und Thoraxbreitenbeurteilung im Kindesalter. (Abhandlungen aus der Kinderheilkunde und ihren Grenzgebieten. Beihefte zum Jahrbuch für Kinderheilkunde, Heft 23). *Berlin, S. Karger, 1929.* iv, 110 pp. Tables, diagrs (orthodiagrams), bibliog. 4to, 26 cms.

A standard reference work on heart size in children, with comprehensive bibliography (pp. 108–10).

BEDFORD (DAVIS EVAN) *b.* 1898 and
TREADGOLD (HENRY ASHBOURNE) 1883–1941

583 The Size of the healthy heart and its measurement. *London, Lancet, 1931.* 20 pp. Tables, diagrs (incl. orthodiagrams), bibliog. 8vo, 22 cms.

Reprinted from *Lancet*, 1931, **2**, 836–42.

NEMET (GEZA) 1895–1936

584 Guide to radiologic diagnosis in heart disease; prepared with the aid of the Committee on Research of the Heart Committee. *New York, New York Tuberculosis and Health Association, 1931.* 25, [9] pp. Diagrs (orthodiagrams). 8vo, 20 cms.

PARKINSON (Sir JOHN) 1885–1976

585 The Radiology of heart disease. *London, British Medical Association, 1933.* 10 pp. Illus (incl. 2 plates). 8vo, 22 cms.

Reprinted from *British medical Journal*, 1933, **2**, 591–4.

586 The Lumleian lectures 1936 on enlargement of the heart, delivered before the Royal College of Physicians of London on March 17th and 19th. [*London, Lancet, 1936*]. 52 pp. Illus, diagrs, bibliog. 8vo, 22 cms.

Reprinted from *Lancet*, 1936, **1**, 1337–45, 1391–1400.
Author's presentation copy to DEB—"with warmest appreciation of your advice and help."

POLEVSKI (JACOB) 1884–1936

587 The Heart visible; a clinical study in cardio-vascular roentgenology in health and disease. *Philadelphia, F. A. Davis, 1934.* xvii, 5–207 pp. Illus, diagrs, bibliog. 8vo, 24 cms.

An early American work on cardiac radiology. The author had worked in Holzknecht's clinic in Vienna.

BREDNOW (WALTER) *b.* 1896

588 Röntgenatlas der Erkrankungen des Herzens und der Gefässe; ein Leitfaden für Arzte. *Berlin und Wien, Urban & Schwarzenberg, 1936.* [v], 155 pp. Illus. 4to, 26 cms.

Second edition, 1939; third edition, 1942; fifth edition, 1951. An important early work on cardiac radiology from Göttingen. Brednow made relief models of the heart using methods of Palmieri, Lysholm, Berg and Shatzki.

EVANS (WILLIAM) *b.* 1895

589 The Course of the oesophagus in health and in disease of the heart and great vessels. (Medical Research Council. Special Report Series, No. 208.) *London, His Majesty's Stationery Office, 1936.* 93 pp. Illus (plates), tables, bibliog. 8vo, 25 cms.

Pp. 1–30 text, pp. 31–93 plates. List of M.R.C. publications (xii pp.) bound in at end.
Evans began noting in detail the normal course of the gullet or oesophagus, the whole length of which passes through the chest in close proximity to the heart, the great vessels and the roots of the lungs, being moulded against these and associated structures. By noticing radiologically small distortions in the course of the oesophagus, and thus changes in outline of the surrounding organs, Evans was able to diagnose early forms of diseases of the heart and great vessels.

KURTZ (Chester Mott) *b.* 1899

590 Orthodiascopy: an analysis of over seventeen hundred orthodiascopic examinations. (Macmillan Medical Monographs). *New York, Macmillan, 1937.* xxiii, 247 pp. Illus (plates), tables, diagrs (orthodiagrams), bibliog. 8vo, 22 cms.

One of the earliest works on the orthodiagraph in English.

PALMER (John Hammond) 1896–1958

591 The Development of cardiac enlargement in disease of the heart: a radiological study. (Medical Research Council. Special Report Series, No. 222). *London, His Majesty's Stationery Office, 1937.* 49 pp. Illus (plates), tables, diagrs (orthodiagrams), bibliog. 8vo, 25 cms.

List of M.R.C. publications (xiv pp.) bound in at end.

Palmer, a Canadian physician working under Parkinson at the London Hospital, investigated the rate of enlargement by serial records in various forms of heart disease.

ROESLER (Hugo) 1899–1961

592 Clinical roentgenology of the cardio-vascular system; anatomy, physiology, pathology, experiments and clinical applications. *London, Baillière, Tindall & Cox, 1937.* xvi, 343 pp. Illus, diagrs (orthodiagrams), bibliog. 4to, 26 cms.

Extensive alphabetical bibliographies at the end of each chapter, brought right up to date with additional references. Well illustrated (199 figures).

Roesler was radiologist at the Herzstation in Vienna and was one of the greatest authorities on cardiac radiology at the time, with an encyclopaedic knowledge of the literature. He left Vienna for U.S.A. with Dressler, his clinical colleague.

SHANKS (Seymour Cochrane) *b.* 1893

593 A Text-book of x-ray diagnosis by British authors. *London, H. K. Lewis, 1938–1939.* 3 vols. Illus, diagrs, bibliog. 4to, 26 cms.

Vol. 1: Thorax (xii, 591 pp.); vols 2–3, wanting. Presentation copy to DEB from Kerley with an autograph letter (1938). Second edition, 1950–1951, and third edition, 1957–1959, and fourth edition, 1969–1972, edited by Shanks and Kerley for same publisher. Kerley's account was the first authoritative British radiological work on the cardiovascular system (pp. 3–96).

LAUBRY (Charles) 1872–1960, and others

594 Radiologie clinique du cœur et des gros vaisseaux. *Paris, Masson, 1939.* 2 tom. (7, 340 pp., continuous pagination). Illus, diagrs, bibliog. Folio, 32 cms.

Laubry's collaborators were: Paul Henri Cottentot (1882–1949), Daniel Routier (*b.* 1887) and Raymond Heim de Balsac (*b.* 1903). Profusely illustrated (over 1000 x-ray photographs with explanatory diagrams). Important bibliography (pp. 319–28). Authors' presentation copy, signed by Laubry and Routier.

This atlas covers the radiological anatomy of the normal and diseased heart based on radio-opaque injections of the right and left cavities of the heart in situ in the cadaver. It represents ten years of work at the Hôpital Broussais, Paris, and is a landmark in radiological knowledge prior to the advent of angiocardiography.

ZDANSKY (Erich) *b.* 1893

595 Röntgendiagnostik des Herzens und der grossen Gefässe. 2e Aufl. *Wien, Springer, 1949.* viii, 434 pp. Illus, diagrs (orthodiagrams), bibliog. 8vo, 25 cms.

Profusely illustrated (397 figures). Author's presentation copy to Sir John Parkinson. Zdansky was radiologist in Wenckebach's clinic in Vienna and his book was later translated and published in U.S.A. in a new enlarged edition (New York, Grune and Stratton, 1963; second American edition, 1965). First edition, 1939.

DOTTER (Charles Theodore) *b.* 1920 and STEINBERG (Israel) *b.* 1902

596 Angiocardiography. (Annals of Roentgenology, vol. 20). *London* [*etc*], *Cassell, 1951.* xix, [i], 304 pp. Illus, tables, diagrs, bibliog. 4to, 27 cms.

The most authoritative work on angiocardiography to date and still very valuable; profusely illustrated.

SCHIROSA (Giuseppe) and TEDESCHI (Azaria)

597 Il Pneumomediastino nello studio radiologico del cuore e dei grossi vasi. Prefazione del Prof. Luigi Condorelli. (*Italian and English*). *Roma, Società Editrice Universo, 1958.* xv, 182 pp. Illus, diagrs, bibliog. Folio, 35 cms.

Profusely illustrated; legends in atlas in 5 languages (Italian, English, French, Spanish, German).

ANGINA PECTORIS, CORONARY DISEASE AND THE CORONARY CIRCULATION

Heberden's "Some account of a disorder of the breast", which he named angina pectoris, is the most precise and concise description of a new disease in the history of medicine.

Odd cases were recorded before Heberden's time (see nos. 603–06), but the only important claim to priority is Rougnon's account of Captain Charles contained in a letter to Lorry and published in Besançon in 1768, shortly before Heberden's account. The case has been much discussed (see nos. 600–01), and incidentally Rougnon's account is probably the rarest medical book, only two copies are known.

Jenner and Parry originated the coronary theory of anginal pain, the neuritic or neuralgic theory became popular in France, painful distension of the left ventricle was sponsored by Lauder Brunton and Merklen; the aortic theory of Clifford Allbutt was important because of his strong opposition to the coronary theory which undoubtedly delayed full recognition of the clinical syndrome of coronary thrombosis and myocardial infarction described by Herrick in 1912 and 1918.

In regard to treatment Heberden advocated alcohol and opium. Lauder Brunton introduced amyl nitrite in 1867 and Murrell nitro-glycerine in 1879, 1882, and these are still effective remedies.

SENECA (LUCIUS ANNAEUS) *c.* 4 B.C.–A.D 65.

MARX (KARL FRIEDRICH HEINRICH) 1796–1877

598 Ueber die Anfälle mit dem Gefühle des Verscheidens, den intermittirenden chronischen Herzschmerz, das Leiden des Philosophen Lucius Annäus Seneca. *Göttingen, Dieterischen Buchhandlung, 1872.* 44 pp. Bibliog. (ftn. refs). 8vo, 24 cms.

Reprinted from *Abhandlunger der königlichen Gesellschaft der Wissenschaften zu Göttingen*, 1872, **17,** 3–44.

Book-stamp: Prof. Dr. E. Leyden (?Ernst von Leyden, 1832–1910).

An account of the angina of Lucius Annaeus Seneca (*c.* 4 B.C.–65 A.D.), philosopher and tutor of the Roman Emperor Nero.

See also *The Workes of Seneca* . . . newly enlarged and corrected by Thomas Lodge (London, [1620], pp. 256–7) (RCP) and Seneca's *Epistolae morales*. (Loeb Classical Library). London, 1925, vol. 1, pp. 360–1 (RCP).

NICHOLLS (FRANK) 1699–1778

599 Observations concerning the body of his late Majesty [George II] . . . to . . . George, Earl of Macclesfield . . .

Extracted from *Philosophical Transactions of the Royal Society* (reprinted at Wittenberg, 1773) 1761, **52,** 127–31. Illus.

Nicholls was an anatomist, and became physician to George II. His Goulstonian Lecture at the College of Physicians was entitled "The structure of the heart and the circulation of the blood (1734)." King George II died from a ruptured heart, haemopericardium and a dissecting aneurysm. The Wittenberg reprint is paged differently from the original (pp. 265–75), and conflicting references to this paper fail to take into account reprintings and abridgements of the *Philosophical Transactions*.

ROUGNON DE MAGNY (NICHOLAS FRANÇOIS) 1727–1799

600 Lettre de M. Rougnon a M. Lorry touchant les causes de la mort de feu Monsieur Charles, ancien Capitaine de Cavalerie, arrivée à Besançon, le 23 Fevrier, 1768. *Besançon, de l'imprimerie de J. F. Charmet, 1768.* 55 pp. 12mo, 13 cms. [*Xeroxcopy*].

Garrison and Morton 2886. Reproduced from photostat copy in the library of the Royal College of Physicians of London, presented by Professor Hans Kohn.

Rougnon's booklet claimed by many French authorities as the first description of angina pectoris was published four months before Heberden's paper, which was read in 1768 but not published until 1772. Only two copies of Rougnon's book are known, one at Besançon, one in the National Library of Medicine at Bethesda, Md., U.S.A. It was abstracted in the *Journal des Scavans* (1768, **33,** 321–37) and by H. El. Nemeri for his Paris thesis (*La première description de l'angine de poitrine: la vie et l'oeuvre de Rougnon*, 1930).

BEDFORD (DAVIS EVAN) *b.* 1898

601 Rougnon's letter to Lorry on the death of Captain Charles: a landmark in the history of angina pectoris. *London, British Medical Association, 1970.* Port., facsim., bibliog. 8vo, 25 cms.

Reprinted from *British Heart Journal*, 1970, **32,** 277–80.

COUTENOT (FRANÇOIS MARIE)

602 Docteur Rougnon de l'Université de Besançon (1727–1799). *Besançon, imprimerie Henri Bosanne, 1895.* vi, 86 pp. Port. (frontispiece), bibliog. (occasional ftn. refs). 8vo, 23 cms.

Biography of Rougnon with portrait and historical review of medicine in 17th and 18th centuries.

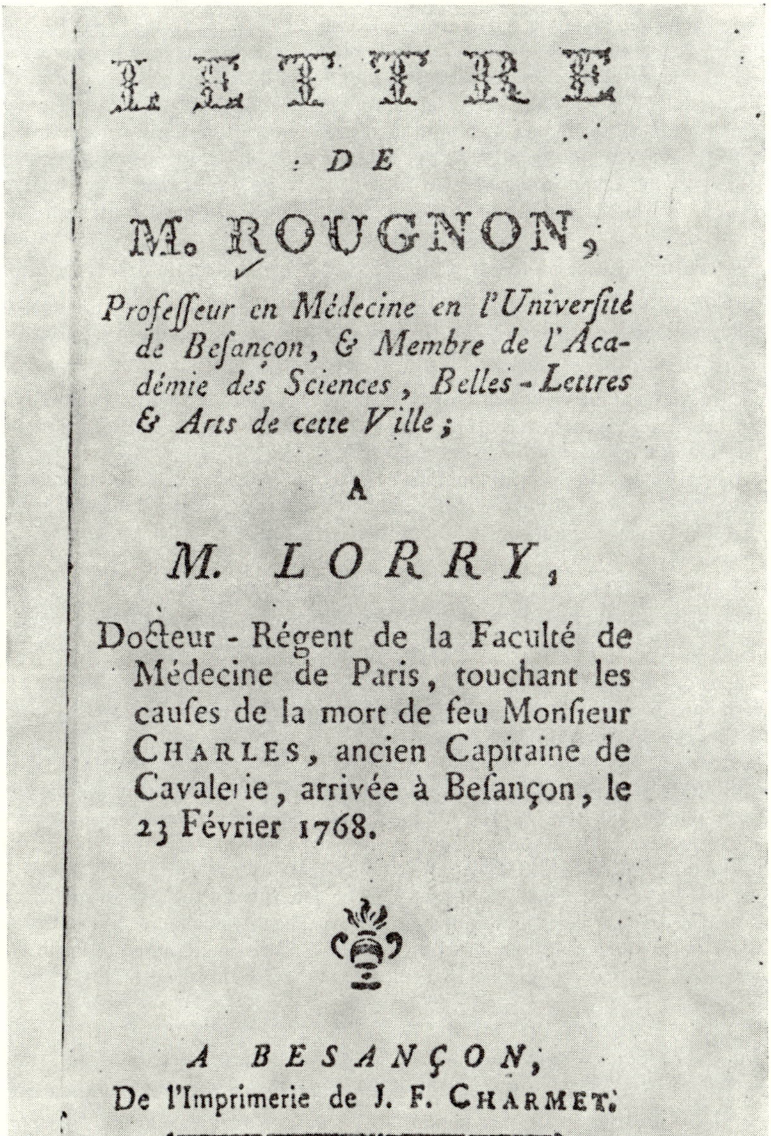

LETTRE

DE

M. ROUGNON,

Profeſſeur en Médecine en l'Univerſité de Beſançon, & Membre de l'Académie des Sciences, Belles-Lettres & Arts de cette Ville;

A

M. LORRY,

Docteur-Régent de la Faculté de Médecine de Paris, touchant les cauſes de la mort de feu Monſieur CHARLES, ancien Capitaine de Cavalerie, arrivée à Beſançon, le 23 Février 1768.

A BESANÇON,

De l'Imprimerie de J. F. CHARMET.

M. DCC. LXVIII.

No. 600. The first description of angina pectoris?

HEBERDEN (WILLIAM) the elder, 1710–1801

[42] Some account of a disorder of the breast.

Pp. 59–67 in ROYAL COLLEGE OF PHYSICIANS OF LONDON. *Medical transactions, published by the College of Physicians in London.* London, S. Baker and J. Dodsley, 1772. Vol. 2 (xv, 533 pp., [i] f). 8vo, 23 cms.

Heberden's paper on angina pectoris covered only nine pages, printed in large type, and probably the most concise and precise original description of a new disease in the history of medicine. It was read on 21st July, 1768, but not published until 1772. Besides effort pain, he described the more prolonged nocturnal attacks and mentioned a case in which pain persisted several days when the patient's life was in peril, obviously a case of cardiac infarction. His next contribution (*ibid*, 1785, **3**, 1–11) (RCP) was the unknown patient who died suddenly, a few weeks later when Hunter performed the necropsy at which Parry was present and stated later that the coronary arteries were not examined.

603 *The same.* An Introduction to the study of physic (now for the first time published) . . . with prefatory essay by Leroy Crummer [1872–1934]; with a reprint of Heberden's Some account of a disorder of the breast. *New York, P. B. Hoeber, 1929.* xi, 159 pp. Illus, port. (frontispiece), facsims, bibliog. 8vo, 20 cms.

This copy has the imprint of London [etc.], Humphrey Milford, Oxford University Press tipped in on the title-page. Prefatory essay, pp. 1–67; An Introduction to the study of physic, pp. 69–149; Some account of a disorder of the breast, pp. 151–9.

Leroy Crummer purchased the unpublished MS in a bookshop in London and subsequently gave it to the Royal College of Physicians (MS 343). Their librarian confirmed that the handwriting was Heberden's. Heberden recommends books on botany, chemistry, pharmacy, anatomy, surgery and various classical works.

604 Commentaries on the history and cure of diseases. *London, T. Payne, 1802.* x, 483 pp. 8vo, 22 cms.

Collations of copies vary, suggesting that contents Latin [1 leaf] and English index [1 leaf] after the preface (pp. iii–v) are not consistently placed or sometimes may be omitted.

Book-stamp: Middlesex Hospital Library (cancelled).

Second edition, 1803 (RCP); third edition, 1806 (RCP); fourth edition, 1816 (RCP). Another edition, Boston, Wells & Lilley, 1818. American edition (American medical library series) Philadelphia, E. Barrington & G. D. Haswell, 1945; original Latin edition, *Commentarii de morborum historia et curatione* [ed. by W. Heberden, the younger] Londini, apud T. Payne, 1802 (RCP); Ed. altera. Londini, T. Payne, 1807 (RCP).

By the time he wrote the manuscript (1782?) Heberden had seen 100 cases of angina and associated it with sudden death. Besides the chapter on angina, Pectoris dolor, pp. 362–9, the *Commentaries* contain one on palpitation, Palpitatio cordis, pp. 336–8. The manuscript notes for the *Commentaries* in Heberden's own hand are preserved in the library of the Royal College of Physicians (MSS 341–2, 344).

605 Gulielmi Heberdeni Opera medica. Recognovit vitam auctoris adjecit atque edidit Ludov. Herm. Friedlaenderus. (Scriptorum classicorum de praxi medica nonnullorum opera collecta, vol. X.). *Lipsiae, sumptibus Leopoldi Vossii [ex officina Hirschfeldii], 1831.* xviii, 291 pp. Bibliog. (occasional ftn. refs). 12mo, 18 cms.

Contents: Editoris praefatio pp. v–vii, Gulielmi Heberdeni vita pp. viii–xiv, Commentarii de morborum historia et curatione, pp. 1–246, Commentarioli quidam Heberdeni anglice conscripti nunc primum ab editore Latine redditi pp. 247–64. The Commentarioli are equivalent to the four papers appended to the second edition of the *Commentaries* (1803) and consist of (1) Praefationis, qua G. Heberdenus Acta Medica (Medical Transactions) anni 1767 auspicaturus erat, adumbratio; (2) De rheumatismo chronico; (3) Observationes de pulsu arteriarum; (substantially the same as no. 42, but with the remark quoted toned down); (4) De vena in haemorrhagis secanda; Index, pp. 265–91. Unidentified final page ("de Thermis Postheniensibus") used as book mark.

BEDFORD (DAVIS EVAN) *b.* 1898

606 William Heberden's contribution to cardiology.

Reprinted from the *Journal of the Royal College of Physicians of London*, 1968, **2**, 127–35. Port., facsims, bibliog.

Written on the bicentenary of the publication of Heberden's paper "Some account of a disorder of the breast".

FOTHERGILL (JOHN) 1712–1780

607 A Case of an angina pectoris with remarks; [*and*] Farther account of the angina pectoris.

Pp. 233–51, and 252–8 in *Medical Observations and Inquiries by a Society of Physicians in London*. London, T. Cadell, 1776, vol. 5 (xv, 405, [26] pp.). 8vo, 21 cms.

The set of six volumes (London, William Johnston and T. Cadell, 1757–1814) (RCP; vol. 6, wanting in this library; vol. 4 has autograph of Geo Roe, 1814) contains papers of interest on many medical and surgical topics, for example, aneurysm, tapping for dropsy, haemopericardium, and Fothergill's paper on lead poisoning in water colour painters. The most important is his case of angina pectoris with ossified coronary arteries. John Hunter performed the post-mortem examination. A pencilled note on p. 252 reads "first published P[ost] M[ortem] in A[ngina] P[ectoris] showing coron[ary] atheroma. DEB."

WALL (JOHN) 1708–1776

608 A Letter to Dr. Heberden on the angina pectoris.

Pp. 324–35 in his *Medical tracts* collected and republished by Martin Wall, M.D. Oxford, D. Prince and J. Cook: London, T. Caddell, 1780. [vi], xxix, iv pp., [1] f., 355 pp., [8] ff. Bibliog. (occasional ftn. refs). 8vo, 22 cms.

Title-page has manuscript correction of motto and an additional quote from Virgil's *Aeneid*. The imprimatur by George Horne, vice-chancellor of Oxford, is dated Jan. 17, 1780. An "Extract from Dr. Nash's History of Worcestershire relative to the Author" (iv pp.) following the preface (p. xxix), appears to be a late addition. It was not found in the copy formerly in the library of the Royal College of Physicians of London, nor in that recorded in the *Index-Catalogue* of the Library of the Surgeon-General's Office. It is not mentioned in the contents list and seems contradicted by the writer of the preface (p. 1, "I shall not in this Place introduce a Panegyric on the Author."). Volume acquired in 1942.

The *Letter* has the note: "Published in a Pamphlet with a few other Tracts, in 1775, when the College of Physicians discontinued the Publication of the Medical Transactions. Those Tracts had been read before the College, and were intended as Part of the Third Volume of the Transactions. Read at the College, Nov. 17, 1772." The pamphlet of 1775 has not been traced, but the third volume of the *Medical Transactions* was eventually published in 1786, and the *Letter* was included, pp. 12–24, and described one of the earliest necropsies, showing ossification of the aortic valves.

PARRY (CALEB HILLIER) 1755–1822

609 Untersuchung der Symptome und Ursachen der Syncope anginosa, gewöhnlich Angina Pectoris genannt. Aus dem Englischer übersetzt und mit einigen Anmerkungen versehen von Friedrich Gotthelf Friese. *Breslau, Hirschberg und Lissa, bei Johann Friedrich Korn dem Aeltern, 1801.* xvi, 160 pp. Bibliog. (ftn. refs). 8vo, 21 cms.

German translation of *An Inquiry into the symptoms and causes of the syncope anginosa, commonly called angina pectoris* (London, Cadell & Davis, 1799) (RCP).

610 *The same.* Recherches sur les symptomes et les causes de la syncope angineuse, vulgairement appelée angine de la poitrine; éclairées par les ouvertures cadaveriques. Mises en

française par A. [Jacques André] Matthey. *Paris, Patris et Gilbert, 1806.* [iii], x, 116 pp. Bibliog. (occasional ftn. refs). 12mo, 19 cms.

The English and French editions are now very rare. Both Parry and Jenner had described the association of angina with coronary artery disease at the Fleece Medical Society, but delayed its publication for fear of alarming John Hunter in whom Jenner had diagnosed angina pectoris (see no. 1092). Jenner's paper was prior to Parry's and he is generally regarded as the originator of the coronary theory. Black (nos. 615–6) had described coronary disease in angina independently of Parry, who cited one of his cases.

MACINTYRE (WILLIAM) 1792?–1857

611 Tentamen medicum inaugurale, de angina pectoris . . . *Edinburgi, excudebat C. Stewart, 1811.* [vii], 22 pp. Bibliog. (occasional ftn. refs). 8vo, 24 cms.

A good example of an Edinburgh University M.D. thesis in Latin, making reference to Black (nos. 615–6), Parry (nos. 609–10), Burns (nos. 263–5), Wall (no. 608), and Fothergill (no. 607).

BLACKALL (JOHN) 1771–1860

612 Observations on the nature and cure of dropsies and particularly on the presence of the coagulable part of the blood in dropsical urine; to which is added an appendix containing several cases of angina pectoris with dissections, etc. 2nd ed., corrected and improved. *London, Longman, Hurst, Rees, Orme and Brown, 1814.* viii, xiii, [14]–416 pp. Bibliog. (ftn. refs). 8vo, 22 cms.

Errata on half-leaf inserted between pp. 14 and 15. First edition, London, Longman [and others], 1813. Callisen records the third edition as 1818 and a German translation from it by "Just. Radius. Pesth (Leipzig), bei Hartlebeni, 1821". Fourth edition, London, Longman [and others] 1824, from which a second American edition was made (Philadelphia, J. Webster, 1825).

Book-stamp: Brighton and Sussex Medico-Chirurgical Society, 1837.

Blackall was physician to the Devon and Exeter Hospital and discovered the association of albuminuria with dropsy before Bright. He collected twenty cases of angina, including four of his own, in which aortic disease was found at necropsy, and may be regarded as the originator of the aortic theory.

JURINE (LOUIS) 1751–1819

613 Mémoire sur l'angine de poitrine, qui a remporté le prix au concours ouvert sur ce sujet par la Société de Médecine de Paris, le 31 octobre 1809, et qui fut adjugé le 2 février 1813. *Paris, J. J. Paschoud, 1815.* 360 (i.e. 362) pp. Bibliog. (ftn. refs). 8vo, 20 cms.

[*and*] DESPORTES (EUGÈNE HENRI) 1782–1875

Traité de l'angine de poitrine, ou nouvelles recherches sur une maladie de la poitrine, que l'on a presque toujours confondue avec l'asthme, les maladies du cœur, etc. *Paris, Méquignon l'ainé, de l'imprimerie de Crapelet, 1811.* [iv], viii, 229 pp. Bibliog. (ftn. refs and in text). 8vo, 20 cms.

614 *The same.*

Pp. 381–474 in RAMAZZINI (Bernardino) 1633–1714. *Traité des maladies des artisans. Traité de la maladie muqueuse*, par [J. G.] Roederer et [K. G.] Wagler (French and Latin); *Mémoire sur l'angine de poitrine*, par Jurine. Paris, Adolphe Delahays, 1855. vii, 479 pp. Bibliog. (ftn. refs). 8vo, 22 cms.

Jurine was professor of anatomy, surgery, and midwifery at Geneva. His treatise on angina pectoris was awarded the prize offered by the Société de Médecine de Paris in 1812, for a "description of the disease designated mainly by English physicians as angina pectoris". The popular theories as to causation were gout, spasm of the heart, asthmatic disease, ossification of the coronary arteries or aortic valve, and neuralgia of the cardiac plexus. Jurine and Desportes supported the neuralgia theory, his main objection to the coronary theory being the occurrence of ossified coronaries at post-mortem in subjects who had not had anginal pain. His comprehensive review was for long cited as one of the classical works on the subject.

BLACK (Samuel) *fl.* 1786–1839

615 History of two cases of angina pectoris . . . communicated to Dr. Curry.

Extracted from *Medico-chirurgical Transactions*, 1816, **7**, 70–83. Bibliog. 8vo, 22 cms.

Dr. Curry was James Curry (*d.* 1819), physician to Guy's Hospital. Black was one of the first to report coronary disease post-mortem in cases of angina pectoris, and an advocate of the coronary theory of anginal pain before Parry and Jenner.

616 Angina pectoris.

Pp. 15–90 in his *Clinical and pathological reports.* Newry, printed by Alexander Wilkinson, and sold by Longman [etc.], London, 1819. xii, vii–xiv, 15–234 pp. 8vo, 24 cms.

The collation of this copy is the same as that of the Manchester University Medical School Library (formerly of the Manchester Medical Society); there is no contents page. Contents are Dedication pp. iii–iv, Preface v–xii, Introduction vii–xiv, Angina pectoris 15–90, Dissections of two habitual drunkards 91–98, Case of gouty affection 99–109, Cases and dissections illustrative of disease of the brain 111–53, Peritonitis chronica 155–79, Otitis 181–95, Diabetes mellitus 197–234.

Author's presentation copy to "the Revd. Mr. Thackeray" (Elias Thackeray, 1771–1854, son of a surgeon and brother to two medical men, retired from service in the Irish Rebellion as major and became chaplain to the Lord Lieutenant of Ireland 1799, vicar of Dundalk and rector of Louth. He is mentioned in the *Irish Sketchbook* of the novelist William Makepeace Thackeray, to whom he was cousin once removed).

Black took his M.D. degree in Edinburgh in 1786, and is last mentioned in the Dublin directories in 1839.

DENOUH (Louis François)

617 Des ruptures du cœur. (Thèse pour le doctorat en médecine 1852. Paris thesis 1852, no. 256, v. 522.). *Paris, Rignoux, imprimeur de la Faculté de Médecine, 1852.* 34 pp. 8vo, 25 cms.

Author's presentation copy: "à Mr. le Dr. Martin Ma[gron], Hommage d'un d[e] ses élèves, L. Denou[h]." The ascription is slightly cropped; the teaching of Dr. Martin Magron (1810–1872) is acknowledged in the thesis.

BRÜCKE (Ernst Wilhelm von) 1819–1892

618 Der Verschluss der Kranzschlagadern durch die Aortenklappen. Eine Entgegnung auf dem vom Herrn Prof. Jos. Hyrtl am 7 December 1854 . . . gehaltenen Vortrag. *Vienna, Carl Gerold, 1855.* 24 pp. 8vo, 22 cms.

[*and*] HYRTYL (Josef) 1810–1894

Über die Selbsteuerung des Herzens: ein Beitrag zur Mechanik der Aortenklappen. *Wien, Wilhelm Braumüller, 1855.* iv, 5–71 pp. Bibliog. (ftn. refs). 8vo, 22 cms.

An English summary (typescript) of the two papers by Dr. Peter Meyer is inserted.

Von Brücke, professor of physiology at Vienna, revived Stroem's hypothesis that the coronary ostia were closed in systole by the aortic semilunar cusps, so that coronary flow was diastolic in time. A stormy dispute arose with Hyrtl, his anatomical colleague, who opposed his theory on anatomical grounds. This controversy was an important one in the history of the coronary circulation (See also James Wilson's *Lectures*, 1819, p. 133, no. 710).

RIDGE (JOSEPH) *d.* 1875

619 Observations on the life, disease and death of John Hunter, in elucidation of the nature and treatment of gout and angina pectoris, being the oration delivered before the Hunterian Society at its thirty-sixth anniversary. *London, John Churchill, 1855.* 47 pp. 8vo, 21 cms.

Ridge reviewed Hunter's illness and the necropsy reported by Home and attributed the arterial disease to gout.

BRUNTON (Sir THOMAS LAUDER) 1844–1916

620 On the use of nitrite of amyl in angina pectoris. [*London, Lancet, 1867*]. 3 pp. 8vo, 21 cms.

Reprinted from *Lancet*, 1867, **2**, 97–8. Author's presentation copy to Dr. Grainger Stewart (later Sir Thomas Grainger Stewart, 1837–1900, professor of the practice of physic and of clinical medicine at Edinburgh University).

[*and*] On the action of nitrite of amyl on the circulation.

Reprinted from *Journal of Anatomy & Physiology*, 1870–1871, **5**, 92–101. Diagrs.

"With the author's best compliments". Brunton first studied the action of amyl nitrite on the small vessels in Carl Ludwig's laboratory in Leipzig, and tried it on angina pectoris with the idea of lowering the blood-pressure.

MURRELL (WILLIAM) 1853–1912

621 Nitro-glycerine as a remedy for angina pectoris. *London, printed by T. Richards, 1880.* 26 pp. Tables, diagrs (tracings). 8vo, 21 cms.

Reprinted from *Lancet*, 1879, **1**, 80–1, 113–15, 151–2, 225–7.

Murrell's original paper on nitro-glycerine (glyceryl trinitrate).

622 Nitro-glycerine as a remedy for angina pectoris. *London, H. K. Lewis, 1882.* [v], 78 pp. Diagrs (tracings). 8vo, 20 cms.

Publisher's catalogue, March 1882, (18 pp.) bound in at end. American edition, Detroit, G. S. Davis, 1882.

Book-stamp: Birmingham Medical Institute; autograph: John Parkinson (Sir John Parkinson, 1885–1976).

Murrell, physician to Westminster Hospital and lecturer on therapeutics, introduced nitro-glycerine as a remedy for anginal pain. He wrote a medical best-seller *What to do in cases of poisoning* (1881) which went through eleven editions.

LEGG (JOHN WICKHAM) 1843–1921

623 Some account of cardiac aneurysms . . . (Bradshaw Lecture, 1883.) *London, J. & A. Churchill, 1884.* ix, 75 pp. Tables, bibliog. 8vo, 21 cms.

Wickham Legg was physician and lecturer on pathology at St. Bartholomew's Hospital. His monograph on cardiac aneurysm was a classic in its day: he regarded it as due to fibrous myocarditis. A full classified bibliography is included (pp. 58–75). He retired from medicine after two attacks of rheumatic fever and became the greatest English authority on liturgiology.

GÉLINEAU (JEAN BAPTISTE EDOUARD) 1827?–1906

624 Traité de l'angine de poitrine. *Paris, Adrien Delahaye et Émile Lecrosnier, 1887.* [iii], iv, 617 pp. 8vo, 24 cms.

Inserted is correspondence with Dr. Samuel Oram on the reference to tobacco angina (pp. 190–205), which he cites at the beginning of his article on the subject (no. 673).

Gélineau was a French naval surgeon whose place in the history of angina pectoris rests on his account of an epidemic of anginal pain in the French corvette, l'Embuscade, in 1858, on a long cruise in the Pacific, during which scurvy, lead colic, fever and dysentery combined to cause a debilitated state of the crew, many of whom smoked incessantly and chewed tobacco. He describes at length every known aetiological variety of anginal pain, and gives an early account of tobacco angina.

Also known as the discoverer of "Gélineau's syndrome" (narcolepsy; see Garrison and Morton 4561), Gélineau is best remembered as a specialist in nerve diseases. According to his Montpellier thesis *Aperçu médical sur l'Ile Mayotte*, 1858 (copies in the British Museum Library and Wellcome Institute of the History of Medicine) and his obituary in *British medical Journal*, 1906, **1**, 778, he was born at Blaye (Gironde) in 1827. *The National Library of Medical catalog* places the *Traité* and other works under Édouard Gelineau, 1828–1906, the form of name under which he usually wrote. The earlier *Index-catalogue of the library of the Surgeon-General's Office* places these under his full names of Jean Baptiste Édouard, but the birth date of 1859, copied by other reference sources, is incorrect.

HALL (FRANCIS DE HAVILLAND) 1847–1929

625 Remarks on angina pectoris and allied conditions with cases. [*London, J. & A. Churchill, 1887*]. 23 pp. Bibliog. (ftn. refs). 8vo, 22 cms.

Reprinted from *Westminster Hospital Reports*, 1887, **3**, 81–103.

Hall concludes his paper by abstaining from the question of the pathology of angina pectoris because "the differences on the subject are so great, and the literature devoted to it so voluminous."

CROCQ (JEAN JOSEPH) 1824–1898

626 Nature et traitement de l'angine de poitrine. Avec une introduction de H. Rendu. *Bruxelles, Henri Lamertin, 1893.* xvi, 243 pp. Tables, bibliog. (ftn. refs). 8vo, 23 cms.

An early monograph on angina with a good historical account and bibliography. Crocq was the first author in French to advocate coronary disease and cardiac ischaemia as the sole cause of anginal pain; the others supported the neuralgic theory or a multiple aetiology. The author was professor of medicine at Brussels University.

OSLER (Sir WILLIAM) 1849–1919

627 Lectures on angina pectoris and allied states. *Edinburgh and London, Young J. Pentland, 1897.* viii, 160 pp. Bibliog. (ftn. refs). 8vo, 23 cms.

Also published New York, D. Appleton, 1897. Appleton's catalogue (8 pp.) bound in at end.

Provenance (autograph): A. P. Beddard (Arthur Philip Beddard, 1867–1939, M.D., F.R.C.P.).

These lectures were originally given at Johns Hopkins Hospital, and were republished with additions and corrections. A classic on angina pectoris.

PORTER (WILLIAM TOWNSEND) 1862–1949

628 The Influence of the heart-beat on the flow of blood through the walls of the heart.

Reprinted from *American Journal of Physiology*, 1898, **1**, 145–63. Illus, diagrs, bibliog. (ftn. refs).

An important paper on the physiology of the coronary circulation, postulating the influence of the systolic squeeze emptying the intramural vessels, confirming the theory of Scaramucci (1689).

PRATT (FREDERICK HAVEN) 1873–1958

629 The Nutrition of the heart through the vessels of Thebesius and the coronary veins.

Reprinted from *American Journal of Physiology*, 1898, **1**, 86–103. Illus, diagrs, bibliog. (ftn. refs).
Pratt showed that in the isolated heart the coronary veins and vessels of Thebesius are capable of nourishing the myocardium via the ventricular cavity and coronary sinus.

GIBSON (GEORGE ALEXANDER) 1854–1913

630 The Nervous affections of the heart . . . (Morison Lectures, Edinburgh, 1902, 1903). 2nd ed. *Edinburgh and London, Young J. Pentland, 1905.* [ix], 106 pp. Illus, diagrs, bibliog. (ftn. refs). 8vo, 23 cms.

Autograph: R. D. Brinton (Roland Danvers Brinton, 1858–1946, M.D., M.R.C.P.).
First edition, 1904. Deals with the nervous connections of the heart and angina pectoris.

TESSIER (JEAN P.) *b.* 1876

631 Le Rôle de la distension cardiaque dans la production de l'angine de poitrine. *Paris, J. B. Baillière, 1905.* 92 pp. Illus, bibliog. 4to, 26 cms.

Reprint of M.D. thesis, Paris, 1905, no. 317.
An important contribution to Lauder Brunton's theory of painful distension of the heart by an assistant of Merklen, who also supported this view in relation to angina complicated by pulmonary oedema.

PEISER (LOUIS)

632 Angina pectoris. *Stuttgart, Ferdinand Enke, 1908.* viii, 106 pp. Bibliog. 8vo, 25 cms.

Peiser was physician to the German Hospital in New York.

BLACKHALL-MORISON (ALEXANDER) 1850–1927

633 The Sensory and motor disorders of the heart: their nature and treatment. 2nd ed. Foreword by Sir John Rose Bradford. *London, Baillière, Tindall & Cox, 1928.* x, 362 pp. Illus, diagrs (tracings), tables, bibliog. (ftn. refs and alphabetical index of authorities). 8vo, 23 cms.

Provenance: presented to DEB; "with kind regards Comyns Berkeley (Sir George Harold Arthur Comyns Berkeley, 1865–1946, M.D.), June 1928."
First edition, 1914. Blackhall-Morison made many contributions to anginal pain and this book, published posthumously, summarised his views on angina pectoris which disagree with Allbutt's "opinion that all classical cases of angina pectoris owe their origin to such an extra cardiac cause" (i.e. aortic disease, p. 80). He also gives an early review of the surgical treatment of angina (chapter 7, pp. 175–86). Blackhall-Morison wrote regularly on angina pectoris, heart failure, cardiac pain and neuro-muscular factors in heart disease.

STERNBERG (MAXIMILIAN) 1863–1934

634 Das Chronische partielle Herzaneurysma. Anatomie, Klinik, Diagnose. *Leipzig und Wien, Franz Deuticke, 1914.* [iii], 76 pp. Illus, bibliog. 8vo, 25 cms.

A classic early work on cardiac infarction and aneurysm, giving the clinical picture and introducing the term pericarditis epistenocardica.

ALLBUTT (Sir THOMAS CLIFFORD) 1836–1925

635 Diseases of the arteries, including angina pectoris. *London, Macmillan, 1915.* 2 vols. Bibliog. (ftn. refs). 8vo, 23 cms.

Vol. 1: xiii, 534 pp.; vol. 2: vi, 559 pp.

Allbutt reviews angina pectoris and arteriosclerosis at length, and puts forward his aortic theory of anginal pain; he was a strong opponent of the coronary theory. He also deals with hyperpiesia and arterial disease.

ROLLESTON (Sir HUMPHRY DAVY) 1862–1944

636 The Right Honourable Sir Thomas Clifford Allbutt, K.C.B., . . . : a memoir by Sir H. D. Rolleston. *London, Macmillan, 1929.* vii, 314 pp. Illus, ports, bibliog. (ftn. refs). 8vo, 23 cms.

This copy includes a photograph of Allbutt in academic dress inside the back cover. Provenance: Presentation copy from Lady Allbutt, presumably to Sir D'Arcy Power to whom it originally belonged.

WILSON (CLAUDE) 1860–1937

637 Aneurysm of the heart without symptoms.

Reprinted from *Lancet*, 1919, **2**, 199–200.
An interest in cardiology led Wilson to study under Schott (no. 933) at Nauheim before he entered general practice at Tunbridge Wells with a special interest in cardiology.

VERDON (HENRY WALTER) 1851–1924

638 Angina pectoris. *Brighton, W. T. Moulton, 1920.* xv, 414 pp. Bibliog. (occasional ftn. refs). 8vo, 23 cms.

Errata leaf inserted between pp. vi–vii.
Advocated a gastro-oesophageal origin of anginal pain and is mentioned by Allbutt (no. 635, vol. 2, pp. 344–5). Of historical interest only.

MACKENZIE (Sir JAMES) 1853–1925

639 Angina pectoris. (Oxford Medical Publications). *London, H. Frowde and Hodder & Stoughton, 1923.* xvi, 253 pp. Illus (3 plates), diagrs (tracings). 4to, 26 cms.

A classic on angina pectoris.

640 *The same.* L'Angine de poitrine; traduit de l'anglais par le Dr. E. Guilleaume. *Paris, Felix Alcan, 1925.* xix, 315 pp. Illus, diagrs (tracings). 4to, 26 cms.

GALLAVARDIN (LOUIS BÉNÉDICT) 1875–1957

641 Les Angines de poitrine. *Paris, Masson, 1925.* [v], 181 pp. Illus, tables, bibliog. 8vo, 25 cms.

Autographed presentation copy from the author, Mar. 1926.
This book is by far the best contemporary work on the subject, based on 791 personal cases, with 20 necropsies. Gallavardin, physician to the Hôtel Dieu Hôpital at Lyon, and one of the leading cardiologists in Europe, became Médecin des hôpitaux in 1902 at the age of 26. From the start he

decided to specialise and became the first provincial cardiologist in France. He had an x-ray installed in his consulting room before the 1914 war, and was the first in France to instal an electrocardiograph (a Cambridge instrument) in his hospital service in 1910.

Not being a professor, he was obliged to retire from hospital at the age of 53, but he continued to practise and to publish important papers, a notable one in 1934 on mitral stenosis with pulmonary oedema.

642 Publications médicales (1898–1945) du Docteur Louis Gallavardin. *Lyon, Société Anonyme de l'imprimerie A. Rey, 1945.* 40 pp. 8vo, 24 cms.

Bibliography of 360 references of many of Gallavardin's important papers on cardiology, especially on angina pectoris.

ANREP (Gleb Vassilievitch von) 1891–1955

643 The Regulation of the coronary circulation.

Reprinted from *Physiological Reviews*, 1926, **6**, 596–629. Tables, bibliog. (132 refs).

Anrep was born in St. Petersburg, the son of the director of the Institute of Experimental Medicine. He studied under Pavlov there and graduated M.D., 1915. After the 1917 Revolution he worked under Starling at University College, London. He was an accomplished lecturer and skilful operator of heart-lung preparations. In 1925 he became lecturer at Cambridge and a Fellow of the Royal Society in 1928. In 1939 he was made professor of physiology at Cairo, where DEB met him in 1943. His chief work was in coronary circulation but the bibliography accompanying his obituary in *Biographical memoirs of Fellows of the Royal Society*, 1956, **2**, 19–34 (with portrait) shows a wide range of interests.

644 Lane medical lectures: studies in cardiovascular regulation. *Stanford University, California, Stanford University Press; London, Humphrey Milford, Oxford University Press, 1936.* 118 pp. Illus, diagrs, tables, bibliog. (ftn. refs). 4to, 26 cms.

Reprinted from *Stanford University Publications, University Series: Medical Sciences*, 1936, vol. 3, pp. 197–312. Five lectures: 1: The proprioceptive mechanism of cardiovascular regulation; 2: The respiratory regulation of the heart rate; 3: The dynamics of coronary circulation; 4: The coronary blood flow; 5: The blood flow through skeletal and plain muscles.

Book-stamp: Cambridge University Library.

ANREP (Gleb Vassilievitch von) 1891–1955 and SEGALL (Harold Nathan) *b.* 1897

645 The Regulation of the coronary circulation.

Reprinted from *Heart*, 1926, **13**, 239–60. Illus, tables, diagrs (tracings), bibliog. (35 refs).

LECLERCQ (Arthur) 1856–?

646 Les Angines de poitrine et leur traitement (Les Maladies de la Cinquantaine, tom. 6). *Paris, Octave Doin, 1926.* 192 pp. Illus, diagr. 8vo, 23 cms.

DANIÉLOPOLU (Daniel) 1884–1955

647 L'Angine de poitrine et l'angine abdominale. *Paris, Masson, [1927].* viii, 443 pp. Illus, diagrs (tracings, orthodiagrams), tables, bibliog. 4to, 27 cms.

Daniélopolu was professor of medicine at Bucharest and an authority on the nervous connections of the heart. He disagreed with Jonnesco's sympathectomy for angina (1916), and advocated section of the centrifugal sensory fibres and depressor nerve. He regarded anginal pain as due to an accumulation of fatigue toxins in an ischaemic myocardium. His book is profusely illustrated by figures of the anatomy of the cardiac nerves, and has a full alphabetical bibliography (pp. 391–435).

LEVINE (SAMUEL ALBERT) 1891–1966

648 Coronary thrombosis: its various clinical features. (Medicine Monographs, vol. 16). *London, Baillière, Tindall & Cox, 1929.* [iv], 178 pp. Illus (coloured plate, frontispiece), diagrs (tracings), bibliog. 4to, 26 cms.

Also published in Baltimore, Williams and Wilkins, 1929. Acquired 1930.

Levine was born in Poland and educated at Harvard Medical School, served in the 1914 war, and became physician to the Peter Bent Brigham Hospital. He was a renowned teacher and his monograph on coronary thrombosis was probably the first book published on the subject.

PEZZI (CESARE) 1874–1945

649 L'Infarto miocardico: studio clinico e elettrocardiografico. *Roma, Amministrazione del giornale "il Policlinico", 1929.* 44 pp. Illus, diagrs (tracings), bibliog. (50 refs). 8vo, 24 cms.

Reprinted from *Cuore e Circolazione*, 1929, **13**, 141–82.

Author's signed copy. An early paper on electrocardiographic changes in myocardial infarction.

LIAN (CAMILLE CONSTANT) 1882–1969

650 L'Angor aigu coronarien fébrile.

Reprinted from *Questions cliniques d'actualité:* leçons professées à la Charité service du Professeur Sergent. Paris, Masson, 1930, tom. 2, pp. 120–47. Diagrs, bibliog. (ftn. refs).

Lian was professor of medicine and physician to the Pitié Hospital. He was one of the leading teachers of cardiology in Paris, published many important papers and was one of the first in France to recognise the clinical features of coronary thrombosis.

651 L'Angine de poitrine; formes cliniques, traitement médical et chirurgical; avec la collaboration de MM. A. Blondel [and others]. *Paris, Masson, 1932.* 429 pp. Tables, diagrs (tracings), bibliog. 8vo, 25 cms.

Author's signed presentation copy to DEB.

BEDFORD (DAVIS EVAN) *b.* 1898

652 Camille Lian 1882–1969. *London, British Medical Association, 1969.* [2 pp.]. Port., bibliog. 8vo, 25 cms.

Reprinted from *British Heart Journal*, 1969, **31**, 789–90; with a signed letter from Lenègre to DEB thanking him for a copy.

[*and*] LENÈGRE (JEAN) 1904–1972

Camille Lian (1882–1969). [*Paris, Masson, 1970*]. 7 pp. Port., bibliog. 8vo, 24 cms.

Reprinted from *Bulletin de l'Académie nationale de Médecine*, 1970, **154**, 102–8.

PADILLA (TIBURCIO) and COSSIO (PEDRO) *b.* 1900

653 Occlusión coronaria, brusca y lenta. *Buenos Aires, "La Semana Médica," [1930].* 268 pp. Illus, diagrs (tracings), bibliog. 8vo, 23 cms.

Signed presentation copy to [Sir] John Parkinson and DEB from the authors, 1931.

An early account of coronary occlusion with a good bibliography (318 references).

CONDORELLI (Luigi) *b.* 1899

654 Die Ernährung des Herzens und die Folgen ihrer Störung. (Ergebnisse der Kreislaufforschung; herausgegeben von . . . Bruno Kisch, Band 3). *Dresden und Leipzig, Theodor Steinkopff, 1932.* xii, 230 pp. Illus, diagrs (tracings), bibliog. (at end of each part). 8vo, 24 cms.

An important early monograph on the coronary circulation and coronary thrombosis. Condorelli was at this time professor at Naples, and later in Rome.

655 Fisiopatologia clinica della stenocardia, con la collaborazione di A. Strano [and others]. *Roma, L. Pozzi, 1965.* viii, 463 pp. Illus, diagrs, tables, bibliog. (ftn. refs). 4to, 26 cms.

Presentation copy to DEB from the author.
Relazione al LXVI Congresso della Società Italiana di Medicina Interna, Catania, 17–20 Ottobre 1965. A comprehensive account of Condorelli's views on coronary physiology, angina of effort, decubitus, and on aortic disease, mitral disease, etc.; bibliography, pp. 449–63.

DELROUS (Yvon)

656 L'Infarctus du myocarde: étude clinique et électrocardiographique. Préface de . . . Prof. [V] Cordier. *Paris, G. Doin, 1932.* 271 pp. Bibliog. 4to, 26 cms.

An early monograph on cardiac infarction from the Lyon school, with a useful classified bibliography of continental papers (pp. 249–70).

HOCHREIN (Max) *b.* 1897

657 Der Coronarkreislauf: Physiologie, Pathologie, Therapie. *Berlin, Julius Springer, 1932.* vii, 227 pp. Illus, diagrs (tracings), bibliog. 4to, 26 cms.

658 Der Myokardinfarkt: Enkennung, Behandlung und Verhütung. (Kreislauf-Bücherei, Band 1). *Dresden und Leipzig, Theodor Steinkopff, 1937.* viii, 196 pp. Illus, diagrs (tracings), bibliog. 8vo, 24 cms.

An important early treatise on cardiac infarction including the electrocardiographic changes.

COELHO (Eduardo) *b.* 1896

659 L'Infarctus du myocarde: étude expérimentale, électrocardiographique et clinique. *Paris, Masson, 1934.* 212 pp. Illus, diagrs (tracings), bibliog. 8vo, 25 cms.

Publisher's catalogue for April 1934 (48 pp.) bound in at end.
Coelho was professor at Lisbon and an early worker on the electrocardiogram in cardiac infarction.

LEVY (Robert Louis) 1888–1974

660 Diseases of the coronary arteries and cardiac pain; ed. by Robert L. Levy. *New York, Macmillan, 1936.* x, 445 pp. Illus, tables, diagrs, bibliog. 8vo, 25 cms.

Contains introduction by Alfred E. Cohn, a historical note by James B. Herrick and five parts. Part 1 on coronary circulation includes sections on anatomy by Joseph T. Wearn, physiology by Carl J. Wiggers, pharmacology by Fred M. Smith, and pathology by William C. von Glahn. Part 2 on cardiac pain is by James C. White and Carl J. Wiggers. Clinical features of diseases of the coronary arteries and cardiac pain (Part 3) are covered by Louis I. Dublin, Robert L. Levy, William J. Kerr, Paul D. White and Frank N. Wilson, their medical treatment (Part 4) by Levy and their surgical treatment (Part 5) by James C. White, Herrman L. Blumgart and Claude S. Beck. (2 copies).

BÉRARD (MARCEL) *b.* 1908

661 Les Méthodes chirurgicales du traitement de l'angine de poitrine; évolution et résultats. Préface par le Professeur René Leriche. *Lyon, Imprimerie A. Rey, 1937.* xvi, 397 pp. Bibliog. 8vo, 25 cms.

Author's presentation copy to DEB.

Bérard, the nephew of Louis Gallavardin and son of a well-known surgeon in Lyon, worked with J. C. White, Cutler and Beck in U.S.A. and with Santy in Lyon. A useful reference work; bibliography, pp. 369–92.

HALLERMANN (WILHELM) *b.* 1909

662 Der plötzliche Herztod bei Kranzgefässerkrankungen. *Stuttgart, Ferdinand Enke, 1939.* vii, 215 pp. Illus, tables, bibliog. 8vo, 25 cms.

Analysis of 783 cases of sudden death from coronary disease. Extensive bibliography (pp. 202–13).

LAUBRY (PIERRE) *b.* 1907

663 Les Coronaires et le problème de la douleur cardiaque. Préface du Professeur Ch. Laubry. *Paris, G. Doin, 1939.* viii, 232 pp. Illus, diagrs, bibliog. 8vo, 24 cms.

Reviews all the theories of anginal pain, coronary, aortic, distension of heart, etc.

LAUBRY (CHARLES) 1872–1960 and
SOULIE (PIERRE LOUIS JEAN) 1903–1970

664 Les Maladies des coronaires: l'infarctus du myocarde, l'insuffisance coronarienne. *Paris, Masson, 1943.* [iv], 432 pp. Illus, tables, diagrs (incl. tracings), bibliog. 8vo, 25 cms.

Tipped in, an autograph letter to DEB from Laubry in reply to greetings on his 80th birthday.

665 *The same.* 2ᵉ éd. *Paris, Masson, 1950.* [iv], 618 pp. Illus, tables, diagrs (incl. tracings), bibliog. 8vo, 24 cms.

Presentation copy signed by authors.

A comprehensive account of the coronary circulation and coronary disease including anatomy, physiology, pathology, clinical and electrocardiographic features. Extensive alphabetically arranged bibliography (pp. 557–604).

CASSIDY (Sir MAURICE ALAN) 1880–1949

666 Coronary disease. (Harveian Oration, 1946). [*London, Lancet, 1946*]. 16 pp. Bibliog. 8vo, 22 cms.

Reprinted from *Lancet*, 1946, **2**, 587–90.

Cassidy gives his personal experience of 1000 cases of angina pectoris—prevalence, diagnosis, aetiology and prognosis.

LOPEZ BRENES (JUAN)

667 Infarto del miocardio. (Congreso nacional de cardiologia, Barcelona, diciembre 1947, 2.). *Barcelona, Editorial "Miguel Servet", [1948?].* [vi], 323 pp. Illus, diagrs (tracings), tables, bibliog. 8vo, 25 cms.

The author gives a comprehensive review to date with an extensive bibliography (pp. 313–23).

GREGG (DONALD EATON) *b.* 1902

668 The Coronary circulation in health and disease. *London, Henry Kimpton, 1950.* 227 pp. Illus, tables, diagrs, bibliog. 8vo, 24 cms.

American edition, Philadelphia, Lea and Febiger, 1950. Acquired 1951.
Important work on the physiology of the coronary circulation.

GERTLER (MENARD MAX) *b.* 1919 and
WHITE (PAUL DUDLEY) 1886–1973

669 Coronary heart disease in young adults: a multi-disciplinary study [with others]. *Cambridge, Mass., Harvard University Press for the Commonwealth Fund, 1954.* xix, 218 pp. Illus, tables, diagrs, bibliog. 8vo, 24 cms.

A research study, conducted at Massachusetts General Hospital and Harvard Medical School, suggesting the possibility of preventive medicine in coronary heart disease. "By taking into consideration sex, body build, morphological characteristics, heredity, serum total cholesterol, serum uric acid, serum total cholesterol/serum lipid phosphorus ratio, CUP index and salivary redox potential, it should theoretically be possible to preselect coronary-prone individuals from the population" (p. 160).

FROMENT (ROGER) *b.* 1907 and GONIN (ANDRÉ)

670 Les Angors coronariens intriqués: étude clinique et expérimentale des inter-réactions neuro et viscéro-coronariennes avec la collaboration des Drs. P. Bruel et R. Mornex. [*Paris*], *Expansion Scientifique Française*, [*1956*]. 175 pp. Illus (x-rays), diagrs (tracings), bibliog. 4to, 28 cms.

Presentation copy to DEB signed by authors, Sept. 1956.
Introduction and individual chapters summarised in English and Spanish. A useful account of anginal pain conditioned by hiatus hernia, peptic ulcer, spondylitis, etc.

MORGAN (ALAN DOUGLAS) *b.* 1910

671 The Pathogenesis of coronary occlusion; with a foreword by John B. Duguid. *Oxford, Blackwell Scientific Publications, 1956.* [vii], 171 pp. Illus, tables, bibliog. 4to, 26 cms.

Based on the author's thesis, University of Aberdeen.
Morgan, professor of pathology at Westminster Hospital, supported the view of John Bright Duguid (*b.* 1895), an authority on arterial diseases and experimental nephritis, on the thrombotic origin of coronary atherosclerotic occlusion.

PRINZMETAL (MYRON) *b.* 1908, and others

672 Coronary artery disease: a simplified summary, by Myron Prinzmetal, Rexford Kennamer, Takashi Wada, Naci Bor. *Institute of Medical Research, Cedars of Lebanon Hospital; University of California Medical School, Duarte, Calif.; City of Hope Medical Center*, [*1959?*]. 67 pp. Illus, port., diagrs (tracings), bibliog. 8vo, 25 cms.

Prinzmetal describes angina pectoris inversa, classic angina, myocardial infarction, accelerated conduction and their electrocardiographic patterns.

ORAM (SAMUEL) *b.* 1913 and SOWTON (GEORGE EDGAR) *b.* 1930

673 Tobacco angina.

Reprinted from *Quarterly Journal of Medicine*, 1963, **32**, 115–43. Tables, diagrs (4 plates of tracings), bibliog.
Provenance: Signed presentation copy from Oram.
Important review with full bibliography.

ROBB-SMITH (ALASTAIR HAMISH TEARLOCH) *b.* 1908

674 The Enigma of coronary heart disease. *London, Lloyd-Luke, 1967.* ix, 150 pp. Tables, diagrs, bibliog. 8vo, 22 cms.

An important pathological, statistical analysis concluding against any increase in coronary disease, 1920–1960.

History and Bibliography

ROLLESTON (Sir HUMPHREY DAVY) 1862–1944

675 The History of angina pectoris. Finlayson Memorial Lecture, 1937. [*Glasgow, Glasgow Medical Journal, 1937*]. [i], 21 pp. Port., facsim., bibliog. 8vo, 25 cms.

Reprinted from *Glasgow medical Journal*, 1937, **127**, 205–25.
Provenance: presentation copy from author ("H.R.").
The best historical account of angina pectoris; text and bibliography cover nomenclature, cases before Heberden's description, forms of angina, the coronary hypothesis and intermittent claudication, diseases of the aorta and other causes of angina pectoris, a doctor's disease, treatment, coronary thrombosis.

ROYAL COLLEGE OF PHYSICIANS OF LONDON. Library

676 Dolor pectoris: an exhibition illustrating the history of angina pectoris. [*London, Royal College of Physicians, 1968*]. pp. 339–58. 4to, 26 cms.

Introduction, 42 items with commentaries. The cover includes overlapping portraits of Jenner, Heberden and Parry on a background of a plate (Tab. vii, fig. 1) from Scarpa's *Tabulae neurologicae* (Pavia, 1794) (RCP).

677 LEIBOWITZ (JOSHUA O.)

The History of coronary heart disease. (Publications of the Wellcome Institute of the History of Medicine, new series, vol. 18). *London, Wellcome Institute of the History of Medicine, 1970.* xvii, 227 pp. Illus, port., bibliog. 4to, 26 cms.

A very comprehensive historical account of arterial disease and coronary heart disease from antiquity to the present time. Bibliography, pp. 186–214.

RHEUMATIC HEART DISEASE

David Pitcairn recognised heart disease due to rheumatism in 1788 and Baillie mentioned this in his *Morbid anatomy*. Jenner read a paper at the Fleece Medical Society in 1789 on heart disease following acute rheumatism but the manuscript was lost. Dundas (1808) described nine cases, but the first full account was published by Wells (1812), and next come Hawkins's Lectures (1826). A very important and overlooked account was given by Joseph Brown (1828) who described the signs of aortic and mitral disease and of pericarditis, and estimated that half of all cases of heart disease were rheumatic. Prior to Laennec, early accounts related mainly to pericarditis, but Bouillaud (1836), who first described endocarditis, employing the stethoscope, finally established the full importance of rheumatic heart disease (Maladie de Bouillaud).

The researches of Poynton and Paine on the rheumatic diplococcus (1903), raised the question of aetiology of rheumatic fever, and their book (1913) reprints most of Poynton's important papers on acute rheumatism and chorea, their treatment and prevention. Carey Coombs's monograph (1924) is really the first systematic study of rheumatic heart disease and was based on his work at Bristol and a follow-up of over 600 cases. Lastly, Parkinson's Harveian Oration (1945) reviews the subject up to date, and includes an important bibliography. He states that the stethoscope was rarely used in children even in Paris before 1839.

WELLS (William Charles) 1757–1817

678 On rheumatism of the heart.

Pp. 373–424, in *Transactions of a Society for the improvement of medical and chirurgical Knowledge*. London, G. & W. Nichol, 1812, vol. 3 (viii, 567, [15] pp.). 8vo, 22 cms.

Appears from pagination to lack half-title page. Final unnumbered pages index. Provenance: Ionian Military Medical Library; book-stamp: Aldershot Military Medical Book Club.

This paper is the first important published account of rheumatic heart disease. Wells was born in America but trained in Edinburgh and practised in London. He was friendly with Pitcairn and Baillie. He also wrote a notable article on dew and this volume includes his papers: "A Case of aneurysm of the aorta, attended by ulceration of the oesophagus and windpipe" (pp. 81–4), and "A Case of aneurysm of the aorta communicating with the pulmonary artery" (pp. 85–90); James Wilson's "An instance of obliteration of the vena cava inferior from inflammation" (pp. 65–80), and John Storer's "An Instance of the entire want of pulsation in the arteries of paralytic limbs" (pp. 448–70).

A bibliography of Wells is appended to an article about him by Frank Lester Pleadwell in *Annals of medical History*, 1934, new series, **6**, 128–42.

HAWKINS (Francis Bisset) 1794–1877

679 Rheumatism, and some diseases of the heart and other internal organs . . . (Goulstonian Lectures, 1826.). *London, Burgess and Hill, 1826.* xiii, 144 pp. Bibliog. (occasional ftn. refs). 8vo, 21 cms.

Book-stamp: Norwich and Norfolk United Medical Book Society.

Hawkins was physician to the Middlesex Hospital and his third lecture deals with rheumatic heart disease, almost all cases having pericarditis with dilatation or hypertrophy. Endocarditis is not mentioned. These were the first lectures to be given in the Royal College of Physicians in Pall Mall East.

BROWN (Joseph) 1784–1868

680 Medical essays on fever, inflammation, rheumatism, diseases of the heart, etc. *London, Longman, Rees, Orme, Brown and Green, 1828.* viii, 309 pp. 8vo, 22 cms.

Half-title (pp. i–ii) ? wanting. Book-stamp and autograph: Hunterian Society, Edinburgh.

Brown was in the Army Medical Service and on Wellington's staff in Spain; his book is dedicated to Sir James McGrigor. His essays on rheumatism and heart disease describe pericarditis, cardiac hypertrophy, and valvular disease complicating rheumatism, and deal with the physical signs of mitral and aortic disease, noting the small pulse of aortic stenosis and attributing the thrill of mitral stenosis to left auricular contraction. Brown's book which has been generally ignored in the literature of rheumatic heart disease, contains important original observations prior to those of Bouillaud and Hope.

BOUILLAUD (JEAN BAPTISTE) 1796–1881

681 Nouvelles recherches sur le rhumatisme articulaire aigu en général et spécialement sur la loi de coincidence de la péricardite et de l'endocardite avec cette maladie, ainsi que sur l'efficacitée de la formule des émissions sanguines coup sur coup dans son traitement. *Paris, J. B. Baillière, 1836.* [i], viii, 162 pp. Table, bibliog. (occasional ftn. refs). 8vo, 21 cms.

Book-stamp: Medical & Chirurgical Society; bookplate: Society of Apothecaries.

A fine copy of Bouillaud's most important contribution to cardiology, published a year after his treatise on heart disease (see no. 375). An English translation by James Kitchen was published in Philadelphia, Haswell, Barrington & Haswell, 1837.

LEES (DAVID BRIDGE) 1846–1915

682 The Treatment of some acute visceral inflammations and other papers. *London, John Murray, 1904.* viii, 300 pp. Illus, diagrs. 8vo, 19 cms.

Contents of cardiological interest are: Carditis and pericarditis, pp. 5–37; Case of malformation of the heart with transposition of the aorta and pulmonary artery. (*Transactions of the Pathological Society of London*, 1879–1880, **31**, 58–62), pp. 101–9; Presystolic apex-murmur due to aortic regurgitation. (*American Journal of the medical Sciences*, Philadelphia, 1890, new ser., **100**, 460–7), pp. 132–47; A Clinical lecture at St. Mary's Hospital on a case of chorea and pericarditis; a case of general paralysis of the insane; a case of mitral disease with spasmodic dyspnoea; a case of cardiac dilatation. (*Clinical Journal*, 1893, **1**, no. 19,), pp. 165–80; Is there a dextrocardiac-respiratory reflex? (*Lancet*, 1893, **2**, 1050–52), pp. 181–91; Acute dilatation of the heart in rheumatic fever. (*Medico-chirurgical Transactions*, London, 1898, **81**, 401–17), pp. 192–214; Rheumatic heart-disease in children: the introduction to a discussion in the section of diseases of children at the Edinburgh meeting of the British Medical Association. (*British medical Journal*, 1898, **2**, 1129–32), pp. 215–30; An address on acute dilatation of the heart in diphtheria, influenza, and rheumatic fever, delivered before the Manchester Medical Society. (*British medical Journal*, 1901, **1**, 7–10), pp. 231–51; A Presidential address on the heart of the child delivered before the Harveian Society. (*Lancet*, 1902, **1**, 279–82), pp. 252–74.

Lees, physician to St. Mary's and Great Ormond Street Hospitals, was an authority on rheumatic heart disease, advocating large doses of salicylate with sodium bicarbonate.

POYNTON (FREDERICK JOHN) 1869–1943 and PAINE (ALEXANDER) 1866–1933

683 Researches on rheumatism. *London, J. & A. Churchill, 1913.* xi, 461 pp. Illus (plates), diagrs, bibliog. 8vo, 24 cms.

Publishers' catalogue, March 1913 (16 pp.), bound in at end.

The book is divided into three parts, the first two containing papers before and after the isolation of the diplococcus rheumaticus respectively, the last results of the previous researches. It includes the authors' papers with D. B. Lees, G. F. Still, W. Vernon Shaw and Gordon F. Holmes. The contents of each part and the sub-groups of part 2 are described in detail, and original references given. Both Poynton and Paine were pupils of D. B. Lees (no. 682), to whom the book is dedicated.

This book not only describes their work on the diplococcus rheumaticus, but includes all Poynton's important papers on rheumatic heart disease and his paper with Gordon Holmes on the pathology of chorea. Poynton was a great pioneer in rheumatic heart disease and inspired many others to work on the subject.

COOMBS (Carey Franklin) 1879–1932

684 Rheumatic heart disease; with an introduction by F. J. Poynton. *Bristol, John Wright, 1924.* xxiii, 376 pp. Illus (20 plates), tables, diagrs, bibliog. 12mo, 19 cms.

Publisher's catalogue (4 pp.) bound in at end.

Carey Coombs had been house physician to D. B. Lees (author of no. 682) at St. Mary's Hospital and this together with his friendship with Poynton started his interest in acute rheumatism and he embarked on a long-term research on the subject at Bristol where he was physician to the Children's Hospital and pathologist to the General Hospital. He organised a follow-up investigation of over 600 cases on which is based his account of the course and prognosis. He was an early advocate of special convalescent centres for rheumatic children. His monograph was the first systematic text-book on rheumatic heart disease.

685 ... On the aetiology of cardiac disease. (Long Fox Memorial Lecture, 1925). *Bristol, [J. W. Arrowsmith, 1926?].* 19 pp. Illus, diagr., tables, bibliog. 8vo, 24 cms.

Also printed (by the same publishers) in the *Bristol medico-chirurgical Journal*, 1926, **43**, 1–19, from which this is possibly a reprint.

Although Aschoff first gave an account of the submiliary nodule, it was the Bristol school who first realised its aetiological importance as a constant feature of active cardiac rheumatism.

WILKINSON (Kenneth Douglas) 1886–1951

686 On rheumatism and its results. (Ingleby Lectures, 1935). *[London, Lancet, 1935].* 20 pp. 8vo, 22 cms.

Reprinted from *Lancet*, 1935, **2**, 411–17. Autograph (initials) presentation copy.

A historical review including a section on the recognition of rheumatism as a cause of heart disease.

SCHLESINGER (Bernard Edward) *b.* 1896

687 On the public health aspect of heart disease in childhood. (Milroy Lectures, 1938). *[London, Lancet, 1938].* 40 pp. Tables, diagrs, bibliog. 8vo, 22 cms.

Reprinted from *Lancet*, 1938, **1**, 593–9, 649–54.

An important review of juvenile rheumatism based on experience at the Children's Heart Hospital, West Wickham, which gives a follow-up of 1000 cases, with a discussion of diagnosis and treatment and after care of these children.

LICHTWITZ (Leopold) 1876–1943

688 Pathology and therapy of rheumatic fever; ed. by William Chester. Foreword by William J. Maloney. *London, William Heinemann (Medical Books), 1944.* xvii, 211 pp. Illus, tables, bibliog. 8vo, 24 cms.

Also published New York, Grune and Stratton, 1944 (both printed in U.S.A.).

Rheumatic heart disease, pp. 38–50; Rheumatic vascular disease, pp. 51–60.

Acquired Alexandria 1945. Lichtwitz postulated the allergic aetiology of rheumatic fever and chorea. The lengthy foreword by Maloney (William Joseph Marie Alois Maloney, 1882–1952) is of interest as he had worked at Great Ormond Street under Poynton and Still, in Paris under Charcot and later in Germany.

PARKINSON (Sir JOHN) 1885–1976

689 Rheumatic fever and heart disease. (Harveian Oration, 1945). [*London, Lancet, 1945*]. 32 pp. Bibliog. 8vo, 22 cms.

Reprinted from *Lancet*, 1945, **2,** 657–63.

Reviews the history of rheumatic heart disease to date, the clinical features and treatment, with an important bibliography (107 references).

PERICARDITIS

ROTCH (THOMAS MORGAN) 1849–1914

690 Absence of resonance in the fifth intercostal space, diagnostic of pericardial effusion . . . reprinted from the Transactions of the Massachusetts Medical Society. *Boston, David Clapp, 1878.* 21 pp. Diagrs. 8vo, 21 cms.

The original account of Rotch's sign of pericardial effusion appeared in the *Boston medical and surgical Journal*, 1878, **99,** 421–9, a journal in which the transactions of the Massachusetts Medical Society seem often to have appeared, and from which this paper may have been reprinted. It was later published in the Society's own *Medical Communications*, 1875–1881, vol. 12 (Boston, 1881).

HARRIS (THOMAS) 1859–1905

691 Indurative mediastino-pericarditis. *London, Smith, Elder, 1895.* 67 pp. Illus, tables, diagrs, bibliog. 8vo, 24 cms.

Reprinted from *Medical Chronicle* (Manchester) 1894–1895, new ser., **2,** 1–12, 87–111, 178–92, 205–62.

"With the author's kind regards."

This rare early work on chronic pericarditis published the year before Pick's paper (1896) describes three cases with necropsy, two being typical Pick's disease, probably tubercular. Harris was physician to the Manchester Royal Infirmary.

BROADBENT (Sir JOHN FRANCIS HARPIN) 1865–1946

692 Adherent pericardium. *London, Baillière, Tindall & Cox, 1895.* 126 pp. 12mo, 19 cms.

Autographs: W. L. Dickinson (William Lee Dickinson, 1863–1904, M.D., F.R.C.P.); bookplate: Terence East (Charles Frederick Terence East, 1894–1967, D.M., F.R.C.P.).

An American edition was published in New York, W. Wood, 1896. A good historical review; Broadbent notes that the heart is not enlarged when constricted by very dense thick pericardium. Broadbent's sign was described by his brother, Walter Broadbent (*Lancet*, 1895, **2,** 200–1).

PICK (FRIEDEL) 1867–1926

693 Uber pericarditische Pseudolebercirrhose chronische, unter dem Bilde der Lebercirrhose verlaufende Pericarditis nebst Bemerkungen über die Zuckergussleber. *Berlin, gedruckt bei L. Schumacher, 1896.* 26 pp. Bibliog. 8vo, 25 cms.

Reprinted from *Zeitschrift für klinische Medicin* (Berlin), 1896, **29,** 385–410.

Pick's original paper on constrictive pericarditis, since known as Pick's disease.

SINNHUBER (FRANZ) 1869–?

694 Die Erkrankungen des Herzbeutels und ihre Behandlung. *Berlin, August Hirschwald, 1911.* vi, 114 pp. Tables, diagrs (tracings), bibliog. 4to, 26 cms.

The early pages wanting up to p. 32 supplied by photostat copies; good bibliography.

BLECHMANN (GERMAIN) 1883–?

695 Les Péricardites aiguës; avant-propos de M. le Professeur Marfan. (Bibliothèque des Connaissances Médicales.) *Paris, Ernest Flammarion, 1922.* 282, [2] pp. Illus, diagrs, bibliog. (occasional ftn. refs). 12mo, 19 cms.

A delightful account of pericarditis with historical account of the various signs, well illustrated, and deals with paracentesis. Blechmann described the "pillow sign" of pericardial effusion. He was interne to Marfan (Antoine Bernard Jean Marfan, 1858–1942, author of no. 698).

BECK (CLAUDE SCHAEFER) *b.* 1894 and GRISWOLD (RETTIG ARNOLD) *b.* 1898

696 Pericardiectomy in the treatment of the Pick syndrome. *Chicago, American Medical Association, 1930.* 48 pp. Illus, diagr., bibliog. (ftn. refs). 4to, 26 cms.

Reprinted from *Archives of Surgery*, 1930, **21**, 1064–1111.

WHITE (PAUL DUDLEY) 1886–1973

697 Chronic constrictive pericarditis (Pick's disease) treated by pericardial resection. (St. Cyres Lecture, 1935.) [*London, Lancet, 1935.*] 48 pp. Illus, bibliog. 8vo, 22 cms.

Reprinted from *Lancet*, 1935, **2**, 539–48, 597–603.
A full historical account of Pick's disease and its surgical treatment, which drew general attention to the diagnosis in England where it was first described by Lower (nos. 213 and 214), Chevers and Wilks (see bibliography, pp. 47–8).

MARFAN (ANTOINE BERNARD JEAN) 1858–1942

698 La Ponction du péricarde, en particulier par voie épigastrique sous-xiphoidienne. *Paris, Masson, 1938.* 75 pp. Illus, bibliog. (ftn. refs). 8vo, 20 cms.

Publisher's catalogue, additional preliminary [6] pp. and final 48 pp. (février 1938).
Marfan introduced the epigastric route for paracentesis in 1911, and it was performed by him and his interne, Blechmann, and this small monograph gives the history of paracentesis and incision as used prior to 1870 when aspiration was introduced by Dieulafoy.

COELHO (EDUARDO) *b.* 1896, and others

699 Estudo da pericardite experimental, por Eduardo Coelho, Artur de Oliveira, Leonel Cabral e Manuel Prates. *Lisboa, [Composio e impresso na Imp. Africana], 1946.* 77 pp. Illus, tables (folding), diagrs (tracings), bibliog. 8vo, 23 cms.

Signed presentation copy to DEB from Leonel Cabral, London, April 1947.
Deals with the electrocardiogram in pericarditis in man and animals.

CONDORELLI (LUIGI) *b.* 1899, and others

700 Fisiopatologia e diagnostica delle pericarditi adesive, con la collaborazione dei dri. A. Turchetti, G. Schirosa, A. Strano, M. Sangiorgi, F. Testoni, G. Filocamo, A. Tedeschi [e Vincenzo Masini]. *Milano, Arrigo Recordati, 1953.* 273 pp. Illus, diagrs, tables, bibliog. 8vo, 25 cms.

Addenda written by collaborators, pp. 125–273; signed presentation copy from Condorelli.

BEDFORD (DAVIS EVAN) *b.* 1898

701 Chronic effusive pericarditis.

Reprinted from *British Heart Journal*, 1964, **26**, 499–572. Illus (radiographs), bibliog.

SPODICK (DAVID HOWARD) *b.* 1927

702 Chronic and constrictive pericarditis. *New York and London, Grune & Stratton, 1964.* xiv, 369 pp. Illus, tables, diagrs, bibliog. 8vo, 23 cms.

A complete review of chronic constrictive pericarditis including history, clinical picture, electrocardiogram, phonocardiogram and treatment, with bibliography of 943 references (pp. 331–60).

ARTERIAL DISEASE, ANEURYSM, HYPERTENSION AND BRIGHT'S DISEASE

Richard Bright, physician to Guy's Hospital published his *Reports of medical cases* (vol. 1) in 1827, describing cases of dropsy, albuminuria and renal disease, illustrating the state of the kidneys by coloured plates. Clifford Allbutt separated hyperpiesia or essential hypertension from Bright's disease; in addition he recognised atheroma and wrote on syphilitic cerebral arterial disease. A raised arterial pressure was suspected before the sphygmomanometer came into use (Von Basch, no. 428). Gallavardin's *Tension arterielle en clinique* (no. 738) gives a good historical account of hypertension, Erichsen deals with the early history of aneurysm (no. 715) and Joseph Hodgson's (no. 706) is a pioneer work on arterial disease.

SCARPA (ANTONIO) 1747–1832

703 Réflexions et observations anatomico-chirurgicales sur l'anéurysme; traduites de l'italien par J. Delpech. *Paris, Migneret, imprimeur, 1809.* vi, 470 pp. Bibliog. (ftn. refs). 8vo, 21 cms.

A French edition of Scarpa's classical work *Sull'aneurisma; riflessioni ed osservazioni anatomico-chirurgiche.* (Pavia, tipog. Bolzani, 1804). A copy in the Library of the Royal College of Physicians of London has the publisher as Mequignon-Mariis and is accompanied by an atlas (1813, folio).

FREER (GEORGE) 1769–1823

704 Observations on aneurism, and some diseases of the arterial system. *Birmingham, [printed by] Knott & Lloyd, 1807.* [viii], 116 pp. Illus (plates), bibliog. (ftn. refs). Folio, 32 cms.

The plates for the book were drawn by Freer's pupil, Joseph Hodgson. There are five numbered plates, four of which are coloured; this agrees with the description of the copy in the *Index-Catalogue of the Library of the Surgeon-General's Office* [1st series], 1884, vol. 5, p. 185. There are in addition four unnumbered, uncoloured plates which are in fact identical to the first four plates, but without captions, numbering of figures and names of artist and engraver; these are probably from an earlier impression of the same plates, before references to numbered plates were inserted in the text. (The author admits the rushed production in his preface.)

Autograph: "Mr. Soden from the Author" (John Smith Soden, 1780–1863, a pupil with Joseph Hodgson of Freer himself).

A rare book dealing mainly with peripheral arterial aneurysm and circoid aneurysm. Freer was surgeon to the General Hospital, Birmingham, from 1793. He inspired his pupils with higher aims than routine practice, for two of them won the Jacksonian Prize Essay in successive years: Soden with "The Bite of a rabid animal" in 1810 and Hodgson with "Wounds and diseases of the arteries and veins" in 1811. Soden became an expert eye surgeon and Hodgson expanded his essay into a full treatise (nos. 706–09).

705 BURNS (ALLAN) 1781–1813

Observations on the surgical anatomy of the head and neck. 2nd ed., with a life of the author, and additional cases and observations by Granville Sharp Pattison. *Glasgow, Wardlow & Cunninghame, 1824.* [i], xxix, 30–511 pp. Illus (10 plates). 8vo, 22 cms.

Acquired 1944. First edition, Edinburgh, T. Bryce, 1811.

Contains much information on aneurysm of the neck and abnormalities of neck arteries.

HODGSON (JOSEPH) 1788–1869

706 A Treatise on the diseases of arteries and veins, containing the pathology and treatment of aneurisms and wounded arteries. *London, Thomas Underwood, 1815.* xix, 604 pp. Bibliog. (ftn. refs). 8vo, 23 cms.

Garrison and Morton 2741 (refers especially to the accompanying atlas, below).

Book-stamp: Norfolk Medical Book Society 1822; bookplate (with regulations): Norwich and Norfolk United Medical Book Society.

Typed note on the Maladie de Hodgson initialled DEB inserted.

707 Engravings intended to illustrate some of the diseases of arteries, accompanied with explanations. *London, Thomas Underwood, 1815.* 27 pp. Illus (separate plates). Folio, 35 cms.

A very rare companion volume to no. 706.

Autograph: E. libris Joannis Ashburner (John Ashburner M.D., M.R.C.P., died November 13, 1878, a confirmed believer in mesmerism).

Inserted is a brief biographical note by B. T. Davis (reprinted from *Queen's medical Magazine*, 1961, **53**, 4–7) with a typescript letter from DEB to Dr Oscar Brenner (1910–1965).

708 *The same.* Von den Krankheiten der Arterien und Venen mit besonderer Rücksicht auf Entwicklung und Behandlung der Aneurysmen und Arterienwunden. Aus dem Englischen übersetzt und mit Dr. Kreysig's sowohl als mit eigenen Anmerkungen, herausgegeben von Dr. F. A. Koberwein. *Hannover, Gebrüdern Hahn, 1817.* xxii, 610 pp. Illus (3 folding plates at end), bibliog. (ftn. refs). 8vo, 21 cms.

Autograph: Tonfick (?) 1875.

709 *The same.* Traité des maladies des artères et des veines . . . traduit de l'anglais et augmenté d'un grand nombre de notes par Gilbert Breschet. *Paris, Gabon, Béchet jeune; Montpellier, Gabon, 1819.* 2 tom. (xx, 416 [1] pp.; [iv], 596 pp.). Bibliog. (ftn. refs). 8vo, 21 cms.

Hodgson was apprenticed to Freer whose book on aneurysm he illustrated. His *Treatise on the diseases of arteries*, published when he was aged 27, gained him an international reputation and was the outstanding work on cardio-vascular disease for almost a century. His atlas with plates engraved from his own drawings portrays infective endocarditis with ruptured aortic cusp, the first published illustration of this condition. He also described cylindrical dilatation of the aorta with relative incompetence (Maladie de Hodgson) which he suspected as syphilitic. He became the leading surgeon in the Midlands and in 1862, the first provincial president of the Royal College of Surgeons. He developed heart-block with a pulse of 40 in 1868.

The discovery of Hodgson's disease or Maladie de Hodgson (aneurysmal dilatation of the aorta seen in the enlargement of the heart) ran counter to the argument of Scarpa, who in his monograph on aneurysm maintained that it was always due to a localised rupture of the inner coat. Allan Burns (1809) found that aneurysm was often a diffuse dilatation of the aorta, without rupture of the coats. Hodgson followed Burns in describing cylindrical dilatation of the aorta without rupture of the coats in the initial stage, admitting that localised rupture of the coats often occurred later. He recognised that diffuse disease of the aortic wall was associated with incompetent or sclerosed aortic valves.

The French separated aortic incompetence into endocarditic (Maladie de Corrigan) and arterial due to diffuse disease of the aortic wall (Maladie de Hodgson).

In Constantin Paul's text-book *Maladies du cœur* (nos. 389 and 390) the terms Maladie de Corrigan and Maladie de Hodgson are used, but who first coined this nomenclature seems difficult to ascertain. The separation of aortic incompetence into the endocarditic and arterio-sclerotic types became general in text-books and only later was syphilitic aortitis separated from atheroma.

WILSON (James) 1765–1821

710 Lectures on the blood, and on the anatomy, physiology and surgical pathology of the vascular system of the human body, delivered before the Royal College of Surgeons of London, in the summer of the year 1819. *London, Burgess and Hill, 1819.* xvi, 429 pp. 8vo, 22 cms.

Book-stamp: Middlesex Hospital Library.

Wilson worked at the Hunterian School of Anatomy, Great Windmill Street, with Hewson and Cruikshank. He noted that the coronary orifices are above the semi-lunar valves, but when the aorta is opened up, they appear to be covered by the cusps—hence the error of Stroem's theory,revived by von Brucke in 1855 (no. 618). An account of the pulse is included (pp. 170–4). Lectures 4–5 (pp. 94–146) deal with the anatomy and physiology of the heart.

BRIGHT (Richard) 1789–1858

711 Original papers of Richard Bright on renal diseases; ed. by A[rthur] A[rnold] Osman. *London, Humphrey Milford [at] Oxford University Press, 1937.* xvi, 172 pp. Illus, port. (frontispiece), facsim. (title-page). 8vo, 25 cms.

Contents: Cases illustrative of some of the appearances observable on the examination of diseases terminating in dropsical effusion (*Reports of medical cases*, London, 1827, [vol. 1], pp. 1–88), pp. 1–92;

Cases and observations, illustrative of renal disease accompanied with the secretion of albuminous urine (*Guy's Hospital Reports*, 1836, **1**, 338–79), pp. 93–131;

Tabular view of the morbid appearances in 100 cases connected with albuminous urine (*Guy's Hospital Reports*, 1836, **1**, 380–400), pp. 132–52;

Gulstonian lecture no. II—On the functions of the abdomen and some of the diagnostic marks of its disease, pp. 153–66. The lectures appeared in *London medical Gazette*, 1833, **12**, 281–7, 312–17, 345–50, 378–84. The latter part of the second lecture (pp. 378–84) only is given in abridged form.

Appendix. Histological sections from the kidneys of three cases of "Bright's disease", originally described by Dr. Bright, by A. Arnold Osman and reprinted with emendations from "Studies in Bright's disease, no. VII" (*Guy's Hospital Reports*, 1933, **83**, 185–93), pp. 167–72, omits references in original paper.

Acquired 1942.

GUY'S HOSPITAL REPORTS

712 Bright centenary double number. (Guy's Hospital Reports, 1927, vol. 77, nos. 3 and 4.). *London, Lancet, 1927.* [ii], 253–502, [4] pp. Illus, ports, tables, plan, diagrs, bibliog. 8vo, 25 cms.

Contents: Richard Bright by W. S. Thayer, pp. 253–301 (Includes chronologically arranged bibliography of 107 references, pp. 298–301. Copious footnotes. Watercolour and photograph of Bright. Portrait with mother in frontispiece.);

The situation of the clinical wards at Guy's Hospital in the time of Richard Bright by H. L. Eason, pp. 302–6;

Chronic Bright's disease without albuminuria: an historical note on the contributions of Bright and his successors of the Guy's School to the study of high blood-pressure and its consequences, by John A. Ryle, pp. 307–13.

Disorders of the kidneys with symptoms of Bright's disease, by Ludwig Aschoff, pp. 314–24 (covers hypertonicity or hypertension and Bright's disease);

Les grands syndromes du mal de Bright. Leçon faite le 8 Juillet, 1927, au Guy's Hospital, by Docteur A. Lemierre, pp. 325–42 (gives an account of the work of his master Widal, who through serious ill-health could not attend to deliver his demonstration);

The process of excretion in the kidney: an account of the work of E. H. Starling and his pupils, by M. S. Pembrey, pp. 343–53 (this contribution was originally to have been written by Starling, but after his death his work was written by his successor Pembrey, also a life-long friend);

Some observations on uraemia, by Sir John Rose Bradford, pp. 354–61;

The urine in latent and sub-acute septicaemia, by F. A. Knott, pp. 490–3.

Purchased by the Society of Apothecaries, July 1927.

713 Special number dedicated to Richard Bright (1789–1858), (Physician to Guy's Hospital 1820–1843) in commemoration of the centenary of his death. (Guy's Hospital Reports 1958, vol. 107, no. 4). *London, Guys's Hospital, 1958.* [vi], 263–543 pp. Illus, port., tables, bibliog. 8vo, 25 cms.

Contents: Richard Bright at Guy's by H. C. Cameron, pp. 263–93;

Richard Bright and his discovery of the disease bearing his name, by Sir William Hale-White, pp. 294–307 (reprinted from *Guy's Hospital Reports*, 1921, **71**, 1–20);

Bright's observations other than those on renal disease by Sir William Hale-White, pp. 308–22 (reprinted from *Guy's Hospital Reports*, 1921, **71**, 143–57);

Bright's disease; the changing concept of a century, by W. N. Mann, pp. 323–347;

A note on albuminuria in Bright's disease, by Christopher Hardwick, pp. 348–52;

Asymptomatic persistent proteinuria: studies by renal biopsies, by Victor E. Pollak, Conrad L. Brandt, Robert C. Muehrcke and Robert M. Kark, pp. 353–72;

Some observations on renal biopsy with reference to Bright's disease, by J. D. Williams, pp. 373–89;

A note on the histological appearances of three kidneys originally described by Richard Bright, by J. B. Cavanagh, pp. 390–8;

The Pathogenesis of chronic pyelonephritis, by S. De Navasquez, pp. 399–404;

Bacteriological conditions leading to destruction of the kidney by R. H. Gorrill, pp. 405–15;

Problems in renal anatomy by G. C. W. Baker, pp. 416–25 (discusses Bright's disease and hypertension, and the lesser circulation of the kidney);

Biochemical changes in acute renal failure by W. H. H. Merivale, pp. 426–32;

Bright's disease and pregnancy by G. F. Gibberd, pp. 433–48;

The problem of pregnancy complicated by systemic lupus erythematosus with renal involvement, by F. A. Murray, pp. 449–53;

Radiological findings in Bright's disease, by J. D. Dow, pp. 454–74;

Urinary excretion of catecholamines in phaeochromocytoma and other abnormal states, by R. H. S. Thompson and J. R. Trounce, pp. 475–85;

The defective absorption of phosphorus and calcium and the effect of vitamin D in the Fanconi syndrome, by H. E. F. Davies, Byron Evans, H. M. N. Rees and P. Fourman, pp. 486–99;

The effect of bed rest on acute haemorrhagic nephritis in children by M. C. Joseph and Paul E. Rolani, pp. 500–14;

The evolution of the treatment of essential hypertension by K. D. Allanby, pp. 515–30;

Richard Bright: a bibliography by William Hill, pp. 531–42 (originally published under the title "Richard Bright—a bio-bibliography" in *Guy's Hospital Gazette*, 1950, **64**, 373–9, 393–7, 419–22, 439–42, 454–7, 472–84, this list is reprinted from pp. 456–7, 472–82).

Special presentation copy.

PIGEAUX (Antoine Louis Jules) 1807–?

714 Traité pratique des maladies des vaisseaux contenant des recherches historiques spéciales. *Paris, Labe, Just Rouvier, 1843.* xvi, 567 pp. 8vo, 22 cms.

Covers history, anatomy, auriculo-ventricular aneurysm, arterio-sclerosis and diseases of veins and lymphatics with a section on the pulse (pp. 499–518). A continuation of his treatise on heart disease of 1839 (no. 379).

ERICHSEN (Sir John Eric) 1818–1896

715 Observations on aneurism, selected from the works of the principal writers on that disease from the earliest periods to the close of the last century, trans. and ed. by John E. Erichsen. (Sydenham Society). *London, The Sydenham Society, 1844.* xii, 524 pp. Bibliog. 8vo, 23 cms.

Contents: Part 1—Symptoms, pathology and causes—consists of extracts in chronological order from Galen, Aetius, Jean Fernel (1497–1558), Jean de Gorris (1505–1577), Ambroise Paré (1510–1590), Jacques Guillemeau (*c.* 1520–1613), Daniel Sennert (1572–1637), Wilhelm Fabricius Hildanus (1560–1634), Richard Wiseman (1622–1676), Lancisi, Alexander Monro, secundus (1733–1817), Jean Louis Petit, père (1674–1760), Haller, William Hunter, William White (1744–1790?), Thomas Armiger (surgeon, *fl.* 1770), and Matthew Baillie.

Part 2—Treatment—has extracts in chronological order from Aetius, Paulus Aegineta, Paré, Guillemeau, Marco Aurelio Severino (1580–1656), Richard Wiseman (1622–1676), Morel, surgeon of the Hôpital de la Charité et Juré in Paris (*fl.* 1681), Royer (*fl.* 1681), Pierre Michon Bourdelot (1610–1685), Barthélemy Saviard (1656–1702), Dominique Anel (*c.* 1679–1730), Lancisi, John Macgill (Edinburgh surgeon, *fl.* 1733), Monro, secundus, Lorenz Heister (1683–1758), Pietro Paolo Molinelli (1702–1764), Hippolito Francesco Albertini (1662–1738), Pierre Foubert (1696–1766), Sauveur François Morand (1697–1733), Morgagni, Richard Lambert (surgeon 1751–1778 at Newcastle upon Tyne Infirmary), James Burchall (surgeon 1752–1779 at Manchester Infirmary), Carlo Guattani (1707–1771), William Bromfield, Charles Leslie (surgeon at Cork, *fl.* 1774), Percivall Pott (1714–1738), Bradford Wilmer (*fl.* 18th cent., 2nd half), Adolph Murray (1751–1803), Everard Home, Pierre Joseph Desault (1744–1795), Joseph François Louis Deschamps (1740–1824), Pierre Guérin (1740–1827) and Barthélemi Lacoste (*fl.* 1799).

Part 3 consists of a chronological bibliography with annotations, pp. 495–518, and a detailed index pp. 519–24.

CRISP (Edwards) 1806–1882

716 A Treatise on the structure, diseases, and injuries of the blood-vessels; with statistical deductions; being the Essay to which the Jacksonian Prize for the year 1844 was awarded by the Royal College of Surgeons of England. With numerous additions. *London, John Churchill, 1847.* xvi, [ii], 354 pp. Illus (plates), tables, bibliog. (ftn. refs). 8vo, 22 cms.

[*and*] Appendix to the Treatise . . . *London, for the Author by H. Teape, 1851.* pp. 355–98. 8vo, 22 cms.

Important early statistics on aneurysms. The appendix covers the information and experience the author has acquired during the four years that have elapsed since the original work was published (p. 357).

RAYNAUD (AUGUSTE G. MAURICE) 1834–1881

717 On local asphyxia and symmetrical gangrene of the extremities . . . trans. by Thomas Barlow.

Pp. v–x, 1–199 in *Selected monographs* (New Sydenham Society, vol. 121). London, New Sydenham Society, 1888. Various paging. 8vo, 22 cms.

Translation of *De l'asphyxie locale et de la gangrène symmétrique des extrémités* (Paris, Rignoux, 1862), Raynaud's original thesis, and his last researches on the subject of local asphyxia in *Archives générales de Médecine*, 1874, **1**, 5, 189. The thesis was the first description of Raynaud's disease (Garrison and Morton 2704).

Also included in the volume (separate pagination) are Klebs and Crudelli *On the nature of malaria*, Marchiafava and Celli *On the origin of melanaemia*, and Neugebauer *On spondyl-olisthesis*.

GULL (Sir WILLIAM WITHEY) 1816–1890

718 [Two reports on aortic disease].

On retroversion of the aortic valves from disease in the sinuses of Valsalva. Reprinted from *Guy's Hospital Reports*, 1859, 3rd series, **5**, 305–6. Illus (1 plate).

Paraplegia from obstruction of the abdominal aorta. Reprinted from *Guy's Hospital Reports*, 1857, 3rd series, **3**, 311–14. Illus. (1 plate).

719 A Collection of the published writings . . . ; ed. by T. D. Acland. (New Sydenham Society 147, 156). *London, New Sydenham Society, 1894–6.* 2 vols. Illus, port., tables, bibliog. 8vo, 22 cms.

Vol. 1 (xii, 600 pp.); Medical papers, of which the following are of cardiological interest: Cases of aneurism of the cerebral vessels, pp. 86–106; On the pathology of the morbid state commonly called chronic Bright's disease with contracted kidney "arterio-capillary fibrosis", pp. 325–74; Clinical lecture on chronic Bright's disease with contracted kidney (arterio-capillary fibrosis), pp. 375–90; On changes in the spinal cord and its vessels in arterio-capillary fibrosis, pp. 391–415; Discussion on the relation of renal disease to disturbances of the general circulation, and to alterations in the heart and blood vessels, pp. 415–21; Chronic nephritis; viz. the relation between the changes of connective tissue, parenchyma, blood-vessels, and heart in this disease, pp. 422–31; Parthenogenetic tumour attached to the muscular tissue of the left ventricle of the heart of a sheep, pp. 432–4; A Case of intermittent haematinuria with remarks, pp. 435–45.

Vol. 2 (lxxii, 184 pp.): Memoirs and addresses, includes a biography with notes and aphorisms, and the Harveian Oration of 1870.

ALLBUTT (Sir THOMAS CLIFFORD) 1836–1925)

720 On the use of the ophthalmoscope in diseases of the nervous system and of the kidneys; also in certain other general disorders. *London & New York, Macmillan, 1871.* xii, [iii], 405 pp. Illus (plates), tables, bibliog. (ftn. refs). 8vo, 23 cms.

Autograph: F. Wright Smith, Ph.D. A pioneer work on the ophthalmoscope in medicine.

721 Arteriosclerosis: a summary view. *London, Macmillan, 1925.* viii, 108 pp. Bibliog. (ftn. refs). 8vo, 19 cms.

Acquired 1942. A review of Allbutt's work in arteriosclerosis.

JOHNSON (Sir GEORGE) 1818–1896

722 Lectures on Bright's disease, with especial reference to pathology, diagnosis and treatment. *London, Smith Elder, 1873.* xi, 152 pp. Illus. 8vo, 21 cms.

American edition, New York, G. P. Putnam's Son, 1874.

An early authority on arterial changes in Bright's disease. Johnson described canter rhythm and was known as "Kidney Johnson".

CHARCOT (JEAN MARTIN) 1825–1893

723 Lectures on Bright's disease of the kidneys, delivered at the School of Medicine of Paris; trans., with the permission of the author, by Henry B. Millard. *London, Baillière, Tindall & Cox; New York, William Wood, 1879.* x, 100 pp. Illus, bibliog. (ftn. refs). 8vo, 25 cms.

According to the title-page this is "(English edition) revised by the author." Errata slip.

Autograph: S. D. Darbishire (Samuel Dukinfield Darbishire, 1846–1892, of Oxford, senior physician at Radcliffe Infirmary, University coroner).

The American edition of the *Lectures* was published a year earlier (New York, W. Wood, 1878) and was a translation of the second part of Charcot's *Leçons sur les maladies du foie, des voies biliaires et des reins* (Paris, 1877). Charcot's *Leçons* were collected and published by his pupils Désiré Magloire Bourneville (1840–1909) and Louis Arthur Sevestre (1843–1907). Millard (1832–1893), the translator, later produced his own *Treatise on Bright's disease* . . . (London, S. Low [and others], 1884).

GOWERS (Sir WILLIAM RICHARD) 1845–1915

724 A Manual and atlas of medical ophthalmoscopy. *London, J. & A. Churchill, 1879.* xii, 352 pp. Illus (16 plates). Bibliog. (ftn. refs). 8vo, 23 cms.

Publisher's catalogue, May 1879 (24 pp.), bound in at end.

Autograph: "Sir William Jenner Bart. with the grateful regards of the author."

A classic on the subject. Second edition, 1882; third edition, 1890; fourth edition, 1904 (all published by Churchill). Second American edition, Philadelphia, P. Blakiston, 1882.

HARRIS (VINCENT DORMER) 1851–1931

725 On Tufnell's treatment of aortic aneurysm.

Reprinted from *St. Bartholomew's Hospital Reports*, 1881, **17**, 13–27. Tables, bibliog. (ftn. refs).

Thomas Jolliffe Tufnell (1819–1885), Dublin surgeon, treated aortic aneurysm by rest and low-calorie diet. Harris maintained that cures by "Tufnell's treatment" were rare, although there was almost certain relief of symptoms. Harris remained at Bart's while filling honorary posts at other London hospitals; he became F.R.C.P. in 1885.

BROWNE (OSWALD AUCHINLECK) 1855–1908

726 Aneurysms of the aorta, with especial reference to their position, direction and effects. Being an exercise for an act for the degree of M.B. in the University of Cambridge. *London, H. K. Lewis, 1885.* [ii], 18, xv pp. Tables, bibliog. (ftn. refs). 8vo, 21 cms.

Historical introduction to the subject pp. 1–3. Browne went on to his M.D., and became F.R.C.P. in 1898. His chief association was with the Royal Hospital for Diseases of the Chest and for the last five years of his life was Assistant Registrar at the Royal College of Physicians of London.

EPPINGER (HANS) 1846–1916

727 Pathogenesis Histogenesis und Aetiologie der Aneurysmen einschliesslich des Aneurysma equi verminosum: pathologisch-anatomische Studien. *Berlin, August Hirschwald, 1887.* [iii], 563 pp. Illus (9 plates), bibliog. (ftn. refs). 8vo, 23 cms.

Forms Supplement-Heft of *Archiv fur klinische Chirurgie*, Berlin, 1887, **35**, Hft 3/4.

FOTHERGILL (JOHN MILNER) 1841–1888

728 Vasco-renal change versus Bright's disease. *London, Baillière, Tindall and Cox, 1887.* xii, 219 pp. Illus (4 plates), tables, 8vo, 22 cms.

Publisher's catalogue (35 pp.), bound in at end. American edition, New York, G. P. Putnam, 1887.
An early work maintaining that high arterial tension precedes renal disease in causing cardiac hypertrophy. One of the earliest works on hyperpiesia.

DA COSTA (JACOB MENDES) 1833–1900

729 Relation of the diseases of the kidney, especially the Bright's diseases, to diseases of the heart. The Middleton Goldsmith Lecture, delivered before the New York Pathological Society, April 18, 1888. [*Philadelphia, H. C. Lea's Son*], *1888.* 37 pp. Illus, bibliog. (occasional ftn. refs). 8vo, 21 cms.

Pp. 3–14 wanting. Reprinted from *Medical News* (Philadelphia), 1888, **52**, 477–86. (Also published in *Medical Record* (New York), 1888, **33**, 485–93).
An important early paper by Da Costa maintaining that chronic Bright's disease is not primarily a renal, but a general arterial disease, often without albuminuria, and he mentions high arterial tension, thus presaging Allbutt's hypothesis. Da Costa studied in Paris and Vienna and became the foremost teacher of physical diagnosis in America. He is best known for his account of heart disease in soldiers, 1867 (Da Costa's syndrome).

BRUCE (JOHN MITCHELL) 1846–1929

730 The Lettsomian Lectures on diseases and disorders of the heart and arteries in middle and advanced life. *London,* [*printed by*] *Harrison & Sons, 1902.* [vii], 50, ix–xii pp. Bibliog. (ftn. refs). 8vo, 22 cms.

Pp. 1–50 appear to be a straight reprint of the lectures in *Transactions of the Medical Society of London*, 1901, **24**, 121–70. The three lectures were also published in the *British medical Journal*, 1901, **1**, 566–9, 700–4, 818–22 and *Lancet*, 1907, **1**, 692–4, 844–8, 991–4.

POTAIN (PIERRE CARL ÉDOUARD) 1825–1901

731 La Pression artérielle de l'homme à l'état normal et pathologique. *Paris, Masson, 1902.* [v], ii, 191 pp. Illus, tables, diagrs. 8vo, 23 cms.

Author's inscription to Marey reproduced before preface. Published posthumously by Pierre Teissier.
Potain's sphygmomanometer was the first handy clinical instrument after von Basch's cumbersome apparatus (no. 428).

JORES (LEONARD ALBERT) 1866–1935

732 Wesen und Entwickelung der Arteriosklerose auf Grund anatomischer und experimenteller untersuchungen. *Wiesbaden, J. F. Bergmann, 1903.* [vii], 172 pp. Illus (4 plates), bibliog. 4to, 26 cms.

Jores was a pioneer worker on arterial disease, who separated senile arteriosclerosis from that associated with hypertension and renal disease. He was much cited by Allbutt, and his book contains 162 references (pp. 162–70).

OLIVER (GEORGE) 1841–1915

733 Studies in blood-pressure, physiological and clinical. 3rd ed., ed. by W. D. Halliburton. *London, H. K. Lewis, 1916.* xxiii, 240 pp. Illus, tables, bibliog. (ftn. refs). 8vo, 21 cms.

Publisher's catalogue (32 pp.) bound in at end.

First edition, 1906; second edition, 1908 (same publisher). Obituary of the author, pp. ix–xiv. For a comparison of the present edition with previous editions see Preface, pp. v–vii.

Oliver of Harrogate, an early worker on blood-pressure, invented an arteriometer. The editor, William Dobinson Halliburton (1860–1931) was famous for his text-books on physiology and biochemistry.

RUSSELL (WILLIAM) 1852–1940

734 Arterial hypertonus sclerosis and blood-pressure. *Edinburgh and London, William Green, 1907.* ix, 194 pp. Illus, tables, bibliog. 8vo, 23 cms.

Text heavily underlined in places. Book-stamp: Alfred Quayle, 7 Scarisbrick New Road, Southport.

An early work on hypertonus of the arterial wall as a factor in measuring blood-pressure.

735 The Sphygmometer; its value in practical medicine. *London, Baillière, Tindall & Cox, 1921.* xi, 145 pp. Illus, tables, diagrs, bibliog. (ftn. refs). 8vo, 23 cms.

Publisher's catalogue (4 pp.) bound in at end. Acquired 1922.

The book in fact covers a wider field than purely sphygmometry, and includes lectures on hypertonus in diseased and normal arteries, estimation of heart power and cerebral angiospasm; also useful for its discussion of terminology.

JOSUÉ (OTTO) 1869–1923

736 Traité de l'artério-sclérose; préface de M. le Professeur Roger. *Paris, J. B. Baillière, 1909.* xii, 404 pp. Illus, tables, bibliog. (ftn. refs). 8vo, 21 cms.

Historical introduction, pp. 1–14.

JOSUÉ (OTTO) 1869–1923 and PARTURIER (MAURICE) *b.* 1888

737 Les Cardio-rénaux: étude théorique et pratique. *Paris, E. Le François, 1921.* 223 pp. Tables, bibliog. (ftn. refs.). 8vo, 20 cms.

Josué was a pioneer worker on arterial disease and produced atheroma in rabbits by injections of adrenalin.

GALLAVARDIN (Louis Bénédict) 1875–1957

738 La Tension arterielle en clinique, sa mesure, sa valeur séméiologique. 2e éd. *Paris, Masson, 1921.* xii, 717 pp. Illus, tables, diagrs, bibliog. 8vo, 25 cms.

This edition was for many years the standard work on blood-pressure and contains a comprehensive bibliography up to that date. Gallavardin gives a good account of left heart failure with "decapitated hypertension." First edition, Paris, G. Steinheil, 1910.

HALL (Francis de Havilland) 1847–1929

739 Lumleian Lectures on intrathoracic aneurysm. (Lumleian Lectures 1913). *London, Lancet, 1913.* 81 pp. Illus, tables, bibliog. 8vo, 22 cms.

Reprinted from *Lancet*, 1913, **1**, 805–9, 869–75, 945–50.

Three lectures with ample bibliographies (39, 41 and 31 references respectively). X-ray photographs.

BISHOP (Louis Faugères) 1864–1941

740 Arterial sclerosis: a consideration of prolongation of life and efficiency after forty. (Oxford Medical Publications). *London, Henry Frowde and Hodder & Stoughton, 1921.* xi, 383 pp. Illus, tables, diagrs, bibliog. (occasional ftn. refs). 8vo, 22 cms.

First published as *Arteriosclerosis . . .* by the same publishers, 1914. The term arteriosclerosis is used throughout the text.

A popular American work by Prof. Bishop of New York.

POULAIN (Pierre)

741 Deux signes sphygmanométriques de rétrécissement aortique: trou auscultatoire et labilité tensionnelle systolique. [Lyon University. Faculté de Médecine Thèse]. *Lyon, imprimerie Express, 1920.* 45 pp. Diagrs, bibliog. (ftn. refs). 8vo, 24 cms.

SHAW (Harold Batty) 1866–1936

742 Hyperpiesia and hyperpiesis (hypertension): a clinical, pathological & experimental study. (Oxford Medical Publications). *London, Henry Frowde and Hodder & Stoughton,* [*1922*]. x, 191 pp. Illus, tables, diagrs, bibliog. (ftn. refs). 4to, 26 cms.

An important contribution to hypertension and its relation to renal disease after Allbutt's work.

BRIN (Louis) *b.* 1883 and GIROUX (Léon) 1876–1934

743 Syphilis du cœur et de l'aorte. *Paris, Octave Doin, 1924.* [iii], ii, 229 pp. Illus, tables, diagrs, bibliog. (ftn. refs). 8vo, 24 cms.

Deals with myocardial and aortic syphilis, aneurysm, heart-block and angina pectoris.

BUERGER (Leo) 1879–1943

744 The Circulatory disturbances of the extremities, including gangrene, vasomotor, and trophic disorders. *Philadelphia and London, W. B. Saunders, 1924.* xiii, 628 pp. Illus, bibliog. (occasional ftn. refs). 8vo, 25 cms.

Autograph: Terence East, D.M. (Charles Frederick Terence East, 1894–1967).

The classical account of Buerger's disease (thromboangiitis obliterans) is described on pp. 213–385. Originally the disease was described in his "Thrombo-angiitis obliterans: the vascular lesions leading to presenile spontaneous gangrene" (*American Journal of medical Science*, 1908, **136**, 567–80) (Garrison and Morton 2912), although F. von Winiwarter described it without the name in 1878 (*Archiv fur klinische Chirurgie, Berlin*, 1878–1879, **23**, 202–25); hence the synonymous name for the disease of Winiwarter-Buerger syndrome.

BENNETT (THOMAS IZOD) 1887–1946

745 On some problems of nephritis. (Goulstonian Lectures 1928). [*London, Lancet, 1928*]. 44 pp. Facsims, tables, diagrs, bibliog. 8vo, 22 cms.

Reprinted from *Lancet*, 1928, **1**, 535–9, 637–47, 741–6. The three lectures are entitled: the problem of uraemia, the problem of oedema, and the problem of blood-pressure in nephritis.

"With the author's compliments."

Bennett's *Nephritis: its problems and treatment* (London, Oxford University Press) followed in 1929.

BERGMANN (GUSTAV VON) 1878–1955

746 Blutdruckkrankheit.

Reprinted from KLEMPERER (Georg) 1865–1946 and KLEMPERER (Felix). *Neue deutsche Klinik*. Berlin, Urban und Schwarzenberg, 1928. Band 2, Lieferung 6, pp. 103–58. Diagrs, bibliog. 8vo, 25 cms.

KAUFFMANN (FRIEDRICH)

747 Pathologie des arteriellen Blutdruckes.

Reprinted from *Handbuch der normalen und pathologischen Physiologie;* herausgegeben von A. Bethe, G. von Bergmann [and others]. Berlin, Julius Springer, [1928]. Band 7, Hälfte 2, Teil 2. pp. 1303–413. Bibliog.

Book-stamp: Dr [later Sir] John Parkinson (1885–1976).

OPPENHEIMER (BERNARD SUTRO) 1876–1958 and
FISHBERG (ARTHUR MAURICE) *b.* 1898

748 Hypertensive encephalopathy. *Chicago, American Medical Association, 1928*. 15 pp. Table, diagr., bibliog. (ftn. refs). 8vo, 25 cms.

Reprinted from *Archives of Internal Medicine*, 1928, **41**, 264–78.

The classic paper separating the cerebral episodes of hypertension from uraemia, and introducing the term hypertensive encephalopathy.

LIAN (CAMILLE CONSTANT) 1882–1969 and BLONDEL (ANDRÉ) *b.* 1897

749 L'Hypotension artérielle permanente d'allure idiopathique. *Montpellier, Librairie Coulet, [1929]*. 148 pp. Diagrs (tracings), bibliog. 8vo, 25 cms.

Although not mentioned as such, this paper is a straight reprint from the proceedings of the *Congrès français de Médecine*, 20e, held at Montpellier in 1929. Bibliography (pp. 134–48) includes "Liste de travaux que nous n'avons pu consulter" (pp. 147–8).

Both authors had written papers with the same or similar titles before this, It was the title of Blondel's Paris M.D. thesis of February 1928 (Paris, A. Legrand, 1928).

750 Syphilis de l'appareil cardio-vasculaire.

Reprinted from JEANSELME ([Antoine] Édouard) 1858–1935. *Traité de la syphilis*. Paris, Gustave Doin, 1934. Tom. 5, fasc. 2, pt. 4, pp. 69–264. Illus, diagrs, bibliog. 8vo, 25 cms.

Deals with aortitis, aneurysm, pulmonary arteritis and myocardial disease. Good classified bibliography, pp. 250–64.

RUSSELL (DOROTHY STUART) *b.* 1895

751 A Classification of Bright's disease. (Medical Research Council. Special Report Series, no. 142). *London, His Majesty's Stationery Office, 1929.* 248, [17] pp. Illus (plates), tables, bibliog. 8vo, 25 cms.

Plates at end interleaved with pages of explanation of figures. List of M.R.C. publications (viii pp.) bound in at end.

A monograph from Professor Turnbull's department at the London Hospital, where Turnbull collected extensive detailed data for many years. These data and others investigated by Dr. Russell form the basis of her conclusions and classification involving evolution and distribution of different types of structural damage, conditions of their occurrence and resulting interferences with function.

OBSERVATIONS

752 Observations on the courses of the different types of Bright's disease, and on the resultant changes in renal anatomy, by D[onald] D[exter] van Slyke and others. (Medicine Monographs, vol. 18). *London, Baillière, Tindall & Cox, 1930.* [iv], 130 pp. Illus, tables, diagrs, bibliog. 8vo, 24 cms.

The authors D. D. van Slyke, Edgar Stillman, Eggert Möller, W. Ehrech, J. F. McIntosh, L. Leiter, E. M. MacKay, R. R. Hannon, N. S. Moore and Christopher Johnston all worked in the Hospital of the Rockefeller Institute for Medical Research, New York. They classify Bright's disease like Volhard and Fahr (Franz Volhard and [Karl] Theodor Fahr. *Die Brightsche Nierenkrankheiten.* Berlin, Springer, 1914), into three types, haemorrhagic glomerular nephritis, hypertensive disease, and nephrosis.

STIEGLITZ (EDWARD JULIUS) 1899–1958

753 Arterial hypertension. *London, Humphrey Milford, Oxford University Press, 1930.* xiii, 280 pp. Illus, diagrs, bibliog. 8vo, 24 cms.

Also published *New York, Paul B. Hoeber, 1930* (our copy printed in the U.S.A.).

A popular work on hypertension much cited in its time, with a bibliography (pp. 233–59) of 1133 references.

SANTOS (REYNALDO DOS) *b.* 1880, LAMAS (A. C.) and CALDAS (J. P.)

754 Artériographie des membres et de l'aorte abdominale. Préface du professeur Leriche. *Paris, Masson, 1931.* xi, 192 pp. Illus. 8vo, 24 cms.

Publisher's catalogue (48 pp.) juin 1931 bound in at end.

Santos introduced arteriography into clinical practice.

COSSIO (PEDRO) *b.* 1900

755 Aortitis sifilitica. *Buenos Aires, El Ateneo, [1932].* 150 pp. Illus (x-ray photographs), diagrs (orthodiagrams), bibliog. 8vo, 22 cms.

Errata slip inserted. Author's signed presentation copy to DEB.

A review of syphilitic aortitis and its history.

LEWIS (Sir THOMAS) 1881–1945

756 Vascular disorders of the limbs described for practitioners and students. *London, Macmillan, 1936.* xi, 111 pp. Diagrs. 8vo, 23 cms.

Second edition, 1946. American edition, New York, 1936.

GOLDBLATT (HARRY) *b.* 1891

757 [Three offprints on experimental hypertension, 1937–1938.]

Experimental hypertension. IV. Clinical and pathologic studies of the eyes: a preliminary report, [by] J. E. L. Keyes and H. Goldblatt. *Chicago, American Medical Association, 1937.* 15 pp. Illus, diagr., bibliog. (ftn. refs). 4to, 26 cms.

Reprinted from the *Archives of Ophthalmology*, 1937, **17,** 1040–54.

Studies on experimental hypertension. VII, The Production of the malignant phase of hypertension.

Reprinted from *Journal of experimental Medicine*, 1938, **67,** 809–26. Illus, bibliog.

Experimental observations on the pathogenesis of essential hypertension. (Mary Scott Newbold Lecture, 1938).

Reprinted from *Transactions and Studies of the College of Physicians of Philadelphia*, 1938, 4th series, **6,** 5–15. Bibliog.

HOLMAN (EMILE FREDERIC) *b.* 1890

758 Arteriovenous aneurysm; abnormal communications between the arterial and venous circulations. (Macmillan Surgical Monographs). *New York, Macmillan, 1937.* xvii, 244 pp. Illus, ports, diagrs, bibliog. 8vo, 22 cms.

Acquired 1942. A pioneer work on arteriovenous fistulae, including those of congenital heart disease, profusely illustrated, and with 205 references.

GILCHRIST (ANDREW RAE) *b.* 1899

759 A Honeyman Gillespie Lecture on the hypertensions. (Honeyman Gillespie Lecture 1941). [*Edinburgh, Oliver and Boyd, 1941*]. [34 pp.] Bibliog. 8vo, 23 cms.

Reprinted from *Edinburgh medical Journal*, 1941, **48,** 752–83.
Presentation copy from the author ("with kindest regards and all good wishes. Xmas 1941. A.R.G.").

WHITE (PAUL DUDLEY) 1886–1973

760 The Heart in hypertension since the days of Richard Bright. (Louis Gross Memorial Lecture, 1945). [*Montreal, Canadian Medical Association, 1946*]. 20 pp. Diagrs, bibliog. 8vo, 21 cms.

Reprinted from *Canadian medical Association Journal*, 1946, **54,** 129–36.
Provenance: initialled "J.P." (Sir John Parkinson, 1885–1976) and "D.E.B.".
White reviews the history of hypertensive heart disease up to that date (1945).

KARSNER (HOWARD THOMAS) 1879–1970 and KOLETSKY (SIMON) *b.* 1910

761 Calcific disease of the aortic valve. *Philadelphia, J. B. Lippincott, 1947.* viii, 111 pp. Illus, tables, diagrs, bibliog. 8vo, 24 cms.

An important contribution to aortic stenosis in which 196 of 200 cases of calcific aortic disease showed pathological evidence of rheumatic aetiology.

REICH (NATHANIEL EDWIN) *b.* 1907

762 Diseases of the aorta; diagnosis and treatment. *New York, Macmillan, 1949.* xv, 288 pp. Illus, tables, diagrs, bibliog. 8vo, 24 cms.

Excellent illustrations (including annotated angiocardiograms). Extensive chapter bibliographies.

RUSKIN (ARTHUR) *b.* 1911

763 Classics in arterial hypertension. (American Lecture Series, no. 290). *Springfield, Ill., C. C. Thomas, 1956.* xxv, 358 pp. Illus, ports, facsims, tables, diagrs, bibliog. 8vo, 24 cms.

An excellent historical review covering all the pioneer contributions in hypertension and sphygmomanometry divided into two parts. Part 1, Methods, includes papers by Stephen Hales (1733), Jean L. M. Poiseuille (1828), Carl Ludwig (1847), Jean Faivre (1856), Etienne J. Marey (1875), Samuel S. K. von Basch (1880), Scipione Riva-Rocci (1896), and Nikolai S. Korotkov (1905). Part 2, Significance, includes papers by Caelius Aurelianus (400), Johann J. Wepfer (1658), Thomas Young (1809), Richard Bright (1827), George Johnson (1852), Ludwig Traube (1856), William W. Gull and Henry G. Sutton (1872), Fred. A. Mahomed (1874), Pierre C. Potain (1875), William R. Gowers (1876), Clifford Allbutt (1896), Robert Tigerstedt and Per C. Bergman (1897), Harvey Cushing (1901), Leo Ambard and Eugene Beaujard (1904), Heinrich E. Hering (1924); Eberhard Kock and Heinz Mies (1929), and Harry Goldblatt and others (1934).

LAMBERT (PIERRE) *b.* 1927

764 Contribution a l'étude de la periarterite noueuse, son aspect général, ses manifestations neurologiques, ses limites nosologiques, sa place dans le cadre de névrites ischémiques. *Paris, Librairie Maloine, 1957.* 234 pp. Illus, tables, bibliog. 8vo, 24 cms.

Paris thesis, but without thesis statement.
Autograph: "A Sir Charles Symonds en respectueux hommage P.L." (Sir Charles Putnam Symonds, *b.* 1890, F.R.C.P.).
Deals with history, pathology, and clinical aspect.

EARLY WORKS ON DROPSY AND HYDROTHORAX

MONRO (DONALD) 1728–1802

765 An Essay on the dropsy, and its different species. 3rd ed. *London, A. Millar, D. Wilson & T. Durham, and T. Payne, 1765.* xiv, 272 pp. Bibliog. (ftn. refs). 8vo, 21 cms.

Autograph: "Ex libris Gulielmi Witwood".
First edition, London, D. Wilson and T. Durham, 1755 (RCP); second edition, 1756.
Deals with dropsy of every part of the body, and classifies it as diffuse or encysted. The *Essay* was first published as Monro's Edinburgh M.D. thesis *Dissertatio . . . de hydrope*, Edinburgi, Hamilton, Balfour et Neill, 1753 (RCP) (reprinted in Smellie's *Thesaurus medicus*, Edinburgi, 1785, vol. 2, pp. 191–248) (RCP).
The book is dedicated to the author's father Alexander Monro (primus, 1697–1767), who was professor of anatomy at Edinburgh. Donald, his second son, was born at Edinburgh on 15 January 1728, became physician at St. George's Hospital and died at his home in Argyle Street 9 June 1802 (see Rex E. Wright-St. Clair. *Doctors Monro; a medical saga.* London, Wellcome Historical Medical Library, 1964). Some confusion concerning his dates has been caused by William Munk, who in his *Roll of the Royal College of Physicians* (1878, vol. 2, p. 294) gave his date of death as ten years earlier.

BACHER (Georges Frédéric) 1709–*c.* 1800

766 Recherches sur les maladies chroniques, particulièrement sur les hydropisies, et sur les moyens de les guérir. *Paris, chez le veuve Thiboust, Didot le jeune, 1776* [iv], xl, 724, xvi, [ii] pp. Bibliog. 8vo, 20 cms.

Autographs: [indecipherable], Office [?] du Santé, 1807. P. [?] Pechot (Prosper Péchot, 1849–1928, was a well-known colonel of artillery, but the ascription is unlikely).

Bacher, Docteur-Régent de la Faculté de Médecine de Paris, introduced a so-called tonic pill for the treatment of dropsy which became a favourite remedy in France; it contained extract of hellebore, myrrh and card. benedictus. His book contains an exhaustive early bibliography of hydropsies (pp. 629–98).

QUIN (Charles Williams) *d.* 1818

767 A Treatise on the dropsy of the brain, illustrated by a variety of cases. To which are added, observations on the use and effects of the digitalis purpurea in dropsies. *Dublin, printed by William Jones, 1790.* 227 pp. 8vo, 21 cms.

Also copies with London imprint, J. Murray, 1790.

Quin studied at Edinburgh where Whytt had written *Observations on the dropsy in the brain*, the first account of tuberculous meningitis, and Quin's cases were mostly examples of this. He also adds an appendix on the use of digitalis in dropsy. Quin's M.D. thesis (see p. 8) was *De hydrocephalo interno* (Edinburgi, Balfour et Smellie, 1779; reprinted in Smellie. *Thesaurus medicus.* Edinburgi, 1785, vol. 4, pp. 135–50) (RCP), and shows an early interest in this field. His *Treatise* was translated into German (Leipzig, C. Fritsch, 1792).

CHARDEL (Frédéric) *d.* 1849

768 Observations sur l'hydropisie de poitrine, sur celle du péricarde, et sur les maladies organiques du cœur. *Paris, Crapelet, an VIII [1800].* [iv], 38 pp. 8vo, 21 cms.

Mentions percussion which "le citoyen Corvisart" has employed with success; this is eight years prior to Corvisart's translation of Auenbrugger.

MACLEAN (Lachlan) of Sudbury, Suffolk, *fl.* 1810

769 An Enquiry into the nature, causes and cure of hydrothorax; illustrated by interesting cases, and many living examples of the success of the mode of treatment recommended. *Sudbury, J. Burkitt, 1810.* xx, 301, 218 pp. Bibliog. (ftn. refs). 8vo, 22 cms.

American edition, Hartford, Hale & Hosmer, 1814. xiii, 187, 176 pp.

Maclean kept careful records of all cases of hydrothorax or hydropsy of the pericardium he saw in practice. In diagnosis neither percussion nor auscultation are mentioned, only the symptoms. He used digitalis freely and also mercury and squills in treatment. The appendix contains details of over 90 personal cases and some with post-mortem from the older literature.

There appear to be several medical men named Lachlan Maclean at this period, and it is impossible to unravel biographical details. According to Callisen Maclean of Sudbury took his M.D. at Edinburgh in 1790, but this qualification is also given to a Lauchlan Maclean who was drowned at Cochin in 1796 (Crawford, D. G. *Roll of the Indian Medical Service 1615–1930.* London, Thacker, 1930. p. 416). The Royal College of Surgeons has an M.R.C.S. of 1816 with this name, who in 1839 gave his address as Liverpool. The name also appears in the 1845 *Medical Directory.*

CRAMPTON (JOHN) *d.* 1840

770 Clinical report on dropsies. In two parts. *Dublin, John Cumming, 1818.* 136 pp. 2 tables (folding plate). 8vo, 22 cms.

Reprinted from *Transactions of the King's and Queen's College of Physicians in Ireland*, 1818, **2**, 140–274. Text begins p. 2; part 2, p. 57 (p. 195 in the original).

Autograph inscription: "For the Library of Steevens Hospital from the Author". Book-stamp: Steevens' Hospital Library (Dr Steevens' Hospital, Dublin, founded 1720).

Crampton, physician to Steevens' Hospital, described 74 cases of dropsy, 21 fatal cases with 15 post-mortems, and 53 other cases treated of which 35 were cured.

COMTE (J. B.) *fl.* 1822

771 De l'hydropisie de poitrine, et des palpitations du cœur, promptement dissipées par la digitale pourprée. 2e ed., considérablement augmentée. *Paris, Croullebois, 1822.* [iv], ii, 180 pp. 8vo, 22 cms.

Comte used percussion, but not the stethoscope in diagnosis, which still depended mainly on symptoms such as orthopnoea. He noted that hydrothorax responded well to digitalis if afebrile, but those with fever indicating an inflammatory condition did not respond. First edition also 1822.

SEYMOUR (EDWARD JAMES) 1795?–1866

772 The Nature and treatment of dropsy; considered especially in reference to the diseases of the internal organs of the body which commonly produce it. Parts I & II. Anasarca and ascites. To which is added an appendix containing a translation of the work of Dr. Geromini on dropsy; from the original Italian. *London, Longman, Rees, Orme, Brown, Green & Longman, 1837.* viii, 218 pp. 8vo, 22 cms.

Seymour, physician to St. George's Hospital, clearly recognised rheumatic heart disease and pericarditis, which he treated with digitalis. He also recognised tuberculous peritonitis as a cause of ascites. The translated work by Felice Giuseppe Geromini (1792–1850) (pp. 111–218) was *Sulla genesi e cura dell'idrope* (Cremona, frat. Manini, 1816). The translator has "retrenched the chapters in refutation of the doctrines" of Brunonianism.

BARIÉ (ERNEST) 1848–1931

773 Les Épanchements pleuraux chez les cardiaques. [*Photostat*].

Reprinted from *La Semaine médicale*, 1902, **22**, 25–7.

An important paper on cardiac hydrothorax.

PULMONARY CIRCULATION AND COR PULMONALE

A good historical review is given by André Cournand in the proceedings of the international symposium sponsored by the Chicago Heart Association (no. 789). Arrilaga's thesis (no. 777) introduced the term Ayerza's disease, so-called "cardiacos negros", which created new interest in pulmonary heart disease. Ljungdahl's is a classic work on pulmonary arteriosclerosis, while Shaw and Ghareeb's is an important pioneer work on bilharzial heart disease in Egypt (no. 783). A comprehensive bibliography is included in Brenner's monograph (no. 781).

EWART (William) 1848–1929

774 The Bronchi and pulmonary blood vessels: their anatomy and nomenclature; with a criticism of Professor Aeby's views on the bronchial tree of mammalia and of man. *London, Baillière, Tindall & Cox, [1889?]*. xvii, 232 pp. Illus (incl. plates), diagrs. 4to, 28 cms.

Also published by A. and C. Churchill. Now a rare book.

Ewart was physician to St. George's and Brompton Hospitals and is best known for his signs of pericarditis.

BLACKHALL-MORISON (Alexander) 1850–1927

775 Passive congestion of the lungs from heart failure, by Alexander Morison. [*London, the Practitioner, 1892*]. 47 pp. Tables, bibliog. (ftn. refs). 8vo, 21 cms.

Reprinted from *Practitioner*, **49**, 1892, 345–61, 420–42; **50**, 1892, 27–35.

Autograph: "With kind regards. A.M." (name not changed to Blackhall-Morison until 1919).

PASTEUR (William) 1855–1943

776 On massive collapse of the lung. (Bradshaw Lecture, 1908). *London, J. Bale and Danielsson, 1908*. 62 pp. Illus, diagrs, bibliog. (ftn. refs). 8vo, 22 cms.

This is the early clinical account of massive collapse of the lung, especially post-operative. Pasteur used a portable orthodiagraph at the Middlesex Hospital, its first use in England. Halls Dally also used the orthodiagraph at the same time. The "Middlesex orthodiagraph" was also used in the Hampstead Military Heart Hospital to measure the heart size in D.A.H. in 1918.

ARRILLAGA (Francisco C.)

777 Esclerosis secundaria de la arteria pulmonar y su cuadro clínico (Cardiacos negros). [Buenos Aires. Universidad Facultad de Ciencias Médicas. Tesis no. 2536, 1912]. *Buenos Aires, "La Ciencia Medica", 1912*. 261, [3] pp. Illus, bibliog. 8vo, 24 cms.

Garrison and Morton 2914. Arrillaga's presentation copy with autograph letter to Parkes Weber (Frederick Parkes Weber, M.A., M.D., F.R.C.P., 1863–1962). Arrillaga refers to Weber's paper Sur la signification pronostique de la polycythémie secondaire dans les affections cardiopulmonaires in *Archives des Maladies du Cœur, des Vaisseaux et du Sang*, 1913, **6**, 265–74; Weber mentioned in a footnote that he had been unable to obtain a copy of Arrillaga's memoir published in *Argentina medica*, 1912, p. 521. Also has cutting from *British medical Journal*, 1920, **2**, 487 on Ayerza's disease, and a review of Arrillaga's *Sclérose de l'artère: rôle de la syphilis* by P. L. Marie from *Société médicale des hôpitaux de Paris*, 29 Fevrier 1924.

Arrillaga's thesis introduced Ayerza's disease into cardiac nosology and reawakened widespread interest in pulmonary vascular disease. In 1901 Abel Ayerza (1861–1918) lectured at the National

University of Buenos Aires on the syndrome of chronic cyanosis, dyspnoea, erythraemia, and sclerosis of the pulmonary artery. The work was not published, and among other synonymous terms, the disease is sometimes called the "Ayerza-Arrillaga" syndrome because of Arrillaga's considerable work on it. According to Garrison and Morton, Corvisart described the condition in 1806. The book is now rare.

778 La Arteritis pulmonar y su cuadro clínico. *Buenos Aires, El Ateneo, 1925.* v, 274 pp. Illus (incl. 2 plates), bibliog. (ftn. refs). 8vo, 24 cms.

Author's signed presentation copy to DEB.

Contains two colour plates of Ayerza's disease (cardiopathia nigra) and the author's further experience since his thesis.

LJUNGDAHL (MALTE) *b.* 1882

779 Untersuchungen über die Arteriosklerose des kleinen Kreislaufs; aus der medizinischen Universitätsklinik zu Lund. *Wiesbaden, J. F. Bergmann, 1915.* vii, 196 pp. Illus (4 plates), bibliog. 4to, 26 cms.

Garrison and Morton 2916. Publisher's catalogue (12 pp.) bound in at end.

A classical work on pulmonary arterial disease from the Pathological Institute at Lund, Sweden. Deals with pulmonary vessels in heart disease, lung disease, chronic nephritis, diabetes and alcoholism, and with primary pulmonary sclerosis. A full bibliography of early literature (pp. 189–96).

WEBER (FREDERICK PARKES) 1863–1962 and BODE (OTTO BERNARD)

780 Polycythaemia, erythrocytosis and erythraemia (Vaquez-Osler syndrome); an epitome based on Parkes Weber's book of 1921 and the recent literature of the subject. *London, H. K. Lewis, 1929.* [iii], 34 pp. Illus (2 plates), bibliog. 8vo, 24 cms.

This epitome deals with polycythaemia in Ayerza's disease, high altitudes, lung disease, etc. An important bibliography (pp. 29–34).

BRENNER (OSCAR) 1901–1965

781 Pathology of the vessels of the pulmonary circulation. *Chicago, Ill., American Medical Association, 1936.* 189 pp. Illus, tables, diagrs, bibliog. (335 refs). 4to, 27 cms.

Reprinted (with additions and modifications) from *Archives of internal Medicine*, 1935, **56**, 211–37, 457–97, 724–52, 976–1014, 1189–1241.

Initialled presentation copy. An important monograph on pulmonary arterial disease, with 335 references, much cited even today.

MILLER (WILLIAM SNOW) 1858–1939

782 The Lung. 2nd ed. *Springfield, Charles C. Thomas, 1950.* xvi, 222 pp. 4to, 26 cms.

Autograph: Walter Somerville, January 1955.

An important work on the anatomy of the lung and its vessels. First edition, C. C. Thomas, and London, Baillière, 1937.

SHAW (ARTHUR FREDERICK BERNARD) 1888–1947 and GHAREEB (A. ABOU)

783 The Pathogenesis of pulmonary schistosomiasis in Egypt with special reference to Ayerza's disease.

Reprinted from *Journal of Pathology and Bacteriology*, 1938, **46**, 401–24. Illus, tables, bibliog.

The classic paper on bilharzial heart disease, describing for the first time the angiomatoid formations around obstructed arterioles, later recognised in severe pulmonary hypertension as plexiform lesions.

BEDFORD (DAVIS EVAN) *b.* 1898, and others

784 Bilharzial heart disease in Egypt: cor pulmonale due to bilharzial pulmonary endarteritis, by D. Evan Bedford, S. M. Aidaros and B. Girgis.

Reprinted from *British Heart Journal*, 1946, **8,** 87–95. Illus, bibliog. 4to, 27 cms.

LENÈGRE (JEAN) 1904–1972 and GERBAUX (A.)

785 La Cœur pulmonaire chronique par thrombose artérielle pulmonaire.

Reprinted from *Archives des Maladies du Cœur*, 1952, **45,** 289–314. Illus, table, diagrs, bibliog.

786 Thrombosis artérielles pulmonaires et embolies pulmonaires.

Reprinted from the proceedings of the *Congrès français de Médecine*, 30e. Alger, 1955, pp. 97–225. Illus, tables, diagrs, bibliog. 8vo, 25 cms. Presentation copy from Lenègre.

An important paper dealing with chronic pulmonary heart disease of thrombo-embolic origin. Bibliography, pp. 215–25.

TOURNIAIRE (A.), and others

787 La Cœur pulmonaire aigu dans l'embolie pulmonaire, par A. Tourniaire, F. Tartulier, F. Deyrieux and J. Blum. *Paris, Expansion Scientifique Française, 1956.* 189 pp. Illus, tables, diagrs, bibliog. 4to, 27 cms.

Covers the clinical, electrocardiographic and radiological diagnosis, and medical and surgical treatments; bibliography, pp. 161–88. A good historical account of pulmonary embolectomy. The authors belong to the Lyon Medical Faculty.

STUART-HARRIS (Sir CHARLES HERBERT) *b.* 1909 and HANLEY (THOMAS) *b.* 1920

788 Chronic bronchitis, emphysema and cor pulmonale, by C. H. Stuart-Harris and T. Hanley. Written in collaboration with Marjorie Clifton [and others]. *Bristol, John Wright, 1957.* vii, 248 pp. Illus, maps, tables, diagrs, bibliog. 8vo, 22 cms.

Pp. [246–8] blank for "Notes".

An account of heart failure from chronic lung disease as encountered in Sheffield and the Midlands.

CHICAGO HEART ASSOCIATION

789 Pulmonary circulation: an international symposium, 1958, sponsored by the Chicago Heart Association; ed. by Wright R[owe] Adams and Ilza Veith. *New York, London, Grune & Stratton, 1959.* xv, 316 pp. Illus, tables, diagrs, bibliog. 4to, 26 cms.

Contains a valuable historical review by André Cournand (The historical development of the concepts of pulmonary circulation, with 38 references, pp. 1–19), and contributions on all aspects of pulmonary circulation and pulmonary vascular disease: physiology, pathology and pulmonary circulation in primary lung disease, congenital and acquired heart disease.

DALEY (RAYMOND) *b.* 1917, GOODWIN (JOHN FORREST) *b.* 1918 and STEINER (ROBERT EMIL) *b.* 1918

790 Clinical disorders of the pulmonary circulation. *London, J. & A. Churchill, 1960.* xii, 364 pp. Illus, tables, diagrs, bibliog. 8vo, 25 cms.

Acquired 1960.

Covers anatomy, physiology, radiology, pathology and clinical aspects of pulmonary heart disease. Contents: Raymond Daley. Anatomy of the pulmonary vasculature, pp. 1–6; Grant de J.

Lee. Physiology and haemodynamics, pp. 7–33; Kenneth W. Donald. Pulmonary function and circulation, pp. 34–56; John Goodwin. The Nature of pulmonary hypertension, pp. 57–79; R. E. Steiner. The Radiology of the pulmonary circulation, pp. 80–135; C. V. Harrison. Pathology, pp. 136–68; John Goodwin. Electrocardiography, pp. 169–96; Mitral valve and left atrial disease, pp. 197–228; and Congenital heart disease, pp. 229–87; J. P. M. Tizard. The Pulmonary hyaline membrane syndrome of the newborn, pp. 288–97; John McMichael. Chronic pulmonary heart disease (Chronic Cor Pulmonale), pp. 298–310; Philip Hugh-Jones. Chronic pulmonary disease, pp. 311–40; Raymond Daley. Pulmonary vascular obstruction; pp. 341–52; and Pulmonary oedema, pp. 353–8.

HARRIS (Peter Charles) *b.* 1923 and HEATH (Donald Albert)

791 The Human pulmonary circulation: its form and function in health and disease. *Edinburgh and London, E. & S. Livingstone, 1962.* xii, 354 pp. Illus, diagrs, bibliog. 8vo, 25 cms.

American edition: Baltimore, Williams and Williams, 1962.

CONGENITAL HEART DISEASE

The history of congenital heart disease by Hahne Heinrich covers the earlier publications. Sandifort gave a famous account of a case of Fallot's tetralogy (no. 792; trans., no. 793). This condition was described by Farre before Peacock whose book (no. 795) became the standard work in this country for many years. Théremin's atlas contains 245 figures from specimens in the stray children's home at St. Petersburg, and Vierordt's monograph is important. When closure of the septal defects by surgery became possible, Rokitansky's book on the subject proved valuable. Maude Abbott's contribution to Osler and McCrae's *System of medicine* (no. 803) is a landmark in her many contributions to the subject; finally Helen Taussig's book is worthy of mention as it led to the surgical treatment by Blalock.

SANDIFORT (Edward) 1742–1814

792 De rarissimo cordis vitio.

Pp. 1–38 in vol. 1 of his *Observationes anatomico-pathologicae.* Lugduni Batavorum, P.v.d. Eyk & D. Vygh, 1777–1781. 4 vols in 1. Illus (plates), bibliog. (ftn. refs). 4to, 26 cms.

Account of a case of Fallot's tetralogy with three engraved plates of the specimen; with autograph letter to DEB from J. W. Brown on this subject, 13.9.47.

Sandifort became professor at Leyden and published works in Latin, Dutch and Swedish.

BENNETT (Lydian Russell)

793 Sandifort's "Observationes" chapter I, concerning a very rare disease of the heart.

Reprinted from *Bulletin of the History of Medicine*, 1946, **20,** 539–70. Illus (3 plates), bibliog.

Translation of Sandifort's account with a bibliography.

Lydian Russell Bennett was a Latin teacher in the East Liverpool, Ohio High School.

FARRE (John Richard) 1775–1862

794 Pathological researches. Essay 1: On malformations of the human heart; illustrated by numerous cases; and preceded by some observations on the method of improving the

diagnostic part of medicine. *London, Longman, Hurst, Rees, Orme and Browne, 1814.* Illus (5 plates). 8vo, 24 cms.

No more *Pathological researches* appear to have been published.

Book-stamp: Steeven's Hospital Med. & Surgical Library 1813 (*sic*).

A very rare book in which Fallot's tetralogy is described and portrayed before Peacock. A founder of Moorfields Hospital, the author is also known for Farre's tubercules of secondary deposits in the liver.

PEACOCK (THOMAS BEVILL) 1812–1882

795 On malformations of the human heart etc., with original cases and illustrations. 2nd ed. *London, J. Churchill, 1866.* xx pp., [8] ff., 204 pp. Illus (8 plates and legends), bibliog. (ftn. refs). 8vo, 23 cms.

Publisher's catalogue, January 1867 (40 pp.), bound in at end.

The first edition (1858) was a smaller work and soon became out of print. The second edition was revised and enlarged and the bibliography expanded. It was the standard work on congenital heart disease for many years.

Peacock was physician to the City of London Hospital for Diseases of the Chest (Victoria Park Hospital) and to St. Thomas's Hospital. He showed many specimens at the Pathological Society of London and presented most of his collection to the Royal College of Surgeons where it was destroyed by bombing in the Second World War. His library is preserved at the Institute of Diseases of the Chest.

BISHOP (PATRICK JAMES) *b.* 1926

796 Thomas Bevill Peacock, 1812–1882: a brief sketch of his life. A brief account of the Peacock Collection.

In *Bulletin of the Library of the Institute of Diseases of the Chest*, 1960, **5**, no. 2, 6–14. Life, pp. 6–8, Collection, pp. 9–14.

Also enclosed is an autographed letter from the author to DEB, together with his: "Thomas Bevill Peacock's library", reprinted from *Circulation*, 1968, **38**, 1011–13. Author's signed presentation copy.

FÖHR (HERMANN)

797 Über stenose der arteria pulmonalis. Eine inaugural-Dissertation zur Erlangung der Doctorwürde in der Medicin und Chirurgie unter dem Praesidium von Dr. W. Griesinger. *Tübingen, Heinrich Laupp, 1859.* 24 pp. 8vo, 22 cms.

FOSTER (BALTHAZAR WALTER) 1st baron Ilkeston, 1840–1913

798 On patency of the foramen ovale, attended with cyanosis and a faint murmur synchronous with the first sound of the heart. *Dublin, John Falconer, 1863.* 16 pp. Bibliog. (ftn. refs). 8vo, 22 cms.

Reprinted from *Dublin quarterly Journal of medical Science*, 1863, 2nd series, **36**, 112–26.

Inscribed on title-page, "With the author's compts".

Deals with familial cyanosis, probably primary pulmonary hypertension.

ROKITANSKY (CARL) Freiherr von, 1804–1878

799 Die Defecte der Scheidewände des Herzens. Pathologisch-anatomische Abhandlung. *Wien, Wilhelm Braumuller, 1875.* [ix], 157 pp. Illus, bibliog. (ftn. refs). Folio, 33 cms.

Rokitansky, professor at Vienna, and co-worker of Skoda's, is best known for his *Handbuch der pathologischen anatomie* (1842–1846), but his book on septal defects is certainly one of his greatest contributions, and his account of atrial septal defect will never be out of date. It ranks as a milestone in the history of congenital heart disease.

VIERORDT (KARL HERMANN) 1853–1944

800 Die angeborenen Herzkrankheiten. *Wien, Alfred Hölder, 1898.* vi, 225 pp. Illus, tables bibliog. 8vo, 25 cms.

Vierordt was professor at Tübingen and his work on congenital heart disease was the first systematic treatise on the subject.

[*and*] SCHRÖTTER VON KRISTELLI (LEOPOLD VON) 1837–1908

Erkrankungen des Herzbeutels. *Wien, Alfred Hölder, 1894.* [iii], 84 pp. Diagr., bibliog. 8vo, 25 cms.

[*and*] Erkrankungen der Gefässe. *Wien, Alfred Hölder, 1901.* iii–x, 569 pp. Illus, diagrs. bibliog. 8vo, 25 cms.

These three items together comprise NOTHNAGEL (Carl Wilhelm Hermann) *Specielle Pathologie und Therapie.* Wien, Alfred Hölder, 1901. Band 15, Theil 2.

CARPENTER (GEORGE) 1859–1910

801 Congenital affections of the heart. *London, John Bale, 1894.* 103 pp. Illus, bibliog. (ftn. refs). 12mo, 18 cms.

Extracts from reviews (2 pp.) tipped in at end.
An early book on congenital heart disease after Peacock by a physician to the Evelina Hospital for Sick Children.

THÉREMIN (ÉMILE)

802 Études sur les affections congénitales du cœur. Planches. *Paris, Asselin & Houzeau, 1895.* 27 ff. Illus (27 plates, 245 figures). Folio, 35 cms.

The text was published separately; there is a copy in the library of the Royal Society of Medicine. The atlas portrays almost every known malformation. Théremin was physician to the Stray Children's Home at St. Petersburg, and examined all the specimens of congenital heart disease preserved there.

OSLER (Sir WILLIAM) 1849–1919 and McCRAE (THOMAS) 1870–1935

803 A System of medicine, by eminent authorities in Great Britain, the United States and the Continent; ed. by William Osler assisted by Thomas McCrae. Vol. 4: Diseases of the circulatory system. Diseases of the blood. Diseases of the spleen, thymus and lymph-glands. (Oxford Medical Publications). *London, Henry Frowde, Hodder & Stoughton, 1908.* ix, 17–865 pp. Illus, tables, diagrs, bibliog. (ftn. refs). 8vo, 25 cms.

This volume, which is notable for Maude Abbott's pioneer contribution on congenital heart disease (pp. 323–425), also contains contributions by Babcock, Osler, A. G. Gibson and others.

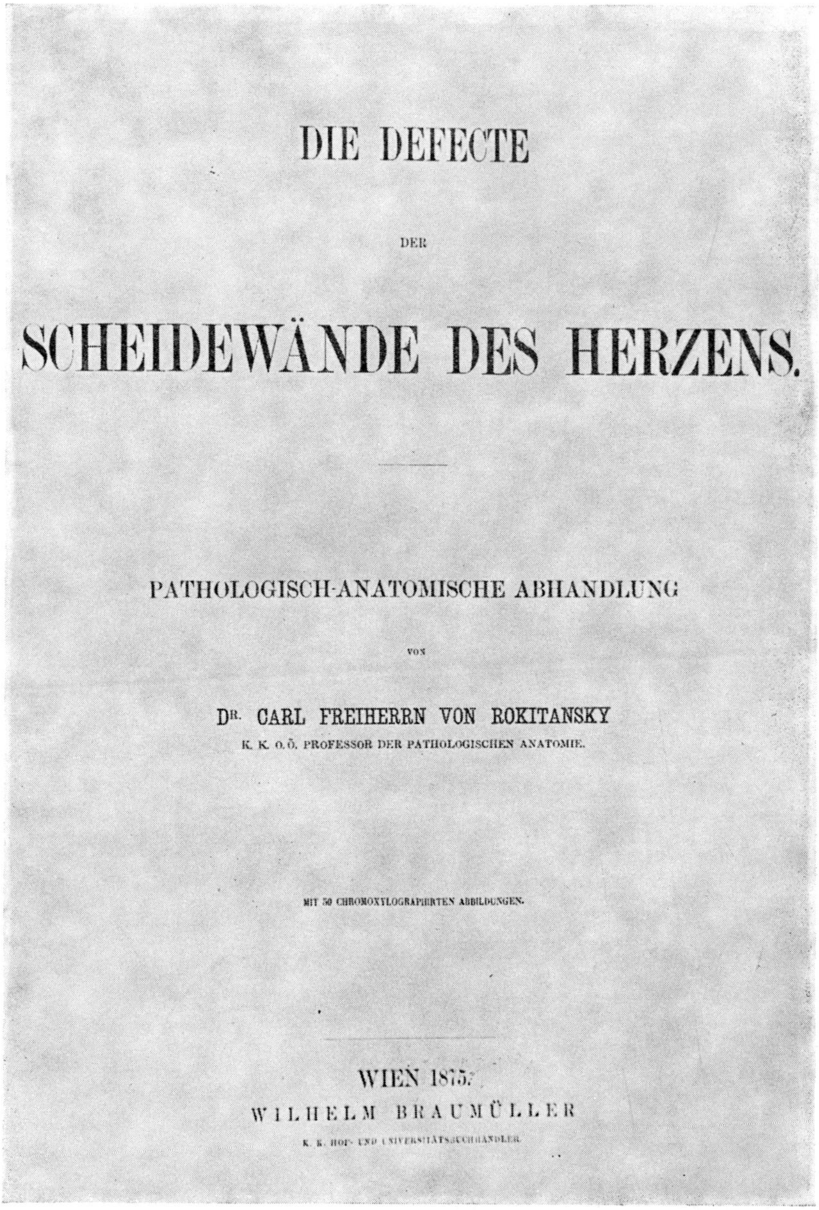

DIE DEFECTE

DER

SCHEIDEWÄNDE DES HERZENS.

PATHOLOGISCH-ANATOMISCHE ABHANDLUNG

VON

DR. CARL FREIHERRN VON ROKITANSKY

K. K. O. Ö. PROFESSOR DER PATHOLOGISCHEN ANATOMIE.

MIT 50 CHROMOXYLOGRAPHIRTEN ABBILDUNGEN.

WIEN 1875.

WILHELM BRAUMÜLLER

K. K. HOF- UND UNIVERSITÄTSBUCHHÄNDLER.

No. 799. A milestone in the history of congenital heart disease

MÖNCKEBERG (Johann Georg) 1877–1925

804 Herzmissbildungen; Ein Atlas angeborener Herzfehler in Querschnitten mit besonderer Berücksichtigung des Atrioventrikularsystems. *Jena, Gustav Fischer, 1912.* 7, [130] pp. Illus (65 plates with facing explanatory text). 4to, 28 cms.

Mönckeberg, professor of pathology at Giessen, was best known for his account of medial sclerosis of the arteries.

NOBÉCOURT (Pierre André Alexandre) 1871–1943

805 Cardiopathies de l'enfance. *Paris, O. Berthier, 1914.* xiv, 260 pp. Illus, diagrs. 8vo, 19 cms.

Publisher's advertisement (2 pp.) bound in at end.
Twelve conferences, two on congenital heart disease in which the term "tetralogie de Fallot" is used, possibly for the first time in French publications.

LAUBRY (Charles) 1872–1960 and PEZZI (Cesare) 1874–1945

806 Traité des maladies congénitales du cœur. Préface de Professeur Vaquez. *Paris, J. B. Baillière, 1921.* xv, 335 pp. Illus, diagrs, bibliog. 8vo, 25 cms.

Acquired 1926.
The first clinical treatise on congenital heart disease to include radiological and electrocardiographic findings. A landmark in this subject. Pezzi of Milan was working in Vaquez's clinic with Laubry.

BLUMENFELDT (Ernst)

807 Die Angeborenen Herz und Gefässkrankheiten.

Reprinted from: Kraus (Friedrich) 1858–1936 and Brusch (Theodor) 1878–1963. Spezielle *Pathologie und Therapie inneren Krankheiten.* Berlin u. Wien, Urban & Schwarzenberg, 1923. Band 4 [Herzkrankheiten], pp. 449–577. Illus, tables, diagrs, bibliog. (pp. 565–77, 530 refs).

ROESLER (Hugo) 1899–1961

808 Beitrage zur Lehre von den angeborenen Herzfehlern: [7 papers].

Reprinted from *Wiener Archiv fur innere Medizin,* 1928, **15,** pp. 487–94, 495–506, 507–20, 521–38; 1929, **16,** 463–82; 1930, **19,** 505–610; 1931, **21,** 271–84. Illus, tables, diagrs, bibliog.
Contents: 1. Über die Röntgenbefunde bei angeborenen Herz- Gefässmissbildungen ("Herzfehlern"). – 2. Untersuchungen zur Ätiologiefrage. – 3. Untersuchungen an einem Fall von Pulmonalstenose. – 4. Untersuchungen an zwei Fällen von Isthmusstenose der Aorta. – 5. (with W. Redisch) Kapillarstudien. – 6. Über die angeborene isolierte Rechtslage des Herzens. – 7. (and A. Kiss) Elektrokardiographische Untersuchungen an 100 Fällen.
The last two papers are signed by the author. Includes Roesler's monograph on dextrocardia (6) and the coarctation of the aorta (4) describing erosions of the ribs in radiographs for the first time.

809 Interatrial septal defect. *Chicago, American Medical Association, 1934.* 42 pp. Illus, tables, bibliog. 4to, 26 cms.

Reprinted from *Archives of internal Medicine,* 1934, **54,** 339–80.
A classic account of atrial septal defect giving the clinical and radiological findings.
Hugo Roesler, born in Vienna, graduated M.D. at the University there in 1923 and was radiologist and physician at the "Herzstation" (Heart Hospital and Polyclinic Hospital) under Rudolf Kaufmann

from 1924 to 1930. A Rockefeller research fellowship (New York University and Boston, 1930–1931) took him to the U.S.A., where he became associate professor of radiology and cardiology at Temple University School of Medicine, Philadelphia from 1932. He compiled *An Atlas of electrocardiography* with Evan Fletcher (Bristol, Wright, 1963) which was published posthumously.

DRESSLER (WILHELM) *b.* 1890 and ROESLER (HUGO) 1899–1961

810 Vorhofseptumdefekt kombiniert mit Mitralstenose und aurikulärem Leberpuls.

Reprinted from *Zeitschrift fur klinische Medizin*, 1930, **112**, 421–36. Illus, diagrs, bibliog.
An important early account of Lutembacher's disease.

ABBOTT (MAUDE ELIZABETH SEYMOUR) 1869–1940

811 Atlas of congenital cardiac disease. *New York, American Heart Association, 1936.* x, 62 pp. Illus, ports, table, diagrs. Folio, 36 cms.

MACDERMOT (HUGH ERNEST) 1888–1963?

812 Maude Abbott; a memoir. *Toronto, Macmillan, 1941.* xiii, 264 pp. Ports, bibliog. 8vo, 22 cms.

Provenance: "From Palmer 1942" (pencilled note on fly-leaf).
Maude Abbott became curator of the McGill Museum in 1899, after two years in Vienna, and was invited by Osler to contribute the section on congenital heart disease in his *System of medicine*. She collected all possible published cases with post-morten diagnosis, and gave an analysis of 412 cases in 1908, later increased to 1000 cases. At the start she was a pathologist, but later became interested in the clinical aspects and in 1929 she spent a time at the Herzstation, Vienna, with Roesler and Dressler. For many years her statistical analysis was a standard reference work.

STANCANELLI (GIOACCHINO)

813 Le Malattie congenite di cuore. *Napoli, Alberto Morano, 1936.* xiii, 460 pp. Illus, tables, bibliog. 8vo, 25 cms.

Acquired 1947. Extensive bibliography, pp. 404–60.

BEDFORD (DAVIS EVAN) *b.* 1898 and BROWN (JAMES WILLIAM) 1897–1958

814 Heart diseases. I.—Congenital diseases. (Butterworth's Medical Publications). *London, Butterworth, 1937.* [i], 206–33 pp. Illus, diagrs, bibliog. 8vo, 25 cms.

Reprinted from *British encyclopaedia of medical practice;* ed. by Sir Humphrey Rolleston, 1937, vol. 6, pp. 206–33.
A concise clinical review of contemporary knowledge of congenital heart disease.

BROWN (JAMES WILLIAM) 1897–1958

815 Congenital heart disease. *London, John Bale, 1939.* xvi, 255 pp. Illus, tables, diagrs, bibliog. 8vo, 23 cms.

Signed presentation copy from author to DEB "with many thanks for thoughts, and valued help in these & other problems—Sept. 22.39."

816 *The same.* 2nd ed. *London, New York, Staples Press, 1950.* xiii, 344 pp. Illus, tables, diagrs, bibliog. 8vo, 23 cms.

Signed presentation copy from the author.

BROWN (JAMES WILLIAM)

817 *The same.* Enfermedades cardiacas congenitas; edición corregida y aumentada por el autor, traducida del inglés por . . . Rodolfo Kreutzer y . . . José Enrique Mosquera. *Buenos Aires, A. Bini; London, Staples Press, 1948.* xviii, 353 pp. Illus, tables, diagrs, bibliog. 8vo, 23 cms.

Author's signed presentation copy.

BEDFORD (DAVIS EVAN) *b.* 1898 and MUIR (DAVID CLARK) *b.* 1931

818 James William Brown. *London, British Medical Association, 1959.* [i], 284–8 pp. Port., bibliog. 8vo, 25 cms.

Reprinted from *British Heart Journal*, 1959, **21**, 284–8.

Brown did most of his work for this book while in general practice in Grimsby, Lincolnshire, where he became pathologist to the hospital, and organised school clinics for children with heart disease in Lincolnshire and worked with Muir in Hull. He was a most versatile man, drew many of the figures in his book and followed almost every case of congenital heart disease in Lincolnshire. Later he abandoned general practice for consulting work, and became regional cardiologist at Sheffield. His book was the most important on congenital heart disease after that of Laubry and Pezzi (1921).

SCHNITKER (MAURICE ARTHUR) *b.* 1905

819 The Electrocardiogram in congenital cardiac disease: a study of 109 cases, 106 with autopsy. *Cambridge, Mass., Harvard University Press, 1940.* [xi], 147 pp. Diagrs, bibliog. 8vo, 25 cms.

Acquired 1944.

820 Congenital anomalies of the heart and great vessels. *New York, Oxford University Press, 1952.* xxiii, 306 pp. Illus, tables, diagrs, bibliog. 8vo, 24 cms.

TAUSSIG (HELEN BROOKE) *b.* 1898

821 Congenital malformations of the heart. *New York, Commonwealth Fund, 1947.* xxxvi, 618 pp. Illus, diagrs, bibliog. 4to, 26 cms.

Acquired 1948. Taussig conceived the idea of anastomosing the subclavian artery to the pulmonary circulation to improve the blood supply to the lungs; the operation was carried out by Alfred Blalock in 1944, and is now known as the Blalock-Taussig operation.

CONGENITAL ANOMALIES

822 Congenital anomalies of the heart and great vessels: clinicopathologic study of 132 cases, by Thomas J. Dry [and others]. (American Lecture Series no. 47). *Springfield, Ill., Charles C. Thomas, 1948.* xiii, 68 pp. Illus, ports, diagrs (tracings), bibliog. 4to, 28 cms.

ŠIKL (HEŘMAN)

823 Vrozené Malformace Srdce. *V. Praze, Ceskoslovenská Kardiologická Společnost, 1948.* vi, 113 pp. Illus, bibliog. 8vo, 25 cms.

Sikl was professor of pathological anatomy at Prague.

COURNAND (ANDRÉ) *b.* 1895, and others

824 Cardiac catheterization in congenital heart disease: a clinical and physiological study in infants and children, by André Cournand, Janet S. Baldwin [and] Aaron Himmelstein. *New York, Commonwealth Fund, 1949.* viii, 108 pp. Illus, diagrs, bibliog. 4to, 29 cms.

MANNHEIMER (EDGAR) *b.* 1904

825 Morbus Caeruleus: an analysis of 114 cases of congenital heart disease with cyanosis, by S. Eek [and others]; ed. by E. Mannheimer. (Bibliotheca Cardiologica, fasc. 4). *Basel, New York, S. Karger, 1949.* 332 pp. Illus, tables, diagrs, bib iog. 8vo, 25 cms.

The text covers history, embryology, radiology, cardiac catheterisation and surgical treatment.

GRAVIER (JEAN) *b.* 1921

826 La "position accroupie" (squatting posture des auteurs americains) dans les cardiopathies congenitales. (Lyon [Université]. Faculté [mixte] de médecine et de pharmacie. Thèse, 1949/50, no. 176). *Lyon, Camille Annequin, 1950.* 115 pp. Illus, diagrs, bibliog. 8vo, 24 cms.

Author's signed presentation copy, 17.9.52.
A useful review of squatting based on 149 cases from Santy's Surgical Clinic in Lyon.

WOOD (PAUL HAMILTON) 1907–1962

827 Congenital heart disease. (St. Cyres Lecture, 1950). *London, British Medical Association, [1950].* 15 pp. Illus (plates), tables. 4to, 28 cms.

Reprinted from *British medical Journal*, 1950, **2**, 639–47, 693–8.
Presentation copy to DEB signed by the author.
An important review of modern techniques of investigation of congenital heart disease.

DE GROOT (J. W. C.)

828 Angiocardiography as a diagnostic aid in congenital heart disease. *Amsterdam, Keesing, 1951.* 108 pp. Illus (plates pp. 90–108), bibliog. 8vo, 25 cms.

Errata slip inserted.
A study of patients at Birmingham Children's Hospital and the University Clinic of Paediatrics, Amsterdam.

LEQUIME (JEAN) and CHARLIER (R.)

829 Clinique et physiopathologie des cardiopathies congénitales opérables. *Bruxelles, Acta Medica Belgica, 1951.* 115 pp. Illus, tables, diagrs, bibliog. 8vo, 24 cms.

Reprinted from *Association belge de chirurgie congrès annuel, 5e*, Bruxelles, 1951. pp. 1–115.
Signed presentation copy to DEB from Lequime.

LEVY (ROBERT LOUIS) 1888–1974

830 Disorders of the heart and circulation; ed. by Robert L. Levy. *New York, Thomas Nelson, 1951.* xv, 944 pp. Illus, tables, diagrs, bib iog. 8vo, 25 cms.

Maude Abbott's original contribution to Nelson's *Loose-leaf medicine* on congenital heart disease is reprinted in this volume (pp. 125–239), which also contains "The physiology of congenital heart disease", by Richard J. Bing (pp. 241–99), and "The Surgical therapy of congenital cardio-vascular defects", by George H. Humphreys (pp. 301–12).

SOULIÉ (PIERRE LOUIS JEAN) 1903–1970

831 L'Angiocardiographie dans le diagnostic des cardiopathies congénitales (à propos de 200 examens), par P. Soulié, A. Piton et M. Touche.

Reprinted from *Archives des Maladies du Cœur*, 1951, **44**, 1057–87. Illus, bibliog. Signed presentation copy from P. Soulié.

832 Cardiopathies congénitales, par P. Soulié avec la collaboration de J. Baillet [and others]. *Paris, Expansion Scientifique Française, [1952]*. 347 pp. Illus, tables, diagrs, bibliog. 4to, 28 cms.

Author's signed presentation copy. Profusely illustrated, with good classified bibliography, pp. 333–45.

SPITZER (ALEXANDER) 1868–1943

833 The Architecture of normal and malformed hearts; a phylogenetic theory of their development; by Alexander Spitzer. With a summary and analysis of the theory by Maurice Lev and Aloysius Vass. *Springfield, Ill., C. C. Thomas, 1951.* xviii, 145 pp. Illus, ports. 8vo, 24 cms.

Translated from the article: "Über den Bauplan des normalen und missbildeten Herzens. Versuch einer phylogenetischen Theorie" in *Virchows Archiv für pathologische Anatomie*, 1923, **243**, 81–201.

Acquired 1952. Spitzer was professor of anatomy at Vienna and wrote in difficult German. His theory of lack of the normal torsion resulting in transposition of the great vessels created much interest and opposition. The translation made in 1936 was shown to Maude Abbott. Spitzer had been assistant to Tandler, author of an important anatomy of the heart.

CAHEN (POL)

834 Angiocardiographie et cathétérisme cardiaque; étude critique de leur apport au diagnostic des cardiopathies congénitales. *Paris, G. Doin, 1952.* xvi, 188 pp. Illus, tables, diagrs, bibliog. 8vo, 24 cms. 188 pp.

Author's signed presentation copy.

CARDIOLOGIA PRATICA

835 Malattie congenite dell'apparato cardio-vascolare. *Firenze, Edizione Cardiologia pratica, [1952]*. 276 pp. Illus, tables, diagrs, bibliog. 8vo, 24 cms.

Signed presentation copy to DEB from the editor, Giuseppe Agostoni.

The whole of this issue of *Cardiologia pratica* (1952, vol. 3, no. 1–2, Febbraio–Aprile) is devoted to congenital cardiovascular disease. Agostoni followed Pezzi at Milan and was in charge of the "Cesare Pezzi" Department of Cardiology. Pezzi was co-author with Laubry of an early treatise on congenital heart disease (no. 806).

DONZELOT (ÉDOUARD AUGUSTE EUGÈNE) 1884–1960 and GAUDART D'ALLAINES (FRANÇOIS LOUIS PAUL DE) *b.* 1892

836 Traité des cardiopathies congénitales, sous la direction de E. Donzelot [et] F. d'Allaines, par R. Heim de Balsac [and others]. *Paris, Masson, 1954.* viii, 1116 pp. Illus, tables, diagrs, bibliog. 4to, 28 cms.

Signed presentation copy to DEB from Heim de Balsac, 10 Dec. 1953.

This monumental review of the subject at this time came from the Centre des Enfants Bleus at the Hôpital Broussais in Paris. Raymond Heim de Balsac (*b.* 1903), one of the chief contributors to this volume, succeeded Chaperon as radiologist in Laubry's clinic at the Broussais, where later the centre for congenital heart disease was established.

BROCK OF WIMBLEDON (RUSSELL CLAUDE BROCK) baron, *b.* 1903

837 The Anatomy of congenital pulmonary stenosis. *London, Cassell, 1957.* xiii, 114 pp. Illus, ports, diagrs, bibliog. 8vo, 25 cms.

Also published by Hoeber [London, 1957].

Deals with embryology, anatomy of right ventricle, varieties of pulmonary stenosis and direct operations.

GASUL (BENJAMIN MORRIS) *b.* 1898, and others

838 The Salient points and the value of venous angiocardiography in the diagnosis of the cyanotic types of congenital malformations of the heart: a ten year study of 421 angiocardiograms done on 283 patients, by Benjamin M. Gasul [and others]. *Springfield, Ill., C. C. Thomas, 1957.* x, 80 pp. Illus, tables, bibliog. 8vo, 24 cms.

KEITH (JOHN DOW) *b.* 1908, and others

839 Heart disease in infancy and childhood, by John D. Keith, Richard D. Rowe [and] Peter Vlad. *New York, Macmillan, 1958.* xv, 877 pp. Illus, tables, diagrs, bibliog. 4to, 26 cms.

Contents include special contributions from J. W. A. Duckworth (Embryology of congenital heart disease, pp. 106–28), Irene Uchida (Familial occurrence of congenital heart disease, pp. 129–32, and Familial incidence of rheumatic fever and rheumatic heart disease, pp. 645–50), and W. T. Mustard and F. G. Dolan (Pre- and post-operative care, pp. 845–50).

Keith was in charge at the Cardiac Clinic, Hospital for Sick Children, Toronto, and an authority on congenital heart disease who, like Mustard, devised the surgical correction of transposition of the great vessels.

ESPINO VELA (JORGE)

840 Malformationes cardiovasculares congénitas. *Mexico, [Instituto Nacional di Cardiología], 1959.* xv, 389 pp. Illus, tables, diagrs, bibliog. 8vo, 25 cms.

Important book on congenital heart disease from the National Institute of Cardiology, Mexico.

FABRICIUS (JORGEN)

841 Isolated pulmonary stenosis: signs and symptoms, course and results of operation in 75 cases, diagnosed at cardiac catheterization; [trans. from the Danish by Axel Andersen]. *Copenhagen, Munksgaard, 1959.* 203 pp. Illus, tables, diagrs, bibliog. 8vo, 24 cms.

Summary in Danish and English (pp. 165–81).

Presentation copy to DEB signed by Professor Erik Warburg and the author.

GUY'S HOSPITAL REPORTS

842 Guy's Hospital Reports. Special number devoted to cardiovascular diseases; [ed. by Sir Russell Brock], 1959, vol. 108, nos. 2 and 3. *London, Guy's Hospital, 1959.* viii, 101–402. Illus, tables, diagrs, bibliog. 8vo, 25 cms.

Autograph: "Best wishes Jane S." (Jane Somerville, F.R.C.P.).

Contains important papers on Fallot's tetralogy, atrial septal defect, aorto-pulmonary defect, coarctation of aorta, and hypothermia by venous cooling.

GROSSE-BROCKHOFF (Franz) *b.* 1907, and others

843 Angeborene Herz und Gefässmissbildungen, von F. Grosse-Brockhoff, F. Loogen und A. Schaede.

Reprinted from *Handbuch der inneren Medizin.* 4 Aufl., herausgegeben von G. von Bergmann [and others]. Berlin, Gottingen and Heidelberg, Springer, 1960. Band 9, pp. 105–652. Illus, tables, diagrs, bibliog. 8vo, 25 cms.

Signed presentation copy from F. Grosse-Brockhoff to DEB

A comprehensive work covering all aspects of congenital heart disease with a classified bibliography of 57 pages.

HAHN (Charles), and others

844 Chirurgie du cœur, par Chs Hahn, A. G. Brom et J. Nauta (Fortschritte der Kardiologie/ Advances in Cardiology/Progrès en Cardiologie, vol. 3). *Bale (Suisse) [et] New York, S. Karger, 1962.* x, 398 pp. Illus, tables, diagrs, bibliog. 8vo, 25 cms.

Foreword and summary (pp. 387–92) in French and English.

Important in regards to congenital heart disease, reporting experience in the Leyden Clinic and including an embryological section by J. Dankmeijer and Los, clinical account by H. A. Snellen, and surgical by Brom. Other contributors are named in the avant-propos.

SHERMAN (Frank Edward) *b.* 1914

845 An Atlas of congenital heart disease; compiled from the Museum of Congenital Heart Disease at Children's Hospital of Pittsburgh. *London, Henry Kimpton, 1963.* 303 pp. 303 pp. Illus, tables, diagrs, bibliog. 4to, 26 cms.

Also published in Philadelphia, Lea & Febiger, 1963.

MICHEL (Dieter)

846 Angeborene Herzfehler; Auskultation, Phonokardiographie Differentialdiagnose. *Berlin, Gottingen, Heidelberg, Springer, 1964.* xii, 302 pp. Tables, diagrs, bibliog. 8vo, 25 cms.

Deals mainly with auscultation and phonocardiography; bibliography with 130 references.

CONDORELLI (Mario)

847 Sulla diagnosi del canale atrio-ventricolare comune.

Reprinted from *Medicina clinica e sperimentale*, 1966, **16**, 101–87. Illus, tables, diagrs, bibliog.

Signed presentation copy from the author.

SELLORS (Sir Thomas Holmes) *b.* 1902

848 Atrial septal defects. (Bradshaw Lecture at Royal College of Surgeons of England, 1969). [*London, Royal College of Surgeons of England, 1969*]. 21 pp. Illus, tables, diagrs. 8vo, 24 cms.

Reprinted from *Annals of the Royal College of Surgeons of England*, 1970, **46**, 1–19.

Author's signed presentation copy inscribed "Evan, without whose skill and help this exercise would not have been possible, Holmes."

A review of 538 cases of atrial septal defect treated surgically.

SOCIETÀ ITALIANA DI CARDIOLOGIA. Congresso 29, Bari, 1968.

849 Atti della Società Italiana di Cardiologia. Vol. 1: Simposii. *Roma, [Società Italiana di Cardiologia], 1970.* 402 pp. Illus, port, facsim., tables, diagrs, bibliog. 8vo, 24 cms.

The President of the Society was Professor Luigi Condorelli, (*b.* 1899), also moderator of the first symposium "Sindromi da errori disembriogenetici degli archi aorbici", pp. 19–288; the second symposium "Censimento campione su base nazionalle delle cardioangiopatie acquisite e congenite", pp. 289–400, had Professor G. Bossa for moderator.

History

HEINRICH (HAHNE)

850 Die Geschichte der angeborenen Herzkrankheiten. *Düsseldorf, G. H. Nolte, 1937.* [vii], 96 pp. Bibliog. 8vo, 22 cms.

Autograph: "James W. Brown, 18.x.38" (James William Brown, 1897–1958, M.D., F.R.C.P.).
A valuable and comprehensive history of congenital heart disease covering cyanosis, foetal endocarditis and the various malformations.

ANATOMY, PHYSIOLOGY, AND PATHOLOGY

Anatomy

The important works on cardiac anatomy are those by Tandler (no. 866) and Walmsley (no. 872). On special subjects, Cyon, Lee and Scarpa deal with the nerves, Gross and Spalteholz with the arteries, and Tawara with the conducting system.

THEBESIUS (ADAM CHRISTIAN) 1686–1731

851 Dissertatio medica de circulo sanguinis in corde. Editio nova correctior. *Lugduni Batavorum, apud Joh. Arnold. Langerak, 1716.* 31, [1] pp. Illus (folding plate, 2 figures). 8vo, 21 cms.

First edition, Lugduni Batavorum, A. Elzevier 1708. Garrison and Morton 763. The original account of the Thebesian circulation.

SCARPA (ANTONIO) 1747–1832

852 Engravings of the cardiac nerves, the nerves of the ninth pair, the glosso-pharyngeal and the pharyngeal branch of the pneumogastric; copied from the *Tabulae neurologicae* of Antonio Scarpa by Edward Mitchell, engraver, with a letterpress description translated from the original Latin by Dr. Knox. 2nd ed. *Edinburgh, Maclachlan & Stewart, 1829.* [95 pp., various paging]. Illus (20 engraved plates and 7 supplementary plates). 4to, 29 cms.

Description of each plate separately paginated. Heart nerves plates II-VI.
The *Tabulae neurologicae* were published in 1794.

LEE (ROBERT) 1793–1877

853 On the ganglia and nerves of the heart.

Reprinted from *Philosophical Transactions of the Royal Society of London*, 1849, **139**, 43–8. Illus (plates).

Lee studied anatomy in Paris, but eventually practised obstetrics and was physician to St. George's Hospital.

BRAUNE (CHRISTIAN WILHELM) 1831–1892

854 An Atlas of topographical anatomy after plane sections of frozen bodies, with 46 woodcuts in text; trans. by Edward Bellamy, F.R.C.S. *London, J. & A. Churchill, 1877*. xii, 200 pp. Illus (34 plates, additional figures). 4to, 27 cms.

Autograph: Edward J. Sidebotham (1860(?)–1929, assistant demonstrator in anatomy at Cambridge, later in practice at Bowdon, Cheshire).

Contains useful cross-section of the thorax (plates Ia, XI–XV, XXV–XXIXa covering the heart and coronary vessels).

Original entitled *Topographisch-anatomischer Atlas. Nach Durchschnitten an gefrorenen Cadavern*. Leipzig, Veit u. Comp., 1867–1872. American edition, Philadelphia, Lindsay & Blakiston, 1877.

SIBSON (FRANCIS) 1814–1876

855 Medical anatomy; or illustrations of the relative position and movements of the internal organs. *London, John Churchill, 1869*. [vii], 44 pp. (i.e. 88 columns). Illus (21 col. plates). Folio, 50 cms.

Issued originally in 7 fascicules.

Autograph: Walter T. Clegg, F.R.C.S.

This copy belonged to Walter Thomas Clegg, F.R.C.S. (1859–1919), surgeon of St. Paul's Eye Hospital, Liverpool, and was mounted on linen and bound in buckram for him, with many inserted anatomical figures. Plates 19–21 on movements, structure and sounds of the heart. Sibson was physician to St. Mary's Hospital and was much cited for his work on pericardial effusion.

SÉE (MARC DANIEL) 1827–1912

856 Recherches sur l'anatomie et la physiologie du cœur, spécialement au point de vue du fonctionnement des valvules auriculoventriculaires. *Paris, G. Masson, 1883*. 86 pp. Illus. (4 plates), bibliog. (ftn. refs). Folio, 32 cms.

First edition, Paris, G. Masson, 1875.

An early important work on the anatomy and functioning of the A-V valves. Cited by Richet.

BENEKE (FRIEDRICH WILHELM) 1824–1882

857 Ueber das Volumen des Herzens und die Umfänge der grossen Arterien des Menchen, in den verschiedenen Lebensaltern. Beiträge zur Physiologie und Pathologie des Menschen. *Cassel, Theodor Kay, 1881*. 56, 48, 64 pp. Tables, diagrs (plates). 4to, 29 cms.

Reprinted from *Schriften der Gesellschaft zur Beförderung der gesammten Naturwissenschaften zu Marburg*, 1879, Bd. 11, Supplementhefte 2, 3, 4. Contents: 1st part (Heft 2): Ueber das Volumen des Herzen und die Weite der Arteria pulmonalis und Aorta ascendens in den verschiedenen Lebensaltern. Ein Beitrag zur Lehre vom Blutdruck, von der Pubertätsentwickelung und Senescenz, sowie zur Pathologie der Carcinome; 2nd part (Heft 3): Ueber die Weite der iliacae communes, subclaviae und carotides communes in den verschiedenen Lebensaltern. Ein zweiter Beitrag . . .; pp. 9–12 are misbound in front of this part; 3rd part (Heft 4): Ueber die Weite der aorta thoracica und aorta abdominalis in den vershiedenen Lebensaltern. Ein dritter Beitrag . . . .

Book-stamp: University Museum, Radcliffe Library, Oxford, 26 Nov [18]80 (*sic*). Bodl[eian] Lib[rary] cancelled.

Tables of measurements made by Beneke in Marburg and Vienna.

KREHL (Ludolf von) 1861–1937

858 Beiträge zur Kenntniss der Füllung und Entleerung des Herzens. *Leipzig, S. Hirzel, 1891.* [i], 24 pp. Illus (plates), bibliog. 4to, 28 cms.

Reprinted from *Abhandlungen der mathematisch—physischen Classe der königlischen sachsischen Gesellschaft der Wissenschaften*, 1891, **17**, 339–63. Seven coloured plates of the anatomy of the heart cavities, with facing explanations. Double pagination (pp. 1–24 inner margin and journal paging).

Provenance: Bodleian Library Oxford [18]91—cancelled.

KEITH (Sir Arthur) 1866–1955

859 Human embryology and morphology. 3rd ed. *London, Edward Arnold, 1913.* viii, 475 pp. Illus, diagrs, bibliog. 8vo, 22 cms.

Publisher's catalogue (8 pp.) bound in at end. Autograph: W.D.S.

First edition, 1901; second edition, 1904; fourth edition, 1921; fifth edition, 1933; sixth edition, 1948.

Chapter 17 (pp. 281–323) deals with the circulatory system including the atrial septum, the Keith-Flack node, and the bulbus cordis on which Keith made notable contributions to congenital heart disease.

KEITH (Sir Arthur) 1866–1955 and FLACK (Martin William) 1882–1931

860 The Form and nature of the muscular connections between the primary divisions of the vertebrate heart.

Reprinted from *Journal of Anatomy and Physiology*, 1907, **41**, 172–89. Illus, bibliog. 8vo, 25 cms.

Garrison and Morton 844. This papers describes their discovery of the sino-auricular node (Keith-Flack node), and confirms Tawara's work on the conducting tissues.

ZUCKERKANDL (Emil) 1849–1910

861 Atlas der topographischen Anatomie des Menschen. *Wien und Leipzig, Wilhelm Braumüller, 1904.* [viii], 845 pp. Illus (636 figures). 8vo, 25 cms.

Figures 240–67 cover the heart and lungs. Zuckerkandl was professor of anatomy at Vienna.

CYON (Élie de) 1843–1912

862 Les Nerfs du cœur; anatomie et physiologie; avec une préface sur les rapports de la médecine avec la physiologie et la bactériologie. *Paris, Félix Alcan, 1905.* xxxiii, 255 pp. Illus, diagrs (tracings). 8vo, 25 cms.

Cyon worked with Ludwig in Leipzig where he first described the cardio-accelerator nerves and with Ludwig the depressor nerve (Nerve of Cyon). He was professor of physiology in St. Petersburg and wrote a treatise on physiology in Russian and many papers in German and French.

TAWARA (K. SUNAO) 1873–1938(?)

863 Das Reizleitungssystem des Säugetierherzens. Eine anatomisch-histologische Studie über das atrioventrikularbündel und die Purkinjeschen Fäden. Mit einem Vorwort von L. Aschoff. *Jena, Gustav Fisher, 1906.* ix, 200 pp. Illus (plates), bibliog. (ftn. refs). 8vo, 25 cms.

Tawara discovered the auriculoventricular node (node of Tawara) and described it in this book (Garrison and Morton 845).

CORNING (HANSON KELLY) 1861–1951

864 Lehrbuch der topographischen Anatomie, fur Studierende und Ärtze. 16. und 17. Aufl. *München, J. F. Bergmann, 1931.* xvi, 817 pp. Illus (677 figures), bibliog. 4to, 28 cms.

Thorax, pp. 248–341, includes section on heart and pericardium (pp. 283–97).
Corning was professor of anatomy at Basel and his classical book on topographical anatomy, first published 1907, is still unsurpassed; 24 Aufl. 1949.

FLACK (MARTIN WILLIAM) 1882–1931

865 An Investigation of the sino-auricular node of the mammalian heart.

Reprinted from *Journal of Physiology*, 1910, **41**, 64–77. Table, diagrs (tracings), bibliog. (ftn. refs).
Flack was demonstrator of physiology at the London Hospital and worked with Sir Arthur Keith. He died of bacterial endocarditis.

TANDLER (JULIUS) 1869–1936

866 Anatomie des Herzens. *Jena, Gustav Fisher, 1913.* viii, 292 pp. Illus, tables, diagrs (pp. 279–92). 4to, 26 cms.

Forms Bd **3**, Abt. 1 of BARDELEBEN (Karl Heinrich von). *Hanbuch der Anatomie des Menschen.*

GROSS (LOUIS) 1895–1937

867 The Blood supply to the heart, in its anatomical and clinical aspects. *London, H. Frowde and Hodder & Stoughton, 1921.* xvi, 171 pp. Illus (incl. 29 plates), tables, bibliog. 4to, 27 cms.

Also published New York, P. B. Hoeber, 1921.
A pioneer work on coronary arterial anatomy studied by radiography of the injected arteries by a standard technique. Gross studied under Horst Oertel (1873–1956), professor of pathology at McGill University and colleague of Maude Abbott.

KROGH (SCHACK AUGUST STEENBERG) 1874–1949

868 The Anatomy and physiology of capillaries (Silliman Memorial Lectures). *New Haven, Yale University Press, 1922.* xvii, 276 pp. Illus, tables, diagrs, bibliog. 8vo, 24 cms.

Autograph: Hector M. Walker (Hector Macdonald Walker, O.B.E., M.D.).
Krogh was a Nobel prizewinner for physiology in 1920.

MOUCHET (AIMÉ)

869 Les Artères coronaires du cœur chez l'homme. 2ᵉ ed. *Paris, Norbert Maloine, 1933.* 64 pp. Illus (17 plates), bibliog. Folio, 32 cms.

First edition, 1922. An important historical review and a detailed anatomical description based on study of 400 hearts by radio-opaque injection, corrosion methods and dissection. "Travaux du même auteur", pp. 5–8.

SPALTEHOLZ (KARL WERNER) 1861–1940

870 Die Arterien der Herzwand. Anatomische Untersuchungen an Menschen und Tierherzen, nebst Erörterung der Voraussetzungen für die Herstellung eines Kollateralkreislaufes. *Leipzig, S. Hirzel, 1924.* viii, 165 pp. Illus (15 plates, figures in text), diagrs, bibliog. 8vo, 25 cms.

Spalteholz worked on coronary arterial anatomy and published his results as early as 1907. His present monograph was completed in 1914, but publication was delayed by the war. He used gelatin coloured by dyes, and cleared the heart with alcohol and oil. He found that the coronary arteries were not end arteries anatomically.

GILIS (JEAN LOUIS PAUL MARIE ANTOINE) 1857–1929

871 Anatomie élémentaire des centres nerveux et du sympathique chez l'homme. *Paris, Masson, 1927.* 232 pp. Illus (35 figures), bibliog. (ftn. refs). 8vo, 20 cms.

Deuxième édition (with Jules Euzières, 1882–1971), Paris, Masson, 1932.

WALMSLEY (THOMAS) 1889–1951

872 The Heart. *London, Longmans, Green, 1929.* vii, 152 pp. 8vo, 25 cms.

Forms vol. 4, part 3 of QUAIN (Jones) 1795–1851. *Quain's Elements of anatomy.* 11th ed., ed. by Sir Edward Sharpey-Schafer, Johnson Symington [and] Thomas Hastie Bryce. London, New York and Toronto, Longmans, Green, 1908–1929.

Comparable with Tandler (no. 866) as a classic on cardiac anatomy.

JONES (EMYR WYN)

873 A Radiographic study of the coronary arteries in health and disease.

Reprinted from *Quarterly Journal of Medicine*, 1931, **24**, 199–217. Illus (plates), bibliog.

An important paper on radiography of the injected coronary vessels.

MAHAIM (IVAN) 1897–1965

874 Les Maladies organiques du faisceau de His—Tawara. Les syndromes coronaires—l'endocardite septale, l'infarctus septal. (Étude Clinique et Anatomique). *Paris, Masson, 1931.* vi, 595 pp. Illus, tables, diagrs, bibliog. 8vo, 24 cms.

Author's signed presentation copy.

A standard work on the subject in its day, with 1032 references. Mahaim worked for many years in Lausanne on the anatomy and histology of the A-V bundle, and mastered the technique of serial sections.

875 Les Nerfs du cœur. *Lausanne, Imprimeries Réunies, 1932.* 16 pp. 8vo, 22 cms.

"Hommage sympathetique, Mahaim."

Inaugural dissertation at Lausanne, 1932. Deals with the neurogenic and myogenic theories, the cardiac nerves and the special conduction system in the heart.

BOSCO (Guillermo Andrés) *b.* 1886

876 Diagnóstico anátomo-topográfico de la obstrucción arterial coronaria. *Buenos Aires, Artes Gráficas Modernas, 1935–1937.* 3 vols. Illus, tables, diagrs, bibliog. 4to, 28 cms.

Contents: [Vol 1], part 1: Descripción anatómica del sistema arterial coronario; part 2: Representación gráfica del sistema arterial coronario; [vol. 2], part 3: Los signos semiológicos topográficos de la obstrucción arterial coronaria; [vol. 3], part 4: El soplo merosistólico; parts 5 and 6, El frote pericárdico and La trombosis arterial subpericárdica izquierda como causa de la isquemia aguda del miocardio, are not in the library.

All volumes author's signed presentation copies to DEB.

Deals at length with the anatomy of the coronary arterial system, profusely illustrated by radio-opaque injections of the various branches, and describes the clinical syndromes resulting from their occlusion. A very useful bibliography.

SYMONDS (Sir Charles Putnam) *b.* 1890

877 The Circle of Willis. (Harveian Oration, 1954). *London, British Medical Association [1955].* 16 pp. Bibliog. 8vo, 22 cms.

Reprinted from *British medical Journal*, 1955, **1**, 119–24.

An important historical account of Willis's *Cerebri anatome*, and of his association with Lower and Wood at Oxford. Discusses carotid artery occlusion and the Circle of Willis.

HENRY (Edmond) *b.* 1910, and others

878 Les Cavités cardiaques. Introduction anatomique à la chirurgie intracardiaque, par E. Henry, R. Courbier et P. Rochu. *Paris, Masson, 1959.* xii, 176 pp. Illus, diagrs. 8vo, 25 cms.

Bought in Rome 1959. A very useful surgical anatomy of the heart.

Physiology

Books and papers dealing with cardiac output, nervous control, with Starling's *Law of the heart.*

PRIESTLEY (Joseph) 1733–1804

879 Experiments and observations on different kinds of air. *London, J. Johnson, 1775.* 2 vols. Illus (plates). 8vo, 22 cms.

Vol. 1 (2nd ed., corrected, 1775) [ii], xxiii, [iv], 324, [4] pp. Vol. 2, 1775, xliv, 399, [21] pp. In both volumes the last 3 pp. and 4 pp. respectively are a catalogue of books written by Priestley.

The arrangement of editions of this work is somewhat complex which explains the confusion in catalogues. Vol. 1 first appeared in 1774 (2nd ed., 1775; 3rd ed., 1781). Vol. 2 appeared in 1775 (2nd ed., 1784). Vol. 3 was added, 1777, vol. 4, 1779, vol. 5, containing an analysis of his previous researches, 1789, and vol. 6, 1786. Vols. 4–6 are entitled *Experiments and observations relating to various branches of natural philosophy, with a continuation of the observations on air.* Collections of volumes of this work are therefore quite often of different editions.

Priestley, a nonconformist minister, discovered oxygen, the significance of which was not realised until the researches of Lavoisier. Because his sympathies with the French revolutionaries led to riots in which his house and belongings were destroyed, Priestley fled from Birmingham and eventually died in America.

TIGERSTEDT (Robert Adolf Armand) 1853–1923

880 Die Physiologie des Kreislaufes. 2 Aufl. *Berlin und Leipzig, Walter de Gruyter, 1921.* Band 2. (viii, 478 pp.). Illus, tables, diagrs, bibliog. (ftn. refs). 4to, 27 cms.

This volume contains book 4 which deals with the innervation of the heart.

First published as *Lehrbuch der Physiologie des Kreislaufes.* (Leipzig, Veit, 1893). This second edition of this authoritative work was in process of appearance when Tigerstedt died. This Finnish physiologist was one of the many distinguished pupils of Carl Ludwig. His extensive writings cover mainly physiology of muscles and nerves, physiology of the circulation, and later respiration and metabolism.

BRAUN (Ludwig) 1867–1936

881 Über Herzbewegung und Herzstoss. *Jena, Gustav Fisher, 1898.* [v], 123 pp. Illus, (incl. 2 folding plates), bibliog. (ftn. refs.). 4to, 26 cms.

Garrison and Morton 838.

Describes the first employment of the cinematograph to record the cardiac changes during phases of the cardiac contraction. Excellent reproductions of films.

FERRIER (Sir David) 1843–1928

882 The Heart and nervous system: being the Harveian Oration . . . 1902. *London, John Bale, Sons & Danielsson, 1902.* 53 pp. Bibliog. (ftn. refs). 8vo, 23 cms.

An important early review of the nervous control of the heart.

ENGELMANN (Theodor Wilhelm) 1843–1909

883 Das Herz und seine Tätigkeit im Lichte neuerer Forschung. *Leipzig, Wilhelm Engelmann, 1904.* 44 pp. 8vo, 25 cms.

Previously published, Berlin, O. Lange, 1903.

GASKELL (Walter Holbrook) 1847–1914

884 The Involuntary nervous system. New ed. (Monographs on Physiology). *London, Longmans, Green, 1920.* ix, 178 pp. Illus, tables, diagrs, bibliog. 8vo, 23 cms.

First edition 1916. This new edition, published posthumously, was "reset without correction," March 1920, and was edited by his son, J. F. Gaskell.

Gaskell was a pupil of Sir M. Foster and had worked in Ludwig's laboratory. His book "sums up the life work of Gaskell, who laid the histological foundation of the modern study of the autonomic nervous system" (Garrison and Morton 1331). His original work on the myogenic theory of cardiac contraction was published in *Philosophical Transactions of the Royal Society of London*, 1882, **173**, 993–1033. Gaskell introduced the term "heart block."

STARLING (Ernest Henry) 1866–1927

885 The Linacre Lecture on the law of the heart, given at Cambridge, 1915. *London, Longmans, Green, 1918.* [iii], 27 pp. Illus, tables, diagrs. (tracings). 8vo, 23 cms.

From experiments with the "heart-lung preparation" Starling showed that the force of cardiac contraction depended on the length of the cardiac muscle fibre in diastole, which was influenced by the diastolic filling pressure.

HALDANE (JOHN SCOTT) 1860–1936

886 Respiration. (Silliman Memorial Lectures). *New Haven, Yale University Press; London, Humphrey Milford, Oxford University Press, 1922.* xviii, 427 pp. Illus, tables, diagrs, bibliog. (ftn. refs). 8vo, 24 cms.

Autograph: Basil Mott; book-stamp: Institution of Civil Engineers, duplicate.

Historical introduction and deals with nervous control of breathing, blood as carrier of O_2 and CO_2, oxygen want, effects of high altitude, etc. Covers 20 years of experimental work.

New edition (with John Gillies Priestly), Oxford, Clarendon Press, 1935.

WIGGERS (CARL JOHN) 1883–1963

887 Modern aspects of the circulation in health and disease. 2nd ed. *Philadelphia and New York, Lea & Febiger, 1923.* viii, 17–662 pp. Illus, tables, diagrs, bibliog. 8vo, 24 cms.

For long the standard work on the physiology of the circulation.

GRELLETY BOSVIEL (PIERRE) *b.* 1891

888 La Circulation veineuse périphérique: recherches physiologiques et cliniques basées sur la mesure de la pression veineuse. *Paris, Amédée Legrand, 1925.* 225 pp. Bibliog. 8vo, 25 cms.

Acquired 1926.

The author, a list of whose writings appears on pp.[11–12], was an interne of Villaret who was a pioneer in the study of venous pressure in France.

CLARK (ALFRED JOSEPH) 1885–1941

889 Comparative physiology of the heart. (Cambridge Comparative Physiology). *Cambridge, University Press, 1927.* [vii], 157 pp. Illus, tables, diagrs, bibliog. 8vo, 23 cms.

Deals with physiology of heart in cold-blooded and warm-blooded vertebrates, nervous control of heart, bodyweight, heart size, pulse rate, etc. An important reference work.

EYSTER (JOHN AUGUSTINE ENGLISH) 1881–1960

890 The Clinical aspects of venous pressure. (Macmillan Medical Monographs). *New York, Macmillan, 1929.* xiii, 135 pp. Illus, tables, diagrs, bibliog. 8vo, 23 cms.

In 1908, Eyster and Hooker described their apparatus for measuring venous pressure by indirect methods. A full bibliography (122 references) is given.

THOMAS (ANDRÉ ANTOINE HENRI) 1867–1963

891 Les Phénomènes de répercussivité. *Paris, Masson, 1929.* i–vi, 7–244 pp. Bibliog. 8vo, 23 cms.

Deals with vaso-motor and other autonomic nervous reactions, angina pectoris, claudication and vascular spasm. André-Thomas was one of the most prolific and versatile French neurologists. His remarkable thesis on the cerebellum appeared in 1897, and his monograph with Déjerine on diseases of the spinal cord is probably the best ever written. In his late seventies his work turned to the neuropsychology of the newborn and young infants.

SAINSBURY (HARRINGTON) 1855–1936

892 The Cardiac cycle. *Bristol, John Wright; London, Simpkin Marshall, 1931.* 79 pp. Diagr., bibliog. (ftn. refs). 8vo, 23 cms.

Sainsbury, physician to the Royal Free Hospital, was mainly interested in cardiology, and his book deals with the cardiac cycle, the pulse and its effect on the lymphatics.

GROLLMAN (ARTHUR) *b.* 1901

893 The Cardiac output of man in health and disease. *London, Baillière, Tindall & Cox, 1932.* xiv, 325 pp. Illus, tables, diagrs, bibliog. 4to, 26 cms.

American edition, Springfield, Ill., Charles C. Thomas, 1930. Contains an important bibliography of 28 pages (483 refs).

HEYMANS (CORNEILLE JEAN FRANÇOIS) 1892–1968, and others

894 La Sinus carotidien et la zone homologue cardio-aortique; physiologie, pharmacologie, pathologie, clinique, par C. Heymans, J. J. Bouckaert, et P. Regniers. *Paris, G. Doin, 1933.* 334 pp. Illus, tables, diagrs, bibliog. 8vo, 24 cms.

A summary of Heymans' researches at the University of Ghent since 1920. An earlier monograph was published in 1929. Heymans was awarded the Nobel Prize for his work on this subject. Full bibliography, pp. 305–25.

WHITE (JAMES CLARKE) *b.* 1895

895 The Autonomic nervous system: anatomy, physiology and surgical treatment. (Macmillan Surgical Monographs). *London, Henry Kimpton, 1935.* xvii, 386 pp. Illus, tables, diagrs, bibliog. 8vo, 24 cms.

Also published in New York, Macmillan, 1935. Second edition, with Reginald Hammerick Smithwick, New York, 1941.

J. C. White, professor at Harvard, worked in France with Leriche and Hovelacque, and gives an account of the anatomy and physiology of the autonomic nervous system, and of the various surgical procedures such as sympathectomy, paravertebral alcohol injections, etc., of which he was a pioneer.

LEQUIME (JEAN)

896 Le Débit cardiaque: études expérimentales et cliniques. *Paris, Masson, 1940.* ix, 223 pp. Tables, diagrs, bibliog. 8vo, 24 cms.

Also published in Liège, Thone, 1940, forming Supplement 107 of *Acta Medica Scandinavica.*
An excellent contemporary review of cardiac output.

Pathology

The foundation of cardiac pathology was Morgagni's *De sedibus* (nos. 898–900); Ziegler's *Lehrbuch* contains a classical description of acute cardiac infarction due to coronary occlusion. Davies's M.D. thesis introduces a new disease, endomyocardial necrosis (no. 913), and is profusely illustrated. DEB had identified this disease in Africans at the Cardiac Society with Konstam.

Important recent books are those by Gould (no. 914) and Hudson (no. 918).

HALLER (Albrecht von) 1708–1777

897 Pathological observations chiefly from dissections of morbid bodies. *London, D. Wilson and T. Durham, 1756.* viii, iii, 197, [2] pp. Illus, (3 folding plates), bibliog. (ftn. refs). 8vo, 21 cms.

Half-title (? pp. i–ii) wanting. First English edition of Haller's *Opuscula pathologica, partim recusa partim inedita quibus sectiones cadaverum morbosorum potissimum continentur.* Lausannae, Bosquet et soc., 1755. (Ed. nova, Lausannae, F. Grasset et soc. 1768).

MORGAGNI (Giovanni Battista) 1682–1771

898 De sedibus et causis morborum per anatomen indagatis libri quinque. Praefatus est S. A. D. Tissot. *Ebroduni in Helvetia, [n.p.], 1779.* 3 tom. Port., bibliog. (incl. ftn. refs). 4to, 28 cms.

Tom. 1: xxxvi, [iv], 544 pp.; tom. 2: [i], 583 pp.; tom. 3: viii, 547, [1] pp. Historia vitae et operum J. B. Morgagni, tom. 1, pp. vii–xxiv; lib. 2 on diseases of the thorax runs from tom. 1, p. 251 to tom. 2, p. 68.

Bookplate: unidentified coat of arms. This excellent edition of Morgagni's great work on pathology was edited by Simon André Tissot (1728–1797). First edition, folio, Venice, 1761.

899 *The same.* The Seats and causes of diseases investigated by anatomy; in five books, containing a great variety of dissections, with remarks. To which are added very accurate and very copious indexes of the principal things and names therein contained. Trans. from the Latin by Benjamin Alexander. *London, A. Millar, T. Cadell, Johnson and Payne, 1769.* 3 vols. Bibliog. (ftn. refs). 4to, 29 cms.

Vol. 1: xxxii, 868 pp.; vol. 2: iv [i.e. vi], 770 pp.; vol. 3: [vi], 604, [150] pp. Book 2, Of diseases of the thorax, containing letters 15–27, is in vol. 1, pp. 355–868.

Autograph (vol. 1 only): W. King 1818 (probably William King, M.A., M.D., F.R.C.P. 1786–1865, of Brighton, who was licensed to practice in 1817 by Cambridge University, was the Harveian Orator 1850, and an active member of Brighton and Sussex Medico-Chirurgical Society. He was, with Robert Owen, one of the founding fathers of the Co-operative Movement).

Book-stamp: Brighton & Sussex Med. Chir. Soc., also book-label with an extract from the regulations of the library.

Benjamin Alexander, M.D., L.R.C.P., the translator, 1735?–1768, "Used to say that he undertook the translation of Morgagni's work in consequence of a taunt from Sir George Baker, but the guinea per sheet from the bookseller was a more probable cause. He was a clever man, but vain of his talents." (Wadd, quoted in Munk, vol. 2, p. 270).

900 *The same.* Recherches anatomiques sur le siége et les causes des maladies. *Paris, Bureau de l'Encyclopédie, 1837.* 2 tom. en 1. Bibliog. (ftn. refs). 8vo, 22 cms.

Tom. 1: [i], ii, iv, 5–546 pp.; tom. 2: [iii], 559 pp. Contains the first 42 letters including those on diseases of the thorax.

This is Destoüet's French translation, first published Paris, Caille & Ravier, 1820–1824. 10 tom., reprinted for the *Encylopédie des sciences médicales. Collection des auteurs classiques.*

BAILLIE (Matthew) 1761–1823

901 The Morbid anatomy of some of the most important parts of the human body. 2nd ed. *London, J. Johnson & C. Nicol, 1797.* [iii], xxxvi, 460 pp. 8vo, 22 cms

Autograph: H. Cowen M.D., 41st Regts. (Henry Cowen, *d.* 1824).

Describes pericarditis, valvular disease, congenital malformation, cardiac aneurysm, etc. Baillie first stated that Pitcairn taught rheumatism as a cause of heart disease. He describes also complete transposition of the great vessels.

First edition, 1793 (RCP). Numerous other editions and translations are also in the RCP together with the atlas (*A series of engravings* . . . 1799–[1802]; 2nd ed., 1812).

902 The Works of Matthew Baillie. To which is prefixed an account of his life, collected from authentic sources by James Wardrop. *London, Longman, Hurst, Rees, Orme, Brown and Green, 1825.* 2 vols. Port. 8vo, 22 cms.

Vol. 1: lxxi, 237 pp.; vol. 2: lxxii, 407 pp., wanting.

Book-stamp: Malta Military Medical Library. Presented to DEB by Brigadier Morrison (William Kenneth Morrison, D.S.O., D.D.M.S., Malta) 1943.

CRUVEILHIER (JEAN) 1791–1874

903 Essai sur l'anatomie pathologique en général et sur les transformations et productions organiques en particulier. *Paris, Crochard, 1816.* 2 tom. Bibliog. (ftn. refs). 8vo, 20 cms.

Tom. 1: xxviii, 400 pp., half-title (? pp. i–ii) wanting; tom. 2: [iii], 461 pp.

This work preceded his illustrated *Anatomie pathologique du corps humain* . . ., Paris, J. B. Baillière, 1829–1842, and was an expansion of his thesis *Essai sur l'anatomie pathologique en général.* Paris, 1816, no. 18, v. 119.

HASSE (KARL EWALD) 1810–1902

904 An Anatomical description of the diseases of the organs of circulation and respiration; trans. and ed. by W. E. Swaine. *London, Sydenham Society, 1846.* xv, 400 pp. Bibliog. (ftn. refs). 8vo, 23 cms.

A translation of Hasse's *Specielle pathologische Anatomie.* Band. 1, *Anatomische Beschreibung der Krankheiten der Circulations—und Respirations—Organe.* Leipzig, W. Engelmann, 1841 (RCP).

Hasse revised and rewrote the section on heart diseases for this English edition. His work was done at Leipzig, but he was professor at Zurich in 1846. Covers lymphatics, veins and arteries and deals with pericarditis, carditis, endocarditis, cardiac rupture and fatty heart. Cardiac infarction had not been recognised by pathologists at this time. The translator, William Edward Swaine (1804–1868) was physician at the German Hospital.

ROKITANSKY (CARL) Freiherr von, 1804–1878

905 Lehrbuch der pathologischen Anatomie. 3 Aufl. *Wien, Wilhelm Braumüller, 1855–1861.* 3 Bde. Illus. 8vo, 24 cms.

Bd. 1: vii, 392 pp.; Bd. 2: [i], 513 pp. (contains section on the pathology of the heart, pp. 231–86); Bd. 3: [i], 558 pp. First edition as *Handbuch der pathologischen Anatomie.* Wien, Braumüller u. Seidel, 1842–1844–1846. 3 Bde.

Bookstamp: Docent Dr. Ludwig Braun, author of no. 881.

Also enclosed LESKY (Erna). An Unknown portrait—Rokitansky as Rector of Vienna University. Extract from *Ciba Symposium*, 1962, **10**, 194–7. Illus., port. (oil portrait by Anton Einsle).

WILKS (Sir SAMUEL) 1824–1911 and MOXON (WALTER) 1836–1886

906 Lectures on pathological anatomy. 3rd ed., revised by Samuel Wilks. *London, Longmans, Green, 1889.* xx, 672 pp. 8vo, 22 cms.

Contains pathological account of hypertrophy of heart in Bright's disease, including Bernheim's syndrome, and describes enlarged right heart and pulmonary artery without lung disease, probably primary pulmonary hypertension, in the section on diseases of the heart (pp. 103–47).

First edition (lectures delivered at Guy's Hospital during the summer sessions of 1857–1858) by Wilks, London, Longman [and others], 1859; second edition, with Moxon, London J. & A. Churchill, 1875.

COHNHEIM (Julius) 1839–1884

907 Untersuchungen ueber die embolischen Processe. *Berlin, August Hirschwald, 1872.* viii, 113 pp. Illus. (col. folding plate), bibliog. (ftn. refs). 8vo, 23 cms.

Garrison and Morton 3010. Cohnheim, professor of pathology at Kiel, in this classic described infarction and embolic abscesses, etc. "Cohnheim developed the doctrine of infarction as a result of occlusion of terminal arteries. He explained the haemorrhagic nature of certain infarcts on the basis of a reflux flow and diapedesis through the altered capillaries of the infarcted area." (Garrison and Morton).

ZIEGLER (Ernst) 1849–1905

908 Lehrbuch der speciellen pathologischen Anatomie. 6 Aufl. *Jena, Gustav Fischer, 1890.* xii, 3–1024 pp. 8vo, 24 cms.

This is Band 2 of his *Lehrbuch der allgemeinen pathologischen Anatomie* in which he describes myomalacia cordis due to coronary occlusion—the classic account of acute cardiac infarction—in the section on the heart (pp. 17–49).

First edition, 1881–1885; eleven editions (last 1905–1906) published by the same publisher.

First translated into English (*A Textbook of pathological anatomy and pathogenesis*), London, Macmillan, 1883–1886. 2 parts in 3 vols.

ASCHOFF (Karl Albert Ludwig) 1866–1942 and TAWARA (K. Sunao) 1873–1938?

909 Die heutige Lehre von den pathologisch-anatomischen Grundlagen der Herzschwäche; kritische Bemerkungen auf Grund eigener Untersuchungen. *Jena, Gustav Fisher, 1906.* [iii], 79 pp. Tables. 8vo, 24 cms.

Deals with the pathology of the myocardium, rheumatic valvular disease, lung disease, acute infections, anaemia, syphilis, etc.

LIBMAN (Emanuel) 1872–1946 and SACKS (Benjamin) *b.* 1896

910 A Hitherto undescribed form of valvular and mural endocarditis. *Chicago, American Medical Association, 1924.* 39 pp. Illus, tables. 4to, 26 cms.

Reprinted from *Archives of internal Medicine*, 1924, **33**, 701–37.

Garrison and Morton 2855. This is the original account of Libman-Sacks disease, often complicated by pericarditis, later regarded as a variety of systemic lupus erythematosus.

CABOT (Richard Clarke) 1868–1939

911 Facts on the heart. *Philadelphia and London, W. B. Saunders, 1926.* [i], 9–781 pp. Illus, tables, diagrs. 8vo, 25 cms.

A classic work which will never become out of date.

BLUMGART (HERRMAN LUDWIG) *b.* 1895, and others

912 Studies on the relation of the clinical manifestations of angina pectoris, coronary thrombosis, and myocardial infarction to the pathologic findings, by Herrman L. Blumgart, Monroe J. Schlesinger and David Davis.

Reprinted from the *American Heart Journal*, 1940, **19**, 1–91. Illus, tables, bibliog.

Bookplate: Medical Women's Federation Reference Library; presented by American War Information Bureau, Oct. 1945.

DAVIES (JOHN NEVILLE PHILLIPS) *b.* 1915

913 "Endo-myocardial necrosis." A heart disease of obscure aetiology in Africans. A dissertation presented at the M.D. examination of the University of Bristol, June 1948. *Bristol, [privately printed], 1948.* 69, [110]ff. Illus (plates), map, tables (folding). Folio, 34 cms. (*Typescript*).

Profusely illustrated with photographs of pathological specimens and sections; these comprise the major portion of the work.

Signed presentation copy from author to DEB, August 1948.

This is the pioneer account of endo-myocardial necrosis in Uganda, previously described briefly by D. E. Bedford and G. L. E. Konstam ("Heart failure of unknown aetiology in Africans." *British Heart Journal*, 1946, **8**, 236–7, in Proceedings of the Cardiac Society of Great Britain and Ireland). The disease, now known as endomyocardial fibrosis or Davies' disease, was further described by the author in *East African medical Journal*, 1948, **25**, 10–14.

GOULD (SYLVESTER EMANUEL) *b.* 1900

914 Pathology of the heart; ed. by S. E. Gould. *Springfield, Ill., Charles C. Thomas, 1953.* xiii, 1023 pp. Illus, ports, facsims, tables, diagrs, bibliog. 4to, 26 cms.

Autograph: Walter Somerville (M.D., F.R.C.P.), January 1955; book-stamp: Department of Cardiology, Middlesex Hospital, W.1.

See especially J. E. Edwards on congenital malformations of the heart and great vessels, pp. 266–503.

WILLIAMS (ARTHUR WARRINER), and others

915 Endomyocardial fibrosis in Africa: its diagnosis, distribution and nature, by A. W. Williams, J. D. Ball and J. N. P. Davies.

Reprinted from *Transactions of the Royal Society of tropical Medicine and Hygiene*, 1954, **48**, 290–311. Illus, tables, bibliog.

Discussion with DEB, A. J. Hawe, I. R. Gray and E. A. Beet.

MASON (JOHN KENYON FRENCH)

916 Aviation accident pathology: a study of fatalities. *London, Butterworth, 1962.* xvi, 358 pp. Illus, tables, bibliog. 4to, 26 cms.

Covers accidents due to coronary disease, etc.

KEAN (BENJAMIN HARRISON) *b.* 1912 and BRESLAU (ROGER CHARLES) *b.* 1932

917 Parasites of the human heart. *New York, London, Grune & Stratton, 1964.* xi, 186 pp. Illus, diagrs, tables, bibliog. 8vo, 24 cms.

Deals with amoebiasis, kala-azar, Chagas' disease, schistosomiasis, filariasis, toxoplasmosis, etc. and includes useful bibliographies.

HUDSON (REGINALD ERNEST BATES) *b.* 1910

918 Cardiovascular pathology. *London, Edward Arnold, 1965–1970.* 3 vols. Illus, diagrs, bibliog. 4to, 26 cms.

Vol. 1: (1965) ix, 1190 pp.; vol. 2: (1965) [vii], 1191–2123 pp.; vol. 3: (1970) x, 1166 pp. (wanting, but copy in RCP).

An invaluable source of reference on all aspects of heart disease. Described as "An epic of the heart" in review in the *British medical Journal*, 1965, **2,** 1480 (cutting inserted).

History

KRUMBHAAR (EDWARD BELL) 1882–1966

919 Pathology (Clio-Medica, 19). *New York, Hafner, 1962.* xvii, 206 pp. Illus, ports. 8vo, 21 cms.

Garrison and Morton 2319. Originally published New York, P. B. Hoeber, 1937.

A history of pathology with list of pathological milestones, and important bibliography.

DIGITALIS AND THERAPEUTICS

Besides William Withering's *Account of the foxglove*, important books on digitalis in this section are those by Cushny (no. 937) and Luten (no. 940). Lauder Brunton's *Therapeutics of the circulation* includes his work on digitalis, amyl nitrite and blood pressure (no. 930).

WITHERING (WILLIAM) 1741–1799

920 An Account of the foxglove, and some of its medical uses; with practical remarks on dropsy and other diseases. *Birmingham, M. Swinney for G. G. J. & J. Robinson (London), 1785.* xxi, 208 pp. Illus (coloured folding plate). 8vo, 23 cms.

Garrison and Morton 1836. Original boards and label in card case: "A bookseller friend sought a copy for me and found one in Charing Cross Road amongst botanical books. It was bought by him for five shillings and sold to me for £4 in 1929." (note from DEB).

921 *The same.* Facsimile edition. *London, Broomsleigh Press (Fudge), [1948?].* xxi, 208 pp. Illus (coloured folding plate). 8vo. 23 cms.

No. 14 in a limited edition of 250 copies. Leaf with imprint inserted between pp. [ii] and [iii].

922 *The same.* Bericht über den Fingerhut und seine medizinische Anwendung mit praktischen Bemerkungen über Wassersucht und andere Krankheiten. Nach der englischen Ausgabe von 1785 ins Deutsche übertragen. *Mannheim, C. F. Boehringer, [1929].* 210 pp. Illus (folding coloured plate), facsim., bibliog. (ftn. refs).

Includes a short history of digitalis (pp. 192–203).

BREDA (CARL FREDRIK VON) 1759–1818

923 [Portrait of William Withering, painted at Edgbaston Hall, now in the National Art Gallery, Stockholm]. *Hälsingborg, Leo Pharmaceutical Products, [1956].* 4to, 28 cms.

Coloured reproduction printed for the 2nd European Congress of Cardiology, Stockholm, 1956.

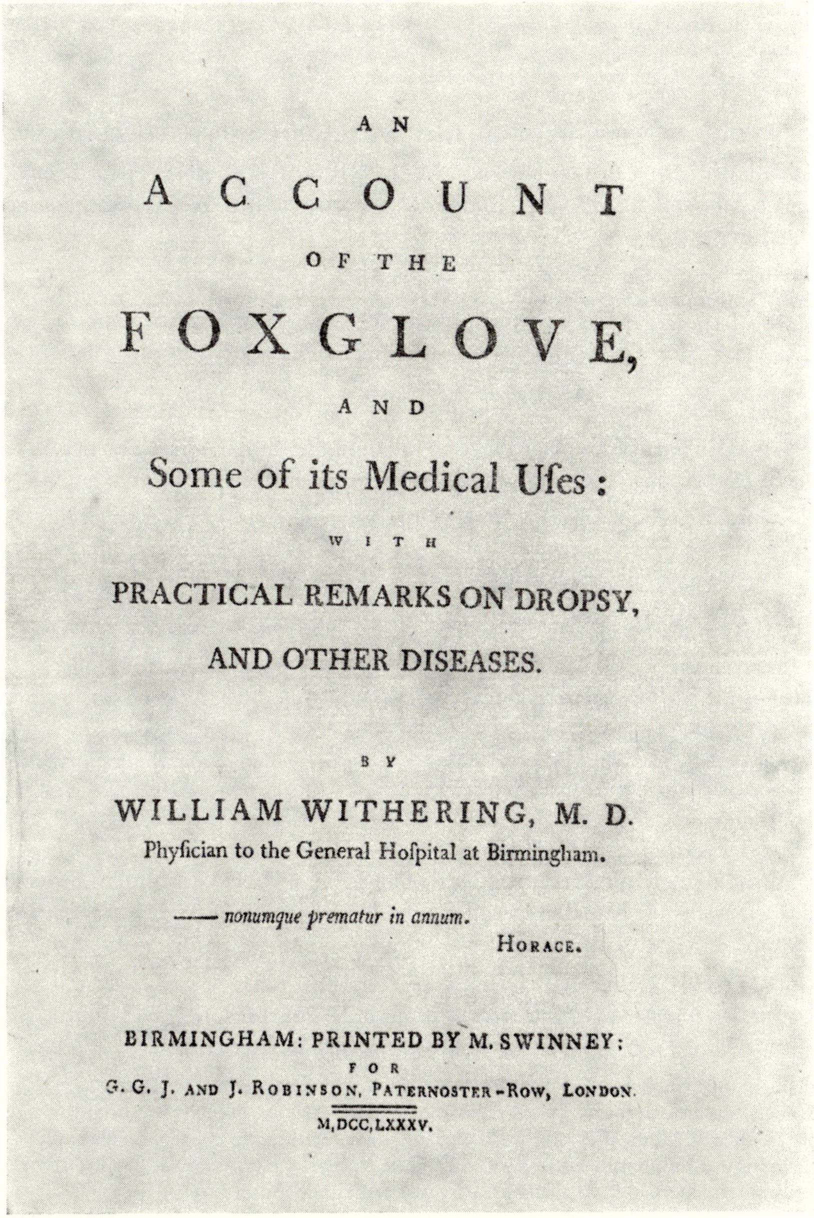

AN

ACCOUNT

OF THE

FOXGLOVE,

AND

Some of its Medical Uſes:

WITH

PRACTICAL REMARKS ON DROPSY,

AND OTHER DISEASES.

BY

WILLIAM WITHERING, M. D.

Phyſician to the General Hoſpital at Birmingham.

—— *nonumque prematur in annum.*

HORACE.

BIRMINGHAM: PRINTED BY M. SWINNEY:

FOR

G. G. J. AND J. ROBINSON, PATERNOSTER-ROW, LONDON.

M,DCC,LXXXV.

No. 920. Introduction of digitalis

WITHERING (WILLIAM)

MCMICHAEL (SIR JOHN) *b.* 1904

924 William Withering in perspective.

Reprinted from *University of Birmingham historical Journal*, 1967, **11**, 41–50. Port, facsims, bibliog. (ftn. refs).

Signed presentation copy to DEB from the author.

PECK (THOMAS WHITMORE) *d.* 1944 and WILKINSON (KENNETH DOUGLAS) 1886–1951

925 William Withering of Birmingham, M.D., F.R.S., F.L.S. *Bristol, John Wright; London, Simpkin Marshall, 1950.* viii, 239 pp. Illus, ports, facsims, maps, plans, diagrs, bibliog. 8vo, 23 cms.

The best biography of Withering and his times in Birmingham.

Extracts from the *British medical Journal* are inserted: an obituary of K. D. Wilkinson (1951, **1**, 890–1) and HOLMES, J. MacD. "Bicentenary of the Staffordshire General Infirmary." (1966, **2**, 1064–5. Ports, plan). William Withering was one of the first physicians at the hospital.

RODDIS (LOUIS HARRY) *b.* 1886

926 William Withering; the introduction of digitalis into medical practice. *New York, Paul B. Hoeber, 1936.* xi, 131 pp. Illus, ports, facsims, bibliog. 8vo, 20 cms.

Reprinted from *Annals of medical History*, 1936, new series **8**, 93–112, 185–201, with additions and corrections.

An historical account with bibliography of Withering's publications.

FERRIAR (JOHN) 1761–1815

927 An Essay on the medical properties of the digitalis purpurea or foxglove. *Manchester, Sowler and Russell for Cadell and Davies (London), 1799.* [iii], iv, 3–66 pp. 12mo, 21 cms.

Bookplate: Ex libris Arpad Plesch. Presented to DEB by Arpad Plesch 1958.

Ferriar used digitalis with opium or Dover's powder to counteract vomiting in pulmonary phthisis. He also used it in palpitation and hydrothorax.

SANDERS (JAMES) 1777–1843

928 Essai sur la digitale pourprée; traduit de l'anglais par A. F. G. Murat . . . avec des notes et des réflexions sur la matière médicale par le traducteur. *Paris et Anvers, Ancelle, 1812.* xl, 98 pp. 8vo, 21 cms.

[*and*] BIDAULT DE VILLIERS (F. T.) 1775–1824

Essai sur les propriétés médicales de la digitale pourprée. 3me éd. *Paris, Mequignon-Marvis, 1812.* xxiv, 168 pp. Bibliog. (ftn. refs). 8vo, 21 cms.

Book-stamp: Cabinet de Lecture rue de l'École de Medecine No. 3.

Sanders of Edinburgh took his M.D. in 1805 and his essay on digitalis was originally published in 1808. He died at Montpellier and was father of William Rutherford Sanders (1828–1881), professor of pathology at Edinburgh University. Bidault de Villiers was physician at Saulieu (Côte d'Or) and spent some time at Galway in Ireland. His *Essai* was first published in 1803.

BRUNTON (Sir THOMAS LAUDER) 1844–1916

929 On digitalis; with some observations of the urine. *London, John Churchill, 1868* viii, 132 pp. Tables, diagrs, bibliog. (ftn. refs). 8vo, 20 cms.

Book-stamp: Kings College London.

930 Therapeutics of the circulation: eight lectures delivered in the spring of 1905 in the physiological laboratory of the University of London. *London, John Murray, 1908.* xii, 272 pp. Illus, diagrs, bibliog. (ftn. refs). 8vo, 22 cms.

Publisher's catalogue (4 pp.) bound in at end. Second edition, 1915. American edition, Philadelphia, P. Blakiston's Son, 1908.

Author's presentation copy. This book includes Brunton's work on digitalis, amyl nitrite and blood-pressure.

FOTHERGILL (JOHN MILNER) 1841–1888

931 Digitalis; its mode of action, and its use: an enquiry illustrating the effect of remedial agents over diseased conditions of the heart. The Hastings prize essay of the British Medical Association for 1870. *London, H. K. Lewis, 1871.* [iii], 89 pp. 8vo, 20 cms.

Presentation copy; autograph: Herbert Davies (1818–1885, physician to London Hospital).

HUCHARD (HENRI) 1844–1910

932 Quand et comment doit-on prescrire la digitale. *Paris, Leclerc [et] Bureaux de la Revue Générale, 1888.* [iii], 136 pp. Bibliog. (ftn. refs). 8vo, 23 cms.

THORNE (WILLIAM BEZLY) *d.* 1917

933 The Schott methods of the treatment of chronic diseases of the heart, with an account of the Nauheim baths, and of the therapeutic exercises. 2nd ed. *London, J. & A. Churchill, 1896.* 84 pp. Illus, tables, diagrs, bibliog. (ftn. refs). 8vo, 23 cms.

Autograph: Thos. G. Emerson, Wantage, Berks. (Thomas Gilbert Emerson, M.D., *d.* 1912).

First published as *A Treatment of chronic diseases of the heart by baths and exercises according to the method of the Drs. [A. and T.] Schott.* London, J. & A. Churchill, 1894; second edition, 1896 (reprinted 1897); third edition, 1899; fourth edition, 1902; fifth edition, 1906; the third, fourth and fifth editions were published in America in the same years by P. Blakiston's Son, Philadelphia.

The percussion outlines of the heart—before and after treatment—are noteworthy. Schott's treatment, a method begun at Bad Nauheim by August Schott (1839–1886) and his brother Theodor (1852–1921), involved "therapy of heart disorders by means of warm saline baths and regulated exercises. This is no longer a treatment of cardiovascular disease, but is a useful means of rehabilitating the patient who is convalescing from cardiac disease." (*British medical dictionary*, ed. by Sir Arthur Salusbury MacNalty. London [etc.], Caxton, 1961, p. 1277).

POWELL (Sir RICHARD DOUGLAS) 1842–1925

934 On the principles which govern treatment in diseases and disorders of the heart. (Lumleian Lectures, 1898). *London, H. K. Lewis, 1899.* [x], 118 pp. Illus (plates), diagrs, bibliog. (ftn. refs). 8vo.

Autograph W. [?]T. Strugnell (possibly Walter Thomas Strugnell, *d.* 1939, M.D.).
See his remarks on angina pectoris with and without organic heart disease.

BRAUN (LUDWIG) 1867–1936

935 Therapie der Herzkrankheiten. *Berlin, Wien, Urban & Schwarzenberg, 1903.* vi, 246 pp. Bibliog. (ftn. refs). 8vo, 22 cms.

Second edition, *Diagnosie und Therapie der Herzkrankheiten*, 1913.

ROBINSON (GEORGE CANBY) 1878–1960

936 The Therapeutic use of digitalis. (Medicine Monographs). *Baltimore, Williams & Wilkins, 1923.* [v], 137 pp. Tables, bibliog. 8vo, 24 cms.

Acquired 1926. An important contemporary account of digitalis and full bibliography.

CUSHNY (ARTHUR ROBERTSON) 1866–1926

937 The Action and uses in medicine of digitalis and its allies. *London, Longmans, Green, 1925.* xi, 303 pp. Port., diagrs, bibliog. 8vo, 23 cms.

Acquired 1925.

HOFFMANN-LA ROCHE

938 Grundlage und Ergebnisse der Digitalistherapie; zum 25 jährigen Jubiläum des Digalen "Roche" 1904–1929. *Berlin, F. Hoffmann-La Roche, 1929.* 95 pp. Illus, ports, diagrs. 8vo, 21 cms.

A good historical and pharmacological review of digitalis.

VAQUEZ (LOUIS HENRI) 1860–1936

939 Préparations galéniques et glucosides de la digitale. *Paris, J. B. Baillière, 1935.* 13 pp. Tables. 8vo, 23 cms.

Reprinted from *Archives des Maladies du Cœur, des Vaisseaux et du Sang,* 1935, **28,** 185–97.

LUTEN (DREW WILLIAM) 1881–1970

940 The Clinical use of digitalis. *Springfield, Ill., and Baltimore, Maryland, Charles C. Thomas, 1936.* xx, 226 pp. Port., facsims, bibliog. 8vo, 24 cms.

Comprehensive bibliography of 10 pages, mainly of contemporary work.

STOLL (ARTHUR) *b.* 1887

941 The Cardiac glycosides: a series of three lectures delivered in the College of the Pharmaceutical Society of Great Britain under the auspices of the University of London. *London, Pharmaceutical Press, 1937.* viii, 80 pp. Illus, port., facsims, diagrs, bibliog. 8vo, 25 cms.

Three lectures on the cardiac glycosides with bibliography and historical essay.

CARDIAC SURGERY

Recent advances in cardiac surgery are not covered; but some of the important early works such as Sir Charles Ballance's Bradshaw Lecture and King's *Surgery of the heart* cover the historical aspects. Frey deals with cardiac surgery up to the 1939 war. Virtue's is a pioneer work on hypothermia and Dubost and Blondeau cover open heart surgery with hypothermia and extracorporeal circulation, while Hardy gives an excellent account of surgery of the aorta and main branches.

BALLANCE (Sir CHARLES ALFRED) 1856–1936

942 The Bradshaw Lecture on the surgery of the heart delivered before the Royal College of Surgeons, December 11th, 1919. *London, Macmillan, 1920.* [iii], 154 pp. Illus, tables, bibliog. (ftn. refs). 8vo, 23 cms.

An early classic on cardiac surgery.

FREY (EMIL KARL) *b.* 1888

943 Die Chirurgie des Herzens. (Neue deutsche Chirurgie, Band. 61). *Stuttgart, Ferdinand Enke, 1939.* xi, 278 pp. Illus, tables, diagrs, bibliog. 4to, 26 cms.

Publisher's catalogue (6 pp.) including list of volumes in the series bound in at end.
Deals with cardiac surgery up to the 1939 war—pericardial and early valve surgery, cardiac aneurysm, sympathectomy, omentopexy, thyroidectomy, etc. Comprehensive bibliography (pp. 240–75).

KING (EDGAR SAMUEL JOHN) 1900–1966

944 Surgery of the heart. *Baltimore, Williams & Wilkins, 1941.* xii, 728 pp. Illus, diagrs, bibliog. 8vo, 24 cms.

Also published in London, E. Arnold, 1941.
Has a useful bibliography of early heart surgery.

GROSS (ROBERT EDWARD) *b.* 1905

945 The Surgical treatment for abnormalities of the heart and great vessels. (Beaumont Lecture. America Lecture Series, no. 3. American Lectures in Surgery). *Springfield, Ill., Charles C. Thomas, 1947.* vii, 72 pp. Illus, diagrs, bibliog. 8vo, 22 cms.

Presented by J. W. Brown, Sept. 1948 (James William Brown, author of no. 815).
Covers surgery of pericardial defects, patent ductus, Fallot's tetralogy and anomalies of the aortic arch and subclavian artery.

GAUDART D'ALLAINES (FRANÇOIS LOUIS PAUL DE) *b.* 1892

946 Chirurgie du cœur: avec la collaboration de E. Donzelot, J. Lenègre, [and others]. *Paris, Expansion Scientifique Française, 1950.* 346 pp. Illus, tables, diagrs, bibliog. 12mo, 19 cms.

A contemporary account of French cardiac surgery.

BAILEY (CHARLES PHILAMORE) *b.* 1910

947 Surgery of the heart. *London, Henry Kimpton, 1955.* 1062 pp. Illus, tables, diagrs, bibliog. 8vo, 24 cms.

Covers anaesthesia and surgery of congenital and acquired heart disease up to 1955, with contributions from Robert S. Litwak on the development of cardiac surgery and hydatid disease of the heart, Kenneth K. Keown on hypothermia and (with Mary Lou Buckley and Henry S. Ruth) cardiac resuscitation, and Charles P. Bailey and Houck E. Bolton on both mitral and aortic stenosis.

VIRTUE (ROBERT WALLACE) *b.* 1904

948 Hypothermic anesthesia. (American Lecture Series no. 275. American Lectures in Anesthesiology). *Springfield, Ill., Charles C. Thomas, 1955.* ix, 62 pp. Illus, tables, diagrs, bibliog. 8vo, 22 cms.

Virtue, working in Denver with Swan, first established safe hypothermia for heart surgery by a technique of surface cooling. They pioneered closing atrial septa defects by open heart surgery.

DUBOST (CHARLES) *b.* 1914 and BLONDEAU (PHILIPPE)

949 Chirurgie à cœur ouvert. *Paris, Masson, 1957.* [iii], 319 pp. Illus, tables, diagrs, (ftn. refs). 4to, 26 cms.

A good historical account of open heart surgery, hypothermia and extracorporeal circulation to date.

NORMAND (JEAN) *b.* 1926

950 Les Rétrécissements aortiques sigmoidiens: indications operatoires actuelles. *Paris, G. Doin, 1957.* 248 pp. Illus, tables, diagrs, bibliog. 8vo, 24 cms.

Author's presentation copy.

Also issued as Lyon M.D. thesis under the title *Formes anatome—cliniques du rétrécissements aortiques sigmoidiens* (Lyon Université. Faculté de médécine et de pharmacie. Thèse, 1956, no. 31).

Deals with experience at Froment's Heart Clinic in Lyon.

COOPER (KEITH EDWARD) and ROSS (DONALD NIXON)

951 Hypothermia in surgical practice. *London, Cassell, 1960.* xi, 116 pp. Illus, diagrs, bibliog. 8vo, 23 cms.

Other contributors: B. A. Sellich, L. S. Walsh, V. Wynn.

Covers surface and blood-stream cooling, and hypothermia with an assisted circulation. Extensive bibliography, pp. 101–7.

HARDY (JAMES DANIEL) *b.* 1918

952 Surgery of the aorta and its branches. *Philadelphia, Lippincott, 1960.* xiii, 386 pp. Illus, tables, diagrs, bibliog. 12mo, 19 cms.

Reprinted from *American Practitioner and Digest of Treatment*, Jan.–July 1960.

An excellent account of clinical diagnosis and surgery of aorta and main branches, with bibliography.

FROMENT (ROGER) *b.* 1907, and others

953 Actualités cardio-vasculaires médico-chirurgicales, publiées sous la direction de R. Froment, A. Gonin [et] P. Michaud; 1ère série: les valvulopathies du cœur gauche et

leur traitement chirurgical (sténose mitrale et commissurotomie exceptées). *Paris, Masson, 1964.* vi, 258 pp. Illus, tables, diagrs, bibliog. 8vo, 25 cms.

Presentation copy from Froment. "Au Docteur Bedford en amical hommage pour sa bibliotheque, Juin 1964."

Contributions by various physicians covering surgery of mitral incompetence, aortic disease, and valve replacement.

History

RICHARDSON (ROBERT GALLOWAY) *b.* 1926

954 The Surgeon's heart: a history of cardiac surgery. *London, William Heinemann Medical Books, 1969.* [vii], 344 pp. Illus, ports, facsims. 8vo, 22 cms.

The story of heart surgery from ancient to modern times, recorded in simple terms.

A copy of the list of references separately produced, [London, the Author, 1972?]. [ii], 133 ff. (Duplicated typescript), is in the RCP Library.

MONOGRAPHS ON SPECIAL SUBJECTS

Heart Disease in Pregnancy

MACDONALD (ANGUS) 1836–1886

955 The Bearings of chronic disease of the heart upon pregnancy, parturition and child-bed. With papers on puerperal pleuropneumonia and eclampsia. *London, J. & A. Churchill, 1878.* viii, 287 pp. Illus, diagrs (tracings). 8vo, 24 cms.

Autograph: David Hank (?).

Macdonald was lecturer on midwifery and diseases of women at Edinburgh, and this pioneer work gives a good historical review of early French and German papers on the subject, then based mainly on post-mortems in women dying in pregnancy.

MACKENZIE (Sir JAMES) 1853–1925

956 Heart disease and pregnancy. (Oxford Medical Publications). *London, Henry Frowde and Hodder & Stoughton, 1921.* xiv, 138 pp. Illus, diagrs (tracings). 8vo, 22 cms.

BRAMWELL (JOHN CRIGHTON) 1889–1976 and BLAKELEY (EDITH ANNIE)

957 Heart disease and pregnancy, by Crighton Bramwell and Edith A. Longson. (Oxford Medical Publications). *London, New York, Toronto, Oxford University Press, 1938.* xii, 194 pp. Illus, tables, diagrs, bibliog. 8vo, 22 cms.

JONES (ARTHUR MORGAN)

958 Heart disease in pregnancy. *London, Harvey & Blythe, 1951.* x, 57 pp. Illus, tables, diagrs. 8vo, 22 cms.

Heart and Athletics

MORGAN (JOHN EDWARD) 1828–1892

959 University oars, being a critical enquiry into the after health of the men who rowed in the Oxford and Cambridge boat-race from the year 1829 to 1869, based on the personal experience of the rowers themselves. *London, Macmillan, 1873.* xvi, 397 pp. Tables, 8vo, 20 cms.

Morgan gives a list of crews in each race and a follow-up which involved a lengthy enquiry. A classic work on rowing and the heart cited by Rolleston.

DEUTSCH (FELIX) 1884–1964 and KAUF (EMIL)

960 Heart and athletics: clinical researches upon the influence of athletics upon the heart. English translation by Louis M. Warfield. *London, Henry Kimpton, 1927.* 187 pp. Tables, diagrs (orthodiagrams), bibliog. 8vo, 21 cms.

Also published Saint Louis, C. V. Mosby, 1927.

Investigation of the heart in athletics at the Vienna Heart Station where Austrian athletes were specially examined. Separates sport for pleasure from competitive athletics. Based mainly on cardiac enlargement determined by orthocardiography. Clinical findings are also considered.

Palpitation and Nervous Heart

SCHENCK (JOHANN THEODOR), praeses, 1619–1671

961 Disputatio inauguralis medica de palpitatione cordis . . . praeside . . . Johanne Theodoro Schenckio . . . , publico eruditorum examini submittit Caspar Gigas . . . *[Jenae], literis Samuelis Krebsii, 1662.* [1] f., 48 pp., [1] f. 4to, 20 cms.

Although theses with which he was involved are listed in the *British Museum Catalogue*, Gigas, the respondent (*fl.* 1662), does not seem to appear in reference works. However, both Werner Rolfinck (1599–1673) who granted his thesis, and Schenck, his praeses, had written on palpitation of the heart, evidently a popular subject at Jena at this time.

BANIZETTE (LAURENT) *fl.* 1807

962 Dissertation sur la palpitation du cœur . . . (Montpellier University. École de Médecine. Thèse). *Montpellier, Auguste Ricard, 1807.* [vi], 35 pp. Bibliog. (ftn. refs). 4to, 26 cms.

WILLIAMS (JOHN CALTHROP) 1801–1856

963 Practical observations on nervous and sympathetic palpitation of the heart, as well as on palpitation the result of organic disease. 2nd ed. *London, J. Churchill; Nottingham, Thomas Forman, 1852.* vii, 207 pp. 8vo, 23 cms.

Churchill's catalogue, August 1852 [32] pp., bound in at end. Author's presentation copy to Rev. Charles [James] Willoughby (1822–1875), rector of Wollaton-with-Cossall, Nottinghamshire, and brother of the 8th baron Middleton. The book is now very rare. First edition, 1836.

Williams was physician to the Nottingham General Hospital and lectured in the Nottingham Medical School which closed down after a few years. In his book he shows that palpitation is often associated with nervous disturbances, dyspepsia, etc., and he mentions pricking praecordial pain. He also describes vaso-vagal attacks with syncope, and angina pectoris which he regarded as a neuralgic disorder. He supports Wardrop's views on the circulation in general (see no. 290).

O'DONOVAN (PATRICK HENRY)

964 Dr. John Calthrop Williams, physician of Nottingham, 1801–1856. *London, Royal Society of Medicine, 1954.* 6 pp. Illus., facsim., bibliog. 8vo, 25 cms.

Reprinted from *Proceedings of the Royal Society of Medicine*, 1954, **47**, 749–54 (Section of the History of Medicine, pp. 23–8). Author's presentation copy.

BLAKE (EDWARD THOMAS) 1842–1905

965 The Inframammary pain. *London, Henry J. Glaisher, 1898.* [i], 15 pp. 8vo, 23 cms.

This is an early account of left mammary pain which the author attributed to toxic absorption from pelvic and uterine infections.

GOWERS (Sir WILLIAM RICHARD) 1845–1915

966 The Borderland of epilepsy; faints, vagal attacks, vertigo, migraine, sleep symptoms and their treatment. *London, J. & A. Churchill, 1907.* vi, 121 pp. 8vo, 23 cms.

Also published Philadelphia, P. Blakiston's Son, 1907.

Deals with the diagnostic difficulty of distinguishing minor epilepsy as cardiac faints, cardiac aura in epilepsy, cardiac discomfort in vagal attacks, etc.

GALLAVARDIN (LOUIS BÉNÉDICT) 1875–1957

967 Formes cliniques des névroses tachycardiques. *Paris, A. Poinat, 1918.* 24 pp. Diagrs (tracings), bibliog. (ftn. refs). 8vo, 22 cms.

Reprinted from *Journal médical Français*, May 1918.

GALLAVARDIN (LOUIS BÉNÉDICT) 1875–1957 and TOURNIAIRE (A.)

968 Les Névroses tachycardiques. (Médecine et Chirurgie Pratiques). *Paris, Masson, 1935.* [viii], 121 pp. Tables, diagrs, bibliog. (283 refs.). 8vo, 20 cms.

Presentation copy signed by authors.

PARKINSON (Sir JOHN) 1885–1976

969 Left scapular pain and tenderness in heart disease and distress. [*London, Lancet, 1919*]. 13 pp. Illus. 8vo, 22 cms.

Reprinted from *Lancet*, 1919, **1**, 550–83.

"With my kind regards. J.P."

A classical account of left chest pain based on experience at military heart centres in the war

WILSON (ROBERT MCNAIR) 1882–1963 and
CARROLL (JOHN HAROLD) 1884–1968

970 The Nervous heart: its nature, causation, prognosis and treatment. *London, H. Frowde, Hodder & Stoughton, 1919.* vii, 136 pp. Illus, diagrs. 8vo, 19 cms.

Wilson worked with Mackenzie on the soldier's heart.

BAKER (DORIS MANNING) 1895–1971

971 Left inframammary pain; with a note by Dr. John Parkinson. [*London, Lancet, 1930*]. 16 pp. Illus, tables, diagr., bibliog. 8vo, 22 cms.

Reprinted from *Lancet*, 1930, **1**, 1280–5.

972 Sighing respiration as a symptom. [*London, Lancet, 1934*]. 8 pp. Diagr., bibliog. 8vo, 22 cms.

Reprinted from *Lancet*, 1934, **1**, 174–7.
"With compliments DMB."

973 Cardiac symptoms in the neuroses. *London, H. K. Lewis, 1942.* v, 49 pp. Illus, tables, diagrs (tracings), bibliog. 12mo, 18 cms.

"With kind regards, DMB" (1942).

974 *The same.* 2nd ed. *London, H. K. Lewis, 1955.* viii, 50 pp. Illus, tables, diagrs, bibliog. 12mo, 19 cms.

Presentation copy from the author, 1955.
Describes left mammary pain, sighing respiration and palpitation, based on experience at the National Heart Hospital. An excellent account which merits wider recognition.

Traumatic Heart Disease

WARBURG (ERIK JOHAN) *b.* 1892

975 Subacute and chronic pericardial and myocardial lesions due to non-penetrating traumatic injuries: a clinical study. [Translated by Hans Anderson and Gerda Seidelin]. With a short biography of Oluff Borch (Olaus Borrichius) by Torben Geill. *København, Levin & Munksgaard; London, Humphrey Milford, (Oxford University Press), 1938.* 147 pp. Illus, port., tables, diagrs, bibliog. 4to, 26 cms.

Also forms *Arbejder fra Rigshospitalets Afdeling B*, Kobenhavn. (1938) 1942, **2**, no. 14.
A pioneer and much quoted work by Professor Warburg of Copenhagen.

GROSSE - BROCKHOFF (FRANZ) *b.* 1907 and KAISER (K.)

976 Herzschädigung durch stumpfe Gewalteinwirkung.

Reprinted from *Handbuch der inneren Medizin;* 4. Aufl., herausgegeben von G. von Bergmann [and others]. Berlin, Springer, 1960, pp. 462–542.
Deals with non-penetrating injury of the heart. Bibliography of 6 pages.

Cardiac Liver

POPPI (ARRIGO), and others

977 Il Fegato dei cardiaci; [da] A. Poppi, G. Labò [e] G. Lenzi. *Bologna, L. Capelli, 1954.* [vi], 291 pp. Illus, tables, diagrs, bibliog.

Presentation copy "With best compliments, Arrigo Poppi."
Summary in English, French and German, with a full bibliography (pp. 279–88).

VAGUE (JEAN) *b.* 1911

978 Le Foie cardiaque. *Paris, Masson, 1939.* 185 pp. Illus, bibliog. 8vo, 20 cms.

Publisher's catalogue, Mai 1939 (48 pp.) bound in at end.
A good historical account and bibliography (pp. 151–82).

Tuberculosis

PIC (FERDINAND ADRIEN) 1862–1943 and
MORENAS (ERNEST FRANÇOIS LÉON) 1891–1949

979 La Tuberculose cardio-vasculaire. Le cœur des tuberculeux. (Bibliothèque de la Tuberculose). *Paris, Gaston Doin, 1930.* xii, 288 pp. Illus, diagrs, bibliog. 8vo, 22 cms.

Deals with pericarditis, endocarditis, myocardial and arterial tuberculosis. An extensive bibliography (pp. 235–68).

Bacterial Endocarditis

PERRY (CHARLES BRUCE) *b.* 1903

980 Bacterial endocarditis; with an appendix on an experimental study of malignant endocarditis, by D. M. Lloyd Jones. *Bristol, John Wright, 1936.* [viii], 137 pp. Illus, tables, diagrs, bibliog. 8vo, 22 cms.

Bibliography, pp. 102–9; appendix, pp. 111–37.

OSLER (Sir WILLIAM) 1849–1919

981 Infectious (so-called ulcerative) endocarditis.

Reprinted from *Archives of Medicine*, 1881, **5**, 44–68. Illus.
An early paper prior to his classical account in the *Quarterly Journal of Medicine*, 1908–1909, **2**, 219–30.

LIBMAN (EMANUEL) 1872–1946 and FRIEDBERG (CHARLES KAYE) 1905–1972

982 Subacute bacterial endocarditis. (Oxford Medical Publications). *New York, London, Toronto, Oxford University Press, 1941.* xiv, 108 pp. Illus, bibliog. 8vo, 24 cms.

Acquired 1944 (Jerusalem). Second edition, New York, Elsevier, 1948.

THIVOLET (JEAN) *b.* 1926

983 Evolution et thérapeutique actuelles de l'endocardite, a propos de 82 observations pérsonelles. (Lyon University. Faculté de Médecine et de Pharmacie. Thèse 1954/55, no. 96). *Lyon, Camille Annequin, 1955.* 272 pp. Illus, tables, bibliog. (pp. 241–70). 8vo, 24 cms.

Author's presentation copy (unsigned).

Smallpox

BOIGEY (MAURICE AUGUSTE JOSEPH) 1877–1952

984 Les Lésions du cœur dans la variole. *Lyon, A. Rey, 1900.* 79 pp. Illus (7 plates with explanatory facing pages), bibliog. 8vo, 25 cms.

Original thesis with same title, Lyon, 1900, no. 22.

"Monsieur le Dr. Meynier (cover), Hommage respectueux, Dr. Boigey." (p. [1]).

There was an epidemic of smallpox in Lyon in 1899. The author examined 30 hearts from fatal cases histologically, and deals with the clinical features of variolous myocarditis.

Heart Disease in the Tropics

(see also no. 987)

GUNEWARDENE (HUGH OLIVER) 1893–1954

985 Heart disease in the Tropics. *Calcutta, Butterworth, 1935.* xi, 101 pp. Illus, diagrs, bibliog. (ftn. refs). 8vo, 23 cms.

Signed presentation copy from author to DEB. This Ceylonese cardiologist describes the diastolic murmur of anaemia.

Cardiac Tumours

MAHAIM (IVAN) 1897–1965

986 Les Tumeurs et les polypes du cœur: étude anatomo-clinique. *Paris, Masson; Lausanne, F. Roth, 1945.* 568 pp. Illus, tables, diagrs, bibliog. 8vo, 24 cms.

Author's presentation copy to DEB, 1946.

A classical monograph on heart tumours and an invaluable source of reference, with 1298 references. Mahaim was born in Belgium and worked in Lausanne where he was associate professor. He was also a great authority on Beethoven and an accomplished violinist.

Cardio-Myopathies

MYOCARDITIS

987 Myocarditis. (St. Cyres Memorial Lectures 1–7). *London, Eyre & Spottiswoode, 1937.* i–ix, [10]–152 pp. Illus, tables, diagrs (tracings), bibliog. 8vo, 22 cms.

Contains: GOODALL (Joseph Strickland) 1874–1934, Some general aspects of myocarditis, pp. 11–29; WENCKEBACH (Karel Frederik) 1864–1940, Heart and circulation in a tropical avitaminosis (beri-beri), pp. 31–45; MOON (Robert Oswald) 1865–1953, Some observations on disease of the myocardium, pp. 47–65; COWAN (John Marshall) 1870–1947, The Fibroses of the heart, pp. 67–99; GOODALL (Joseph Strickland) 1874–1934, The Right side of the heart, pp. 103–22; HAY (John) 1873–1959, Certain aspects of coronary thrombosis, pp. 123–52. The fifth lecture was delivered by Sir Thomas Lewis (1881–1945), but no record is available.

PERRIN (A.), and others

988 Insuffisance cardiaque des jeunes sujects par sclérose myocardique dense et diffuse d'origine tuberculeuse, incertaine ou inconnue. Le probleme des myocardites subaiguës primitives de Josserand et Gallavardin, par A. Perrin, R[oger] Froment et J[ean] Lenègre.

Reprinted from *Cardiologia*, 1953, **22,** 257–365. Illus, bibliog.

BRIGDEN (Wallace William) *b.* 1916

989 Uncommon myocardial diseases: the non-coronary cardiomyopathies. (St. Cyres Lecture, 1956). [*London, Lancet, 1957*]. 35 pp. Illus, diagrs, bibliog. 8vo, 22 cms.

Reprinted from *Lancet*, 1957, **2,** 1179–84, 1243–9. "With kind regards, W.B."

CIBA FOUNDATION

990 Ciba Foundation Symposium [on] cardio-myopathies, ed. by G. E. W. Wolstenholme and Maeve O'Connor. *London, J. & A. Churchill, 1964.* xiii, 428 pp. Illus, tables, diagrs, bibliog. 8vo, 21 cms.

PERIODICALS

AMERICAN HEART JOURNAL

991 American heart journal; under the editorial direction of the American Heart Association. *St. Louis, C. V. Mosby, 1926–1971.* Vols 1–82. 4to, 26 cms.

Vol. 1, nos 3–5, February, April, and June, 1926, pp. 257–670; and vol. 21, no. 1, January 1941, pp. 1–132, wanting.

ARCHIVES DES MALADIES DU CŒUR

992 Archives des maladies du cœur, des vaisseaux et du sang. *Paris, J. B. Baillière et fils, 1908–1968.* Vols 1–61. 8vo, 24 cms.

"Publiées sous la direction du Dr H. Vaquez."

Library also has 1961, suppts nos. 1–2, and 1964, suppts nos. 1–3, issues of *Revue de l'Athérosclérose*, which began in 1957. A list of "Communications de la Société de l'Athérosclérose" for 1960 and 1963 is inserted in 1961, suppt no. 1, and 1964, suppt no. 2 respectively.

BRITISH HEART JOURNAL

993 British heart journal, for the study of cardiology and the circulation. *London, British Medical Association, 1939.* Vol. 1 to date. 8vo, 25 cms.

Editors: Maurice Campbell and D. Evan Bedford, 1939–1947; Maurice Campbell, 1948–1958; K. Shirley Smith, 1959–1972; Walter Somerville, 1973–.

994 Cumulative index, vols 1–17, 1939–1955. *London, British Medical Association, 1957.* 67 pp. 8vo, 25 cms.

995 Cumulative index, vols 18–29, 1956–1967. *London, British Medical Association, 1968.* 81 pp. 8vo, 25 cms.

HEART

996 Heart: a journal for the study of the circulation. *London, Shaw & Sons, 1910–1933.* 16 vols. 8vo, 24 cms.

Edited by Thomas Lewis. Continued as *Clinical Science*, 1933–.

HISTORY OF CARDIOLOGY

COCKLE (John) 1813?–1900

997 Lectures upon the historic literature of the pathology of the heart and great vessels. Part 1, From the earliest authentic records to the close of the Arabian epoch. *London, [printed by] T. Richards, 1860.* [i], 52 pp. Bibliog. (ftn. refs). 12mo, 19 cms.

No more parts appear to have been published.
Presentation copy to Sir George Johnson.
An important review of the earliest literature on heart disease.

BIANCHON (Horace), *pseudonym*

998 Nos grands médecins d'aujourd'hui. [Redigé par Henry Labonne. Préface de Maurice de Fleury]. Illustrations par F. Desmoulin et Profit. *Paris, Société d'Editions Scientifiques 1891.* [vii], x, 492 pp. Ports (64 plates), bibliog. 8vo, 25 cms.

No. 91 of a limited number of 100 "exemplaires sur japon."

These intimate sketches of prominent French medical men were published seriatim in *Le Figaro*, and collected in this volume. The portraits are excellent. It includes the following physicians who contributed to cardiology in the last century: Dieulafoy, Fauvel, Francois-Franck, Huchard, Jaccoud, Letulle, Peter, Potain, Richet (translator of Harvey) and Germain Sée.

"Horace Bianchon, physician, is a character in Balzac's *Comédie humaine*" (note in the entry in *Index-catalogue of the Library of the Surgeon-General's Office, 2nd series*).

AORTIC INCOMPETENCE

999 Corrigan and the history of aortic incompetence. 7 reprints. 1894–1967.

Agnew (Robin Alan Leslie). The Achievement of Dominic John Corrigan. Reprinted from *Medical History*, 1965, **10,** 230–40. Bibliog. Author's presentation copy to DEB with correspondence.

Bedford (Davis Evan) *b.* 1898. An Early account of aortic incompetence by Thomas Cuming (1798–1887). Reprinted from *Medical History*, 1967, **11,** 398–401. Bibliog.

Bramwell (Edwin) 1873–1952. Corrigan's original description of aortic regurgitation: a reference to some matters of historical interest. Reprinted from *Edinburgh medical Journal*, 1933, **40,** 13–19. Author's signed copy. Purchased from David Low, 1947. (5/-).

Huchard (Henri) 1844–1910. I. Une Rectification historique en faveur de Vieussens au sujet du pouls et de la maladie dite "de Corrigan." II. Sur les signes d'affaiblissement du cœur dans les fièvres. Paris, G. Masson, 1894. 16 pp. Bibliog. (ftn. refs). 8vo, 24 cms. Reprinted from *Bulletins et Mémoires de la Société médicale des Hôpitaux de Paris*, 1894, 3e série, **11,** 489–504.

Mulcahy (Risteárd). Sir Dominic John Corrigan. Reprinted from *Irish Journal of medical Science*, 1961, No. 430, October, 454–63. Port., bibliog.

Mulcahy (Risteárd). The Early descriptions of aortic incompetence. Reprinted from *British Heart Journal*, 1962, **24,** 633–6. Bibliog. Author's signed complimentary copy.

Rolleston (Sir Humphry Davy) 1862–1944. History of aortic regurgitation. Extract from *Annals of medical History*, 1940, 3rd series, **2,** 271–9. Ports, bibliog.

WILKS (Sir SAMUEL) 1824–1911

1000 A Memoir by Sir Samuel Wilks, Bart., M.D., LL.D., F.R.S., on the new discoveries or new observations made during the time he was teacher at Guy's Hospital. *London, Adlard, 1911.* [v], 200 pp. Port. 8vo, 22 cms.

Running title and title on cover and spine: Biographical Reminiscences of Sir Samuel Wilks.

Contains much of importance in Bright's disease, chorea, etc., in abstracts from *Guy's Hospital Reports.*

LEA (CHARLES EDGAR) 1882–1919

1001 Heart: past and present. *London, Baillière, Tindall and Cox, 1919.* viii, 300 pp. Table, bibliog. (ftn. refs). 12mo, 19 cms.

The first part, the historical section (pp. 1–85), includes chapters on Corvisart, Laennec and Stokes.

FLINT (HORACE LANCE) 1881–1945

1002 The Heart: old and new views. *London, H. K. Lewis, 1921.* xii, 177 pp. Illus, diagrs, bibliog. (marginal refs) . 8vo, 22 cms.

A useful reference work on early views, especially a note on Gilles de Corbeil and his poem on the pulse from a MS in the Bodleian Library.

Flint worked under Sir Thomas Lewis after being wounded in the First World War. "On returning to practice in 1919 he was the first physician in Nottinghamshire to own an electrocardiograph, and was frequently called in in consultation in the county. Considerable interest was aroused in the town [Mansfield] when a hunter owned by one of the Royal Family arrived at his house to be electrocardiographed (the first time this had been done on a horse); it was found to be suffering from complete heart-block and had to be destroyed." (*British medical Journal*, 1945, **1**, 681). His many years at Mansfield General Hospital were overshadowed by increasingly frequent anginal attacks after an attack of coronary thrombosis in 1937.

BISHOP (LOUIS FAUGÈRES) 1864–1941 and NEILSON (JOHN) *jr. b.* 1897

1003 History of cardiology. *New York, Medical Life Press, 1927.* 71 pp. Ports, facsim. 8vo, 22 cms.

A comprehensive synopsis of pioneers in cardiology.

MOON (ROBERT OSWALD) 1865–1953

1004 Growth of our knowledge of heart disease. *London, Longmans, Green, 1927.* x, 86 pp. Bibliog. (ftn. refs). 12mo, 19 cms.

A brief scholarly review from Aristotle and Galen to Corvisart and Bouillaud, inspired by the tercentenary of the publication of the *De motu cordis.*

ROLLESTON (Sir HUMPHRY DAVY) 1862–1944

1005 Cardio-vascular diseases since Harvey's discovery. The Harveian Oration delivered before the Royal College of Physicians on 18 October 1928. *Cambridge, University Press, 1928.* [vii], 149 pp. Bibliog. 12mo, 19 cms.

An important review of cardiology since Harvey's day with valuable bibliographies.

MAJOR (RALPH HERMON) 1884–1970

1006 The History of taking the blood pressure. *New York, Paul B. Hoeber, 1930.* [i], 47–55 pp. Illus, port., bibliog. 4to, 28 cms.

Reprinted from *Annals of medical History*, 1930, new series, **2,** 47–55.

1007 Classic descriptions of disease with biographical sketches of the authors. *Springfield, Ill., C. C. Thomas, 1932.* xxvii, 630 pp. Illus, ports, facsims, bibliog. (ftn. refs). 4to, 26 cms.

Contains pioneer contributions to cardiology, with biographical notes.

Part 4, Diseases of the circulatory system, includes descriptions of heart block (Marcus Gerbezius, *d.* 1718, Morgagni, Thomas Spens, 1769–1842, Robert Adams, 1791–1875, William Burnett, 1824, and William Stokes, 1804–1878), Aortic insufficiency (William Cowper, 1666–1709, Vieussens, Morgagni, Thomas Hodgkin, 1798–1866, Hope, Corrigan, Austin Flint, 1812–1886, Heinrich Quincke, 1842–1922, and Paul L. Duroziez, 1826–1897), Mitral stenosis (Vieussens, Morgagni, Corvisart, Laennec, Bertin, Hope, S. A. Fauvel, 1813–1884, and Graham Steell 1851–1942), Pulmonary stenosis (Hope), Pulsus alternans (Traube), Gallop rhythm (Potain), Auricular fibrillation (H. E. Hering, 1903, and James Mackenzie, 1853–1925), Extra-systoles (Mackenzie), Paroxysmal tachycardia (William Stokes 1804–1878, Richard Cotton, 1820–1877, and L. Bouveret, 1889), Pericarditis (Guillaume de Baillou, 1538–1616, Lower, Haller, Auenbrugger, Thomas Rotch, 1849–1914, Sir William Broadbent, and Walter Broadbent), Angina pectoris (Earl of Clarendon, 1609–1674, Heberden, Fothergill, and John Hunter), Coronary occlusion (Adam Hammer, 1818–1878, George Dock, 1860, Osler, and James B. Herrick), Aneurysm (Jean Fernel, 1506–1588, Ambroise Paré, 1510–1590, Richard Wiseman, 1622–1676, Lancisi, Morgagni, Corvisart, and W. S. Oliver, 1878), Apoplexy (Johann Jakob Wepfer, 1620–1695), Raynaud's disease (Maurice Raynaud, 1834–1881), Buerger's disease (Leo Buerger, *b.* 1879), Erythomelalgia (S. Weir Mitchell, 1830–1914).

Also of cardiological interest are descriptions of rheumatic fever and hyperthyroidism, chronic nephritis (Bright's disease) (Guglielmo Salicetti, 1210–1280, Frederik Dekkers, 1648–1720, Domenico Cotugno, 1736–1822, William Charles Wells, 1757–1817, John Blackall, 1771–1860, and Bright); Cheyne-Stokes respiration (Hippocrates, John Cheyne, 1777–1836, and William Stokes, 1804–1878); Bronchial cast (Nicholas Tulp, 1593–1674, and R. Warren, 1767); and Skodaic resonance (Josef Skoda, 1805–1881).

WHITNEY (ROBERT)

1008 The Place of hearts: being a history of the National Hospital for Diseases of the Heart, Westmoreland Street, London, 1857–1937. *London, [privately printed], 1937.* 44 pp. Illus. 8vo, 22 cms.

An amusing but well-documented history of the Heart Hospital by Capt. Whitney, the secretary from 1912. A typescript list of St. Cyres Lectures, 1927–1962 is inserted. Another copy (2 parts in 1) (RCP) takes story down to 1957. See also Robert Marshall, "Early days in Westmoreland Street", *British Heart Journal*, 1964, **26,** 140–5.

WILLIUS (FREDERICK ARTHUR) *b.* 1888 and KEYS (THOMAS EDWARD) *b.* 1908

1009 Cardiac classics: a collection of classic works on the heart and circulation with comprehensive biographic accounts of the authors: fifty-two contributions by fifty-one authors. *London, Henry Kimpton, 1941.* xix, 858 pp. Illus, ports, facsims. 4to, 26 cms.

Garrison and Morton 3158; also published St. Louis, Mosby, 1941.

Contains works by the following authors with biographies and portraits: Harvey, Pierre Gassendi (1592–1657), Malpighi, Niels Stensen (1638–1686), William Cowper (1666–1709), Leeuwenhoek, Hales, Sénac, Haller, Morgagni, Auenbrugger, Heberden, Withering, Baillie, John Hunter, Corvisart, Wells, John Cheyne (1777–1836), Laennec, Parry, Robert Adams (1791–1875), Hope,

Corrigan, Bouilland, Stokes, William Senhouse Kirkes, Paul Louis Duroziez (1826–1897), Austin Flint (1812–1886), Potain, Brunton, Heinrich Irenaeus Quincke (1842–1922), Wilks, Traube, Gowers, Cohnheim, Roger, Murrell, Waller, John Alexander MacWilliam (1857–1937), Steell, Etienne Louis Arthur Fallot (1850–1911), Wilhelm His *jr.* (1863–1914), Francis Henry Williams (1852–1936), Broadbent, Einthoven, Aschoff, Keith and Flack, Mackenzie, Osler, and Herrick.

HERRICK (JAMES BRYAN) 1861–1954

1010 A Short history of cardiology. *Springfield, Ill., Charles C. Thomas, 1942.* xvi, 258 pp. Illus, ports, facsim., bibliog. (ftn. refs). 8vo, 23 cms.

Garrison and Morton 3159. Herrick, professor of medicine at Chicago, had studied literature at Michigan before his medical training and this book, published when he was aged over 80, exemplifies his erudition and charming literary style. He made many important contributions to medicine, notably on sickle-cell anaemia and coronary occlusion.

HINSDALE (GUY) 1858–1948

1011 Our medical debt to France.

Reprinted from *Annals of medical History*, 1942, 3rd series, **4**, 154–66. Ports.
Deals with Corvisart, Laennec, Andral, Trousseau, Dieulafoy, amongst others.

NEUBURGER (MAX) 1868–1955

1012 British medicine and the Vienna School: contacts and parallels. *London, William Heinemann Medical Books, 1943.* 134 pp. Illus, ports, bibliog. 8vo, 23 cms.

Acquired Jerusalem, 1944.
Deals with the Vienna School of Skoda and Rokitansky, and mentions many British authorities on the heart and visitors to Vienna, notably Sir William Wilde, Osler, and H. Davies.

WILLIUS (FREDERICK ARTHUR) *b.* 1888 and DRY (THOMAS JAN) *b.* 1903

1013 A History of the heart and circulation. *Philadelphia & London, W. B. Saunders, 1948.* xvii, 456 pp. Illus, ports. 8vo, 24 cms.

Garrison and Morton 3160. Contents: Part 1, The chronologic presentation of knowledge relating to the heart and circulation 5000 B.C. to 1925 A.D., is largely biographical history with portraits. Part 2, Special biographies, includes Hippocrates, Ibn an-Nafis, Servetus, Caesalpinus, Harvey, Malpighi, Morgagni, Auenbrugger, Withering, Laennec, Joseph Skoda (1805–1881), Brunton, Wilhelm Konrad Roentgen (1845–1922), Francis Henry Williams (1852–1936), Rudolph Matas (1860–1957), Willem Einthoven (1860–1927), Wenckebach, Mackenzie, Osler, and Lewis. Part 3, The chronologic presentation of data according to subjects.
A most useful reference work, profusely illustrated.

BEDFORD (DAVIS EVAN) *b.* 1898

1014 Publications on the history of cardiology: fourteen papers. 1951–1972.

The Ancient art of feeling the pulse.

Reprinted from *British Heart Journal*, 1951, **13**, 423–37. Illus, ports, facsims, bibliog.

La Palpation du pouls radial à travers les âges.

Reprinted from *Livre jubilaire de la Sociéte Belge de Cardiologie*, 1959. pp. 23–33. Illus, ports, facsims. A paper read to the 25th Anniversary of the Belgian Society of Cardiology, Brussels, 1959.

BEDFORD (DAVIS EVAN)

New lamps for old in cardiology. (Annual Oration, Medical Society of London, 1958). *London, The Medical Society, 1958.* 13 pp. 8vo, 22 cms.

Reprinted from *Transactions of the Medical Society of London*, 1957–1958, **74**, 190–202.

New ways for old in cardiology.

Reprinted from European Congress of Cardiology, 3rd. Rome 1960. *Acta tertii Europaei de cordis scientia conventus.* [Amsterdam], Excerpta medica, [1960]. pp. C9–C42. Text in English, Italian, French and German.

A Selection from the library: some early 19th century textbooks on heart disease. [Editorial].

Reprinted from *Circulation*, 1966, **34**, 945–7. Bibliog.

An Early account of aortic incompetence by Thomas Cuming. (1798–1887).

Reprinted from *Medical History*, 1967, **11**, 398–401. Bibliog.

The Surgeon cardiologists of the 19th century.

Reprinted from *British Heart Journal*, 1967, **29**, 461–8. Illus, ports, facsim., bibliog. Allan Burns (1781–1813), Joseph Hodgson (1788–1869), Robert Adams (1791–1875), James Wardrop (1782–1869), O'Bryen Bellingham (1805–1857).

William Heberden's contribution to cardiology.

Reprinted from *Journal of the Royal College of Physicians of London*, 1968, **2**, 127–35. Ports, facsims, bibliog.

Harvey's third circulation: de circulo sanguinis in corde. (Harveian Oration, 1968). [*London, British Medical Association, 1968*]. 15 pp. Bibliog.

Reprinted from *British medical Journal*, 1968, **4**, 273–7.

Cardiology in Italy.

Paper contributed to Professor Condorelli's 70th bithday volume. *Aloiseo Condorelli LXX aetatis annum feliciter conficienti ex omnibus nationibus docti viri scripta ad medicinam pertinentia honoris causa collecta* [edita ab Antonio Strano]. Romae, 1969, pp. 15–20.

Rougnon's letter to Lorry on the death of Captain Charles: a landmark in the history of angina pectoris.

Reprinted from *British Heart Journal*, 1970, **32**, 277–70. Port., facsim., bibliog.

Auenbrugger's contribution to cardiology: history of percussion of the heart.

Reprinted from *British Heart Journal*, 1971, **33**, 817–21. Illus, port., facsim., bibliog.

On Collecting a cardiological library.

Reprinted from *Journal of the Royal College of Physicians of London*, 1972, **6**, 227–34.

The Story of fatty heart: a disease of Victorian times.

Reprinted from *British Heart Journal*, 1972, **34**, 23–8. Illus, ports, bibliog. With a letter to DEB from Dr. Joshua O. Leibowitz (author of no. 677), 28 July 1972.

GRIFFENHAGEN (GEORGE BERNARD) *b.* 1924 and HUGHES (CALVIN H.)

1015 The History of the mechanical heart. (Smithsonian Institution Publication 4241). *Washington, Smithsonian Institution, 1956.* [i], 339–56. Illus, bibliog. 8vo, 23 cms.

Reprinted from Smithsonian Report, 1955, 339–56. Garrison and Morton 3160.1.

O'FARRELL (Patrick Theodore Joseph) 1889–1968

1016 A Famous cardiac controversy: Hope v. Williams.

Reprinted from *Irish Journal of medical Science*, 1957, no. 378, June, 278–85. Bibliog.
Williams and Hope made experiments on asses relative to the heart sounds and murmurs and a dispute arose as to priority in their books. Sir Benjamin Brodie was arbitrator, but his verdict was indecisive.

EAST (Charles Frederick Terence) 1894–1967

1017 The Story of heart disease. The FitzPatrick Lectures for 1956 and 1957 given before the Royal College of Physicians of London. *London, William Dawson*, 1958. 148 pp. Illus, ports, facsims, bibliog. 8vo, 22 cms.

Garrison and Morton 3160.2. Four lectures: 1. Diagnosis—2. Lessons of the deadhouse—3. Coronary circulation and its disorders—4. Failure of the circulation and its treatment.
East was physician to Kings College Hospital and a bibliophile.

SOCIÉTÉ BELGE DE CARDIOLOGIE

1018 Livre Jubilaire publié à l'occasion du xxvme anniversaire de la fondation de la Société Belge de Cardiologie, 1934–1959. *Brussels*, [*Société Belge de Cardiologie*], *1960*. [viii], xxxiii, 171 pp. Illus, ports, facsims, diagrs, bibliog. 8vo, 24 cms.

Séance Académique includes the presidential address by Paul Regniers; Historique de la Société Belge de Cardiologie 1934–1959 by Fr. Van Dooren; and La palpation du pouls radial à travers les âges (Evan Bedford).
Conférences include papers by P. Rijlant on the evolution of the electrocardiogram, and J. Lequime on evolution of the knowledge of haemodynamics over the past twenty years.

MULCAHY (Risteárd)

1019 The Views of the 19th century Irish cardiologists on coronary artery disease.

Reprinted from *Irish Journal of medical Science*, 1963, no. 445, Jan., 35–44. Bibliog.
Signed presentation copy from the author.

CHAVEZ (Ignacio) *b.* 1897

1020 El Instituto Nacional de Cardiología en 1964 (a los veinte anos de su fundación). *México, Instituto Nacional de Cardiología*, [*1965*]. 80 pp. Illus, ports, map, tables, diagrs. Folio, 34 cms.

No. 46 of a limited edition of 300 copies. Author's signed presentation copy to DEB.

MEDICAL HISTORY AND BIOGRAPHY
with a few ancient texts

Medical History

Biographies of physicians, both collected and individual, are important sources of information and are, therefore, included with histories of medicine, except when they can be included in any other section following works written by the subject of a biography. Ancient medical texts often include historical introductions by the translator or editor; these will also be found in this section.

DAVACH DE LA RIVIERE (JEAN)

1021 Le Miroir des urines, par lesquels on voit & connoît les différens tempéramens, les humeurs dominantes, les sièges & les causes des maladies d'un chacun. 4me éd., revûe & corrigée, & augmenteé d'une ample table pour trouver toutes sortes de maladies, signifiées par les urines. *Paris, Cavelier, Delaguette, D'Houry fils, 1752.* [12] ff., 315 pp. 12mo, 17 cms.

This work on uroscopy deals with diagnosis from inspection of the urine as widely practised in the Middle Ages together with feeling the pulse. First edition, Paris, chez l'auteur, 1696; a sixth edition was published, Paris, 1803.

LE CLERC (DANIEL) 1652–1728

1022 Histoire de la médecine, ou l'on voit l'origine & les (*sic*) progrès de cet art, de siècle en siècle; les sectes, qui s'y sont formées; les noms des médecins, leurs découvertes, leurs opinions, & les circonstances les plus remarquables de leur vie . . . Nouvelle édition, revue, corrigée & augmentée par l'auteur en divers endroits, & sur tout d'un plan pour servir à la continuation de cette histoire dépuis la fin du siècle II jusques au milieu du XVII. *Amsterdam, aux dépens de la Compagnie, 1723.* [9] ff., 820 pp., [10] ff. Illus (extra title-page, 8 plates), table (folding), bibliog. (ftn. refs). 4to, 26 cms.

Garrison and Morton 6379.

Autograph: James Vaughan (possibly James Vaughan (1740–1813), M.D., of Leicester, father of Sir Henry Halford, President of the Royal College of Physicians).

Le Clerc's is the first large modern history of medicine. The first edition (Geneva, 1696) is very rare. An English translation *The History of physick* (London, 1699) (RCP) was made from this.

A further edition *Histoire de la médecine* . . . (Amsterdam, 1702) was later followed by our edition (1723) and this latter by another in 1729. As Garrison notes, "later editions are more useful."

Critical mention of Le Clerc in Freind's *History of physick* (1725–1726) called forth *An Answer* (London, 1728), written by Jean Le Clerc, Daniel's brother.

QUINCY (JOHN) *d.* 1722

1023 Lexicon physico-medicum: or, A New medicinal dictionary; explaining the difficult terms used in the several branches of the profession, and in such parts of natural philosophy as are introductory thereto: with an account of the things signified by such terms Collected from the most eminent authors; and particularly those who have wrote upon mechanical principles. 6th ed. *London, T. Longman, 1743.* xvi, 480 pp. Tables, diagrs. 8vo, 21 cms.

Autograph: Matthew Metcalf, Jan. 13th, 1764. "Presented to me by Dr J. L. Morton who died aged over 100 years in 1970": note by DEB (John Leyden Morton, M.D., 1869–1970, was one of the first practitioners in London to recognize the clinical features of coronary thrombosis).

First edition, 1719. This edition (reprinted in 1749) is "with new improvements from the latest chymical and mechanical authors".

FREIND (John) 1675–1728

1024 The History of physick; from the time of Galen to the beginning of the 16th century, chiefly with regard to practice. *London, J. Walthoe, jun., 1725–1726.* 2 vols. Bibliog. (ftn. refs). 8vo, 20 cms.

Vol. 1 [iv], 312 pp.; vol. 2 [i], 415, 72 pp.

Autograph: Chs. Austin Jesu Coll. Cant. (Charles Austin, 1799–1874, distinguished scholar, conversationalist and lawyer).

"Freind was the first English historian of medicine; his book is the best English work on the period of which it treats." (Garrison and Morton 6378). It is Freind's principal work and was intended as a sort of continuation of Daniel Le Clerc's *Histoire*, which he praises at the commencement, but pointed out various imperfections in his plan for a continuation. Freind never replied to the defence by Le Clerc's brother.

There were five editions in English (5th ed. 1758), and translations in Latin and French.

BARTHEZ (Paul-Joseph) 1734–1806, and others

1025 Consultations de médecine de M. Barthez . . . et de MM. Bouvart, Fouquet, Lorry et Lamure. *Paris, Leopold Collin, 1807.* 2 tom. in 1. 8vo, 21 cms.

Tom. 1: [iii], xvi, 478 pp.; tom. 2 [iii], 535 pp.

Barthez of Montpellier was a leading vitalist of this period and physician to Napoleon. Michel-Philippe Bouvart (1711–1787) was physician at the Charité and professor at the Faculty of Medicine. Fouquet is best known for his *Traité sur le pouls* (nos 37 and 38). Rougnon's letter on Captain Charles (no. 600) was addressed to Lorry.

The most important work of François de Bourguignon Buissière de Lamure (1717–1787), dean of the medical professors at Montpellier, was his *Recherches sur la pulsation des artères* . . . Montpellier, 1769, in which without knowing he duplicated the results of Haller.

SPRENGEL (Kurt Polykarp Joachim) 1766–1833

1026 Histoire de la médecine, depuis son origine jusqu'au dix-neuvième siècle. Traduite de l'allemand sur la seconde édition par A. J. L. Jourdan . . ., et revue par E. F. M. Bosquillon . . . *Paris, Deterville [et] Th. Desoer, Bechet; Montpellier, A. Gabon, 1815–1820.* 9 tom. Bibliog. (ftn. refs). 8vo, 21 cms.

The first seven volumes were published in 1815 by Deterville and Desoer, tom. 8 (1820) and 9 (1820) being published by Bechet and Gabon.

A monument of historical scholarship and an invaluable source of reference, originally appearing as *Versuch einer pragmatischen Geschichte der Arzneikunde* (Halle, J. J. Gebauer, 1792–1803).

MAPLESON (Thomas)

1027 A Treatise on the art of cupping in which the history of that operation is traced, the complaints in which it is useful indicated, and the most approved method of performing it described. 2nd ed. *London, the Author and J. Callow, 1821.* [viii], 94 pp. 8vo, 20 cms.

Autograph: Walker.

First edition, London 1813. According to Callisen, Mapleson was at Westminster Hospital. Mr. Gower, the archivist, can find no trace of him, but the cupper in fact kept the surgical implements there.

CROSSE (John Green) 1790–1850

1028 Sketches of the medical schools of Paris. *London, J. Callow, 1815.* xv, 208 pp. Bibliog. (ftn. refs). 8vo, 22 cms.

Book-stamp: Birmingham Medical Institute.

Visits to various Paris hospitals, mostly surgical clinics, but mentions "Percussion de la poitrine" as widely practised at that time (p. 202).

DAGIER (Etienne)

1029 Histoire chronologique de l'Hôpital Général et Grand Hôtel-Dieu de Lyon, depuis sa fondation; melée de faits historiques concernant l'aumone générale et la ville de Lyon. *Lyon, M. P. Rusand, 1830.* 2 tom. 8vo, 23 cms.

Tom. 1 xvi, 462 pp.; tom. 2 [iii], 551, [1] pp.

A fascinating history of the Hôtel-Dieu, one of the oldest hospitals in France. Rabelais was a physician there, and more recently Gallavardin had his cardiological clinic there. DEB visited it in 1926 for a time. Dagier, or Dagiez (Callisen) was archivist at Hôtel-Dieu.

DAREMBERG (Charles Victor) 1817–1872

1030 Histoire des sciences médicales, comprenant l'anatomie, la physiologie, la médecine, la chirurgie et les doctrines de pathologie générale. *Paris, J. B. Baillière, 1870.* 2 tom. (xxviii, 580, [iii], 577–1303 pp.). Illus, bibliog. (ftn. refs). 8vo, 22 cms.

The most important work of the great French medical historian. For his translation of Galen and of Rufus of Ephesus, see nos. 1073 and 2.

MONTEIL (Amans Alexis) 1769–1850

1031 La Médecine en France. Hommes et doctrines depuis l'antiquité jusqu'à nos jours, avec introduction, notes et supplément par A. le Pileur. *Paris, Bibliothèque Nouvelle, P. Dupont, P. Daffis, [1874].* [iii], 438, [2] pp. Bibliog. (ftn. refs). 8vo, 19 cms.

Includes Corvisart and Laennec, and describes the appalling conditions in Hôtel Dieu Hospital with four to six patients in a bed.

GAIRDNER (Sir William Tennant) 1824–1907

1032 The Physician as naturalist: addresses and memoirs bearing on the history and progress of medicine chiefly during the last hundred years. *Glasgow, James Maclehose, 1889.* x, 436 pp. Bibliog. (ftn. refs). 8vo, 20 cms.

Autograph: R. Cormon Robertson.

Includes *The Progress of pathological science; John Baptist Morgagni and his successors* (pp. 294–310). For a life of Sir W. T. Gairdner with selection of his papers by Gibson, see no. 292.

WITHINGTON (Edward Theodore) 1860–1947

1033 Medical history from the earliest times: a popular history of the healing art. *London, Holland Press, 1964.* viii, 424 pp. Table, bibliog. 8vo, 22 cms.

A reprint of this important history first published, London, Scientific Press 1894. Garrison and Morton 6395.

HOLMES (Oliver Wendell) 1809–1894

1034 Medical essays 1842–1882. *Boston and New York, Houghton, Mifflin and Company, 1896.* xvii, 445 pp. Port., bibliog. (ftn. refs). 8vo, 20 cms.

Garrison and Morton 6390. An early important American work dealing with various subjects in the history of medicine.

ALLBUTT (Sir Thomas Clifford) 1836–1925

1035 The Historical relations of medicine and surgery to the end of the sixteenth century. *London, Macmillan, 1905.* xvi, 125 pp. Bibliog. 12mo, 19 cms.

Acquired 1942. Autograph: W. H. Coupland (William Henry Coupland, *d.* 1943) with various insertions without references, except an abstract of Allbutt's "Address on the historical relations between surgery and medicine" (*British medical Journal*, 1904, **1**, 789–92).

1036 Greek medicine in Rome: the FitzPatrick Lectures on the history of medicine delivered at the Royal College of Physicians of London in 1909–1910; with other historical essays. *London, Macmillan, 1921.* xiv, 633 pp. Bibliog. (ftn. refs). 8vo, 23 cms.

Covers Greek and Roman medicine, libraries, pulse doctrines, Archigenes, Rufus, Galen, Herophilus, etc. Reprinted, New York, Blom, 1970.

DELAUNAY (Paul) 1878–1958

1037 Le Monde médicale Parisien au dix-huitième siècle. (Faculté de Médecine de Paris. Thèse pour le doctorat en médecine, 1905, no. 68). *Paris, Jules Rousset, 1905.* viii, 460, lxxvii pp. Ports, bibliog. 8vo, 25 cms.

Pp. i–iv wanting. Deals with royal physicians, hospitals, library, phlebotomy, etc. Good bibliography.

ATLAS

1038 Atlas of ancient and classical geography. (Everyman's Library, no. 451). *London, J. M. Dent: New York, E. P. Dutton, 1907 (rep. 1942).* xiii, 268, 4 pp. Maps, plans. 12mo, 17 cms.

Acquired 1944. A useful atlas in relation to classical medicine.

MOORE (Sir Norman) 1847–1922

1039 The History of the study of medicine in the British Isles; the FitzPatrick Lectures for 1905–1906, delivered before the Royal College of Physicians of London. *Oxford, Clarendon Press, 1908.* viii, 202 pp. Facsims, bibliog. (ftn. refs). 8vo, 23 cms.

This is a very important historical work.

CAMAC (CHARLES NICOLL BANKER) 1868–1940

1040 Epoch-making contributions to medicine, surgery and the allied sciences, being reprints of those communications which first conveyed epoch-making observations to the scientific world, together with biographical sketches of the observers, collected by C. N. B. Camac. *Philadelphia and London, W. B. Saunders, 1909.* x, 435 pp. Ports, facsims, bibliog. 8vo, 24 cms.

Autograph and bookplate of Sir John William Moore, 1845–1937, with his review from *Dublin Journal of medical Science*, 1909, **128,** 120–1 pasted on front end-paper.

Contains extracts from works and biographies of Lister, Harvey, Auenbrugger, Laennec, Edward Jenner, W. T. G. Morton, Horace Wells, John C. Warren, J. Y. Simpson, and O. W. Holmes.

CABANES (AUGUSTIN) 1862–1928

1041 Les Morts mystérieuses de l'histoire. Nouvelle édition. *Paris, Albin Michel, [1910–1911?].* 2 tom. 8vo, 19 cms.

Tom. 1: Rois, reines et princes français de Charlemagne à Louis XIII ([iii], 440 pp.); tom. 2: Louis XIII à Napoléon III ([iii], 443 pp.).

First edition (subtitle "Souverains et princes français de Charlemagne à Louis XVII") Paris, A. Maloine, 1901.

MEUNIER (LEON JOSEPH) 1856–1911

1042 Histoire de la médecine depuis ses origines jusqu'a nos jours. *Paris, J. B. Baillière et fils, 1911.* [iii], vi, 642 pp. 8vo, 20 cms.

Garrison and Morton 6407.

DELMAS (PAUL) 1880–1929

1043 L'Éclosion d'une faculté de province. Comment s'est constituée l'ancienne école de médecine de Montpellier. *Montpellier, Coulet et fils, 1913.* 47 pp. Illus, ports, maps, facsims. 8vo, 25 cms.

GARRISON (FIELDING HUDSON) 1870–1935

1044 An Introduction to the history of medicine, with medical chronology, suggestions for study and bibliographic data. 3rd ed. *Philadelphia and London, W. B. Saunders, 1921.* 942 pp. Illus, ports, bibliog. 8vo, 24 cms.

First edition, 1913; second edition, 1917; fourth edition, 1929.

CONTRIBUTIONS

1045 Contributions to medical and biological research, dedicated to Sir William Osler, Bart., M.D., F.R.S., in honour of his seventieth birthday, July 12, 1919, by his pupils and co-workers. *New York, Paul B. Hoeber, 1919.* 2 vols. Illus, ports, facsims, tables, diagrs, bibliog. 8vo, 25 cms.

Vol. 1: xxi, 649 pp.; vol. 2: xiii, 651–1268 (continuous pagination).

Many of the contributions are on subjects connected with the history of medicine. Note Servetus notes by Mackall, vol. 2, p. 767 as an important bibliography. Of cardiological interest are: Marginal sounds by George E. Bushnell, Visual disturbances in polycythemia vera by Harry Friedenwald, Congenital arterio-venous and lymphatico-venous fistulae, unique clinical and experimental observations by William Stewart Halsted, Clinical features of acute obstruction of the coronary arteries by James B. Herrick, The Intimate relationship of chorea, rheumatism, and cardiac disease by Henry Koplik, On contra-lateral representation in the cerebral cortex of the peripheral blood vessels by S. P. Kramer, Clinical and developmental study of a case of ruptured aneurysm of the right anterior aortic sinus of Valsalva by Maude E. Abbot, The conditions presented in the heart and kidneys of old people by W. T. Councilman, Symptomless obliteration of the superior vena cava by Thomas B. Futcher, Aneurysm of the middle cerebral artery of a child nine and one-half years old by Fritz B. Talbot, The Cardiovascular defective by Louis M. Warfield, A Case of Ayerza's disease by Aldred Scott Warthin, Some experiences and observations in the treatment of arterio-venous aneurysms by Rudolph Matas, and Studies on the potency of digitalis leaves from various sources by Joseph H. Pratt.

Of historical interest are: The Oxford University Museum by T. D. Acland, The Oxford Medical School in the eighteenth century by Arnold Chaplin, Antonius Musa: his practice and patients by Raymond Crawfurd, Some personal reminiscences of Sir William Osler by J. Beattie Crozier, Sweating sickness in modern times by Michael G. Foster, The Cradle of the Hunterian School by Arthur Keith, Thomas Trotter, M.D. by Sir Humphry Rolleston, On a miniature ascribed to Mantegna of an operation by Cosmas and Damian by Charles and Dorothea Singer, Some seventeenth century writings on diseases of children by George F. Still, Galen, Plato and immortality by E. T. Withington, Fragment of a Persian primer of the institutes of medicine by R. Ramsay Wright, The Innate heat by Sir T. Clifford Allbutt, The Schematic drawing of the eye in its historic development by Mortimer Frank, Physicians' letters by Fielding H. Garrison, Sir William Osler and the Johns Hopkins Hospital by Henry M. Hurd, Edward Jenner, a student of medicine, as illustrated in his letters by Henry Barton Jacobs, and Influence of English medicine upon American medicine in its formative period by William H. Welch.

CAMPBELL (DONALD) *d.* 1949

1046 Arabian medicine and its influence on the Middle Ages. (Trubner's Oriental Series). *London, Kegan Paul, Trench, Trubner, 1926.* 2 vols. Bibliog. 8vo, 21 cms.

Vol. 1: xv, 208 pp.; vol. 2: [v], 235 pp. Garrison and Morton 6509.

An important bibliography of Arabic medicine, and the history of its transmission to the West. Vol. 2 consists of two appendices: I: Latin translators of the Arabic work; II: An Investigation of the date and authorship of the Latin versions of the works of Galen, with a full bibliography.

CUMSTON (CHARLES GREENE) 1868–1927

1047 An Introduction to the history of medicine, from the time of the Pharaohs to the end of the eighteenth century. With an essay on the relation of history and philosophy to medicine by F. G. Crookshank. (The History of Civilization). *London, Kegan Paul, Trench & Trubner; New York, Alfred A. Knopf, 1926.* xxii, 390 pp. Illus, ports, facsim. 8vo, 24 cms.

An excellent history dealing especially with the different schools of medical thought. It was reprinted in 1968.

CASTIGLIONI (ARTURO) 1874–1953

1048 Histoire de la médecine; éd. française établie par les soins de l'auteur. Traduction par J. Bertrand . . . et F. Gidon. (Bibliothèque Médicale). *Paris, Payot, 1931.* 781 pp. Illus, ports, facsims, bibliog. 8vo, 25 cms.

Originally published in Italian (Milan, 1927); English translation, second edition, London, 1947.

COMRIE (JOHN DIXON) 1875–1939

1049 History of Scottish medicine to 1860. (Research Studies in Medical History no. 4). *London, Baillière, Tindall & Cox, for Wellcome Historical Medical Museum, 1927.* 301 pp. Illus, ports, facsims, bibliog. (ftn. refs). 8vo, 23 cms.

Second edition, 1932 in two volumes (RCP).

SINGER (CHARLES JOSEPH) 1876–1960

1050 A Short history of medicine: introducing medical principles to students and non-medical readers. *Oxford, Clarendon Press, 1928.* xxiv, 368 pp. 8vo, 21 cms.

Book-stamp: Hammersmith Public Libraries.
Garrison and Morton 6421. The best short history of medicine.

BROCK (ARTHUR JOHN) 1879–1947

1051 Greek medicine; being extracts illustrative of medical writers from Hippocrates to Galen; trans. and annotated by Arthur J. Brock. (Library of Greek Thought). *London, & Toronto, J. M. Dent; New York, E. P. Dutton, 1929.* xii, 256 pp. 8vo, 20 cms.

After a general historical introduction (pp. 1–34), the author translates extracts from Hippocrates, Thucydides, Plato, Aristotle, Rufus of Ephesus, Galen, Diodorus and Aetius. Of cardiological interest are Rufus's case of Myron the wrestler (pp. 117–18), why arteries are joined to veins by Galen (pp. 157–60), and aneurysms by Aetius (pp. 247–8).

FOSSEYEUX (MARCEL)

1052 Il y a cent ans: Paris médical en 1830. *Paris, le François, 1930.* 104 pp. Illus, ports, bibliog. (ftn. refs). 8vo, 20 cms.

Interesting details on Chomel, Piorry, Andral, Bertin, Bichat, Broussais, Cruveilhier, Laennec, Magendie, Pinel, Portal, Raige-Delorme, and others; also on medical societies and booksellers.

ROLLESTON (Sir HUMPHRY DAVY) 1862–1944

1053 The Cambridge Medical School; a biographical history. *Cambridge, University Press, 1932.* ix, 235 pp. Ports (21 plates), facsim., bibliog. 8vo, 22 cms.

Includes biographies of Allbutt, Caius, Gaskell, Glisson, Heberden, Sir Michael Foster and others.

DUMESNIL (RENÉ) 1879–?

1054 Histoire illustrée de la médecine. *Paris, Plon, 1935.* 264 pp. Illus, ports, facsims, bibliog. (ftn. refs). 8vo, 25 cms.

Garrison and Morton 6428. A good survey of the development of medicine especially in France.

MAHFOUZ (NAGUIB) 1882–1974

1055 The History of medical education in Egypt. *Cairo, Government Press, 1935.* xiii, 121 pp. Illus (plates), ports, plans, tables, bibliog. 4to, 25 cms.

Acquired Cairo, July 1943.
Mahfouz, an authority on gynaecological pathology, was professor of gynaecology and obstetrics at the Kasr-el-Aini Hospital, Cairo. The Mahfouz Museum there contains a magnificent collection of drawings and paintings by Stackalovsky, the famous Kasr-el-Aini medical artist.

THOMSON (HERBERT CAMPBELL) 1870–1940

1056 The Story of the Middlesex Hospital Medical School, written at the request of the Council of the Medical School on the occasion of the centenary. *London, John Murray, 1935.* xiii, 182 pp. Illus, ports, bibliog. (ftn. refs). 8vo, 23 cms.

Campbell Thomson was dean of the medical school and neurologist to the Middlesex Hospital, where DEB was a resident and registrar and finally emeritus consulting physician.

ABRAHAM (JAMES JOHNSTON) 1876–1963

1057 The Early history of syphilis. (Vicary Lecture 1943–44). *Bristol, John Wright, 1944.* 43 pp. Illus, ports, facsims, bibliog. 12mo, 15 cms.

Reprinted from *British Journal of Surgery*, 1944, **32,** 225–37.
Author's copy to Dr. Norman (Hubert James Norman, 1881–1948).

GUTHRIE (DOUGLAS JAMES) 1885–1975

1058 A History of medicine. *London, [etc.], Nelson, 1945 (reprinted 1946).* xvi, 448 pp. Illus, ports, facsims, map, bibliog. 8vo, 23 cms.

1059 The Medical School of Edinburgh. *Edinburgh, [printed by] George Waterston [1959].* 32 pp. Illus, ports, map. 8vo, 20 cms.

Published on the occasion of the B.M.A.'s joint meeting with Canadian Medical Association, 1959.

MAJOR (RALPH HERMON) 1884–1970

1060 A History of medicine. *Oxford, Blackwell Scientific Publications, 1954.* 2 vols. Illus, ports, facsims, bibliog. 8vo, 22 cms.

Vol. 1: xxv, 563 pp.; vol. 2: xiii, 565–1155 pp. Also published Springfield, Ill., C. C. Thomas, 1954.
Covers the dawn of medicine down to the 20th century.

Bibliography

CHOULANT (JOHANN LUDWIG) 1791–1861

1061 Handbuch der Bücherkunde für die altere Medicin . . . *Graz, Akademische Druck-u. Verlagsanstalt, 1956.* xxii, 434 pp. 8vo, 17 cms.

Facsimile reprint of the second edition (Leipzig, 1841). First edition, 1828. Garrison and Morton 6753.

PAULY (ALPHONSE)

1062 Bibliographie des sciences médicales. *London, D. Verschoyle, 1954.* [iv], iii–xx pp., 1758 cols, [80] pp. 8vo, 25 cms.

Facsimile reprint; originally published Paris, Tross, 1874.

FINLAYSON (JAMES) 1840–1906

1063 [Bibliographical demonstrations].
Celsus.

Reprinted from *Glasgow medical Journal*, 1892, **37,** 321–48.

FINLAYSON (JAMES)

Hippocrates.

Reprinted from *Glasgow medical Journal*, 1892, **37**, 253–71.

Herophilus and Erasistratus.

Reprinted from *Glasgow medical Journal*, 1893, **39**, 321–52. Autograph: Charles Singer (Charles Joseph Singer 1876–1960, medical historian).

Useful bibliographical details of early texts of these authors. Finlayson, physician to the Glasgow Western Infirmary and to the Royal Hospital for Sick Children, was honorary librarian to the Faculty of Physicians and Surgeons, Glasgow.

GARRISON (FIELDING HUDSON) 1870–1935 and
MORTON (LESLIE THOMAS) *b.* 1907

1064 Garrison and Morton's medical bibliography: an annotated check list of texts illustrating the history of medicine by Leslie T. Morton. 2nd ed. rev. *London, Andre Deutsch, 1965.* xiii, 655 pp. 8vo, 22 cms.

First edition, London, Grafton, 1943; second edition, 1954; third edition, London, Deutsch [Grafton], 1970.

GOLDSCHMIDT (ERNST PHILIP) 1887–1954, and others

1065 A Doctor and his books: Harvey Cushing and his library.

Reprinted from *Journal of the History of Medicine and Allied Sciences*, 1945, **1**, 229–53.

Presentation copy from E. Weil.

Contents: Recollections of Harvey Cushing and his book-collecting, by E. P. Goldschmidt, pp. 229–34; The formation of the Harvey Cushing Collection, by E. Weil, pp. 234–46; Harvey Cushing and his books, by Geoffrey Jefferson, pp. 246–53.

HAHN (ALFRED ANDRÉ) *b.* 1900 and DUMAITRE (PAULE)

1066 Histoire de la médecine et du livre médical, à la lumière des collections de la Bibliothèque de la Faculté de Médecine de Paris [par] André Hahn [et] Paule Dumaitre, avec la collaboration de Janine Samion-Contet. *Paris, Olivier Perrin, [1962].* 430, [4] pp. Illus, ports, facsims, bibliog. 4to, 28 cms.

The most magnificently illustrated history of medical books yet published, with considerable bibliography of sources (pp. 377–94) and descriptions of illustrations (pp. 395–418).

Individual Biographies with some ancient texts

HIPPOCRATES *c.* 460–377 B.C.

1067 The Genuine works of Hippocrates; trans. from the Greek with a preliminary discourse and annotations by Francis Adams. *London, Sydenham Society, 1849.* 2 vols. Illus (plates), bibliog. (ftn. refs). 8vo, 23 cms.

Vol. 1: x, 468 pp.; vol. 2: vii, 469–874 pp. Garrison and Morton 14.

Autograph: J. P. Wall, 6 Mount Street, Grosv'r Sq., London, Nov. 1849 (John Pritchard Wall, *d. c.* 1853?, surgeon, father of Alfred John Wall, 1847–1898, F.R.C.S.).

The standard English edition of Hippocrates limited to the so-called "genuine works".

1068 The Medical works of Hippocrates: a new translation from the original Greek made especially for English readers, by the collaboration of John Chadwick and W. N. Mann. *Oxford, Blackwell Scientific Publications, 1950.* vii, 301 pp. Port. 8vo, 22 cms.

Presentation copy to DEB initialled by W. N. M[ann] (F.R.C.P.).

1069 The Aphorisms of Hippocrates and the sentences of Celsus; with explanations and references to the most considerable writers in physick and philosophy, both ancient and modern. To which are added aphorisms upon the small-pox, measles and other distempers, not so well known in former more temperate ages, by C. J. Sprengell. *London, Bonwick, Freeman and others, 1708.* [5] ff., xiv, 349 pp., [13] ff. Ports. 8vo, 20 cms.

Inscribed "James Moore Esq. M.D. to Thomas M. Parr L.R.C.P. & S.Ed., Belfast, October 1883."
Second edition London, R. Wilkins [and others] 1735.
Sir Conrad Joachim Sprengell (*d.* 1740), the translator, a native of Leipzig, knighted by George I, was a Fellow of the Royal College of Physicians and of the Royal Society.

ARISTOTLE, 384–322 B.C.

1070 On youth & old age, life & death and respiration; trans. with introduction and notes, by W. Ogle. *London, Longmans, Green, 1897.* vii, 135 pp. Bibliog. (ftn. refs). 8vo, 23 cms.

CELSUS (Aulus Aurelius Cornelius) *fl.* 1st cent. A.D.

1071 Of medicine in eight books; trans., with notes, critical and explanatory, by James Greive, M.D. Carefully revised, with additional notes by George Futvoye. 3rd ed. *London, H. Renshaw, T. Hill, T. Burgess, E. Cox and C. Daly, 1838.* xxviii, 468 pp. Bibliog. (ftn. refs). 12mo, 18 cms.

First edition of this translation, London, D. Wilson and T. Durham, 1756; new edition, Edinburgh, University Press, 1814.
Autographs: [undecipherable]; Dr. George Duncan, West Gurty, 7 Octr. 1844; W. Catesby, London, 1883.
The translator James Greive, M.D., F.R.C.P., F.R.S. (*d.* 1773) graduated from Edinburgh in 1752, became physician at St. Thomas's Hospital and Charterhouse, and was tutor to Lettsom. Munk's spelling of his surname is corroborated by his signature in the Royal Society's charter book; though Greive's biography is correct, the spelling "Grieve" adopted by D.N.B. belongs to the Scot James Grieve (graduated M.D., Edinburgh, 1733) who was physician to the Tsarina Elizabeth.

1072 A Translation of the eight books of Aul. Corn. Celsus on medicine. 2nd ed., revised and improved by G. F. Collier. *London, Simpkin & Marshall, 1831.* xx, 363 pp. Illus, plan. 8vo, 21 cms.

Autograph: Julius Kohn.
First edition of this translation: London, S. Highley, 1830; third edition, London, Longman, 1840.

GALEN *c.* 130–*c.* 200

1073 Oeuvres anatomiques, physiologiques et medicales de Galien, traduites sur les textes imprimés et manuscrits, accompagnées de sommaires, de notes, de planches, et d'une table des matières, précédées d'une introduction, ou étude biographique, littéraire et scientifique sur Galien par le dr. Ch. Daremberg. *Paris, J. B. Baillière, 1854–1856.* 2 tom. Bibliog. (ftn. refs). 8vo, 23 cms.

Tom. 1: [iii], xvi, 706, [2] pp.; tom. 2: [iii], 786, [1] pp.

1074 Galen on the natural faculties, with English translation by Arthur John Brock. (Loeb Classical Library). *London, W. Heinemann; Cambridge, Mass., Harvard University Press, 1916.* lv, 339 pp. Bibliog. 12mo, 17 cms.

1075 Galen on medical experience: first edition of the Arabic version with English translation by R. Walzer. *London, New York, Toronto, Oxford University Press, 1944.* xi, 164 pp. Bibliog. (ftn. refs and notes). 4to, 26 cms.

Translation title: Galen's Treatise on medical experience. Translation by Hunain from Greek into Syriac, and translation by Hubaish from Syriac into Arabic.

Galen's original text, written in Pergamum before A.D. 150, has been lost. This ninth-century Arabic translation was discovered in Constantinople in 1931 by Dr. H. Ritter, and is a translation from the Syriac translation of Hunain ibn Ishaq by his nephew and disciple (*c.* 850 A.D.) Hubaish ibn al-Hasan al A'sam. It agrees with a Greek fragment discovered by Hermann Schöne in 1901 and part of a Latin version thought originally to have been an unknown work by Galen.

AVICENNA, 980–1037

AFNAN (SOHEIL MUHSIN)

1076 Avicenna: his life and works. *London, George Allen & Unwin, 1958.* 298 pp. Bibliog. 8vo, 22 cms.

Includes a selective bibliography of works on Avicenna, and a chapter on medicine and the natural sciences (pp. 201–32).

SALERNUM. SCHOLA MEDICA

1077 The School of Salernum. Regimen Sanitatis Salernitanum; the English version by Sir John Harington. History of the School of Salernum by Francis R. Packard, M.D., and a note on the prehistory of the Regimen Sanitatis by Fielding H. Garrison, M.D. *London, Humphrey Milford, 1922.* [i], 216 pp. Illus, ports, bibliog. (ftn. refs). 8vo, 21 cms.

Autograph: Hubert Norman (Herbert James Norman, 1881–1948). Acquired 1942.

Garrison and Morton 51. The English text of Sir John Harington (1561–1612) was first published in 1607. A handbook of domestic medicine written in verse and dating from the eleventh, or more probably the twelfth century.

PARACELSUS (PHILIPPUS AUREOLUS THEOPHRASTUS) 1493–1541

1078 The Life of Philippus Theophrastus Bombast of Hohenheim, known by the name of Paracelsus, and the substance of his teachings concerning cosmology, anthropology, pneumatology, magic and sorcery, medicine, alchemy, and astrology, philosophy and theosophy. Extracted and translated from his rare and extensive works and from some unpublished manuscripts by Franz Hartmann. 2nd ed. *London, Kegan Paul, French, Trübner & Co., [1896].* xv, 311 pp. 8vo, 22 cms.

PARE (Ambroise) 1510–1590

1079 Œuvres complètes. Revues et collationnées sur toutes les editions, avec les variantes . . . accompagnées de notes historiques et critiques, et précédées d'une introduction sur l'origine et les progrès de la chirurgie en Occident du sixième au seizième siècle, et sur la vie en les ouvrages d'Ambroise Paré, par J.-F. Malgaigne. *Paris, J. B. Baillière, 1840–1841.* 3 tom. Bibliog. (ftn. refs). 4to, 27 cms.

Garrison and Morton 64.

VESALIUS (Andreas) 1514–1564

1080 The Illustrations from the works of Andreas Vesalius of Brussels with annotations and translations, a discussion of the plates and their background, authorship and influence, and a biographical sketch of Vesalius, by J. B. de C. M. Saunders and Charles D. O'Malley. *Cleveland and New York, World Publishing Co., 1950.* 248 pp. Illus, port., plates, facsims. Folio, 31 cms.

"The anatomical illustrations in this volume have been reproduced from *Andreae Vesalii Bruxellensis Icones Anatomicae*, published jointly by the Library of the University of Munich and the New York Academy of Medicine."

BALL (JAMES MOORE) *jr.* 1862–1929

1081 Andreas Vesalius, the reformer of anatomy. *St. Louis, Medical Science Press, 1910.* xviii, 149 pp. Illus, ports, bibliog. (ftn. refs). Folio, 33 cms.

GALILEI (Galileo) 1564–1642

CHASLES (VICTOR EUPHÉMION PHILARÈTE) 1798–1873

1082 Galileo Galilei, sa vie, son procès et ses contemporains d'après les documents originaux. *Paris, Poulet-Malassis, 1862.* [iv], viii, 287 pp. 8vo, 19 cms.

HAMEY (Baldwin) 1568–1640

KEEVIL (JOHN JOYCE) 1901–1957

1083 Hamey the stranger. *London, Geoffrey Bles, 1952.* xvi, 192 pp. Illus, port, plan, facsims, bibliog. 8vo, 22 cms.

Keevil also wrote a sequel *The Stranger's son* (London, Bles, 1953) (RCP) on Baldwin Hamey, junior, 1600–1676.

SYDENHAM (Thomas) 1624–1689

1084 The Whole works of that excellent practical physician Dr. Thomas Sydenham. Wherein not only the history and cures of acute diseases are treated of, after a new and accurate method; but also the shortest and safest way of curing chronic diseases. 6th ed. corrected from the original Latin by John Pechey. *London, R. Wellington, 1715.* [8] ff., 453, [3] pp. 8vo, 21 cms.

Page facing p. 1 and last two pages publisher's catalogue.

Pechey's translation was first published in 1696, and went through eleven editions (11th ed. 1740) until superseded by that of John Swan in 1742.

For a biography of John Pechey (1665–1718) see *Janus*, 1918, **23**, 121–41.

SYDENHAM (THOMAS)

1085 Selected works of Thomas Sydenham, M.D., with a short biography and explanatory notes by John D. Comrie. (Bale's Medical Books and Journals). *London, John Bale, Sons & Danielsson, 1922.* viii, 153 pp. Illus, port., facsim., bibliog. 12mo, 19 cms.

BOERHAAVE (HERMANN) 1668–1738

1086 Aphorisms concerning the knowledge and cure of diseases; trans. from the last edition printed in Latin at Leyden, 1728. *London, A. Bettesworth, C. Hitch, W. Innys and R. Manby, 1735.* [8] ff., 444, [4] pp. 8vo, 21 cms.

Bookplate: Will: Cotton (on verso of A3).

First Latin edition, *Aphorismi de cognoscendis et curandis morbis* (Lugduni Batavorum, J. Van der Linden, 1715.); an earlier translation was made by J. Delacoste (London, B. Cowse & W. Innys, 1815).

Boerhaave, professor of medicine at Leyden, was the foremost physician of his time.

PRINGLE (Sir JOHN) 1707–1782

1087 Observations on the diseases of the army. 3rd ed. enlarged. *London, A. Millar, D. Wilson and T. Durham and T. Payne, 1761.* xvi [i.e. xxvii], 435 [i.e. 436] pp., 18 ff. 8vo, 22 cms.

Two pages numbered 164; subsequent pages misnumbered.

Signature: "John Soden [in different hands], Birmingham" (John Smith Soden, 1780–1863, F.R.C.S., was apprenticed to the surgeon, George Freer of Birmingham; does this explain why Soden is written above a deleted surname, which could be Freer?); book-stamp: Bath Medical Library (Soden practised in Bath).

First edition London, A. Millar & D. Wilson, 1752. Eight English editions (last 1810) and one American edition were published; the book was also translated, at least twice each, into German, Dutch, and French. Deals mainly with various fevers and gives an account of acute rheumatism in the army.

HUNTER (WILLIAM) 1718–1783

FOX (RICHARD HINGSTON) 1853–1924

1088 William Hunter, anatomist, physician, obstetrician (1718–1783), with notices of his friends Cullen, Smellie, Fothergill, and Baillie. *London, H. K. Lewis, 1901.* viii, 75 pp. Illus, ports, bibliog. 8vo, 22 cms.

HUNTER (JOHN) 1728–1793

KOBLER (JOHN)

1089 The Reluctant surgeon: the life of John Hunter. *London [etc.], Heinemann, 1960.* 359 pp. Bibliog. 8vo, 23 cms.

OPPENHEIMER (JANE MARION) *b.* 1911

1090 New aspects of John and William Hunter. *London, Heinemann, 1946.* xix, 188 pp. Illus, ports, facsims, bibliog. 8vo, 21 cms.

Contains 1. Everard Home and the destruction of the John Hunter manuscripts. 2. William Hunter and his contemporaries.

JENNER (Edward) 1749–1823

1091 An Inquiry into the causes and effects of the variolae vaccinae, a disease discovered in some of the western counties of England, particularly Gloucestershire, and known by the name of the cow pox. [*Milan, R. Lier, 1923*]. iv, 75 pp., [2] ff. Illus (col.). 4to, 28 cms.

Facsimile reprint of first edition (London, printed for the author, by Sampson Low, 1798); to mark the centenary of Jenner's death; one of 500 copies.

Enclosed are extracts from the *London Medical Review and Magazine*, 1801, vol. 6, on vaccination, consisting of:

Observations on the utility of inoculating for the variolae vaccinae, or cow-pox. By Edward Gardner [review] pp. 25–6.

Extract of a letter from Dr. De Carro to Dr. Jenner, dated Vienna, 14th February, 1801, giving an account of the progress of vaccine inoculation in Germany and Italy pp. 152–3.

Extract of a letter on the Jennerian disease, from Dr. J. H. Marshall to Mr. Ring, dated La Valette January 21, 1801, pp. 153–4.

On the cow-pock inoculation at Vienna, Hanover and Berlin; from *Hufeland's Journal* pp. 225–8.

Notice of the vaccine disease introduced at Jamaica. Communicated to the Editors by Mr. Ring, p. 228.

On the origin of the vaccine inoculation. By Edward Jenner [Review] pp. 313–16.

BARON (JOHN) 1786–1851

1092 The Life of Edward Jenner, M.D.; with illustrations of his doctrines and selections from his correspondence. *London, Henry Colburn, 1827*. xxiv, 624 pp. Port. 8vo, 23 cms.

Contains Jenner's letter to Heberden on the diagnosis of coronary disease in John Hunter (pp. 39–40), and Sir Everard Home's letter to Jenner confirming the diagnosis at necropsy (pp. 104–5).

This first part was reprinted as volume 1 with a new title-page in 1838, when the second volume appeared. This two volume set is in RCP.

DREWITT (FREDERIC GEORGE DAWTREY) 1848–1942

1093 The Life of Edward Jenner, M.D., F.R.S., naturalist and discoverer of vaccination. *London, [etc.], Longmans, Green, 1931*. vii, 127 pp. Port., bibliog. (ftn. refs). 8vo, 20 cms.

BICHAT (Marie François Xavier) 1771–1802

1094 Recherches physiologiques sur la vie et la mort. 5me éd., revue et augmentée de notes pour la deuxième fois par F. Magendie. *Paris, Béchet jeune, Gabon, 1829*. xxvi, 528 pp. 8vo, 21 cms.

First edition, Paris, Brosson, Gabon an VIII [1800].

TURNER (Sir William) 1832–1916

TURNER (ARTHUR LOGAN) 1865–1939

1095 Sir William Turner, K.C.B., F.R.S., . . . a chapter in medical history. *Edinburgh and London, William Blackwood, 1919*. xvii, 514 pp. Ports, bibliog. 8vo, 23 cms.

Turner was professor of anatomy, principal and vice-chancellor of the University of Edinburgh.

TEISSIER (Louis Anne Marie Joseph) 1851–1926

LIVRE JUBILAIRE

1096 Livre jubilaire: memoires originaux dédiés a M. J. Teissier, professeur de clinique médicale à l'Université de Lyon à l'occasion du xxve anniversaire de son professorat: pathologie interne—clinique médicale 1884–1909. *Lyon, A. Rey, 1910.* [v], 664 pp. Illus, port, tables, diagrs, bibliog. 4to, 29 cms.

Book-stamps: Radcliffe Library Oxford 16 Sep. 1919. Bodl[eian] Lib[rary] cancelled.
Seventy-four memoirs by distinguished physicians including Alexis Carrel, H. Frenkel, W. His, P. Marie, M. Raynaud, F. Widal, Francois Frank and Louis Gallavardin. Teissier was physician to the Hôtel Dieu Hospital and one of the most renowned teachers of Lyon. Of cardiological interest are: Baccelli (Guido)—Tachycardie paroxystique essentielle et injections intraveineuses de strophantine, pp. 33–43; Bard (L.)—Du rôle des contractions latentes dans la séméiologie cardiaque, pp. 45–51; Bret (J.)—Note sur l'état du cœur dans l'asystolie chronique de la myocardite interstitielle d'origine cardiaque, pp. 87–96; Carrel (Alexis)—Anévrismes et chirurgie expérimentale de l'aorte thoracique, pp. 107–9; Gallavardin (Louis)—Mesure de la pente de la tension dans un même territoire vasculaire; ses résultats, ses causes d'erreurs, pp. 247–55; Garel (J.)—Paralysie récurrentielle et rétrécissement mitral: histoire et pathogénèse, pp. 257–64; Henrijean (F.)—Recherches expérimentales sur les médicaments cardio-vasculaires, pp. 307–18; Péhu (M.)—Remarques sur la topographie périvasculaire de la tuberculose intestinale dans le premier âge, pp. 503–8; Teissier (P.)—Les troubles de rythme cardiaque dans la scarlatine, pp. 621–9.

RAMON Y CAJAL (Santiago) 1852–1934

WILLIAMS (JOHN HARGREAVES HARLEY) 1901–1974

1097 Don Quixote of the microscope: an interpretation of the Spanish savant Santiago Ramon y Cajal (1852–1934). *London, Jonathan Cape, 1954.* 255 pp. Illus, port., bibliog. 8vo, 21 cms.

Author's signed presentation copy to DEB, 1965.

DAWSON OF PENN (Bertrand Edward Dawson), Viscount, 1864–1945

WATSON (FRANCIS) *b.* 1907

1098 Dawson of Penn. *London, Chatto & Windus, 1950.* viii, 344 pp. Port. 8vo, 23 cms.

Medical Biography

MACMICHAEL (William) 1784–1839

1099 The Gold-headed cane. [*anon.*]. [3rd ed.]. ed. by William Munk. *London, Longmans, Green, 1884.* xvi, 246 pp. 8vo, 21 cms.

Autograph: "To Father B. [?] W. Kelly from B.[?] G. Munk" (most probably Beatrice G. Munk, William Munk's daughter; two of her autograph letters are in the library of the Royal College of Physicians).
The cane belonged successively to Radcliffe, Mead, Askew, William and David Pitcairn and Matthew Baillie; Munk adds chapters on Halford, Paris and Mayo. First edition, 1827, Garrison and Morton 6709.

1100 Lives of British physicians [*anon.*]. *London, John Murray, 1830.* [viii], 341 pp. Ports. 12mo, 15 cms.

Bookplate: Walter Burnell Tubbs.

Includes biographies of Linacre, Caius, Harvey, Browne, Sydenham, Radcliffe, Mead, Huxham, Pringle, Fothergill, Heberden, Cullen, William Hunter, Warren, Baillie, Jenner, Parry, and Gooch.

DEZEIMERIS (JEAN EUGÈNE) 1799–1852, and others

1101 Dictionnaire historique de la médecine ancienne et moderne, ou précis de l'histoire générale, technologique et littéraire de la médecine, suivi de la bibliographie médicale du dix-neuvième siècle, et d'un répertoire bibliographique par ordre de matières; par MM. Dezeimeris, [Charles Prosper] Olliver (d'Angers) et [Jacques] Raige-Delorme. *Paris, Béchet jeune, 1828–1839.* 4 tom. Bibliog. 8vo, 21 cms.

Bookplate: Ex libris Dis. E. T. Hamy, and book-stamp: Ernest Hamy. (Most probably Jules Théodore Ernest Hamy, 1842–1908, French anthropologist, ethnologist and archaeologist, who started as a doctor, but later became professor of anthropology at the Musée du Trocadéro).

Tom. 1 (1828, 1831; 2 parts) xxiv, 446, [6], 447–902 pp.; tom. 2 (1834, 1835; 2 parts) xiv, 374, [4], 375–690 pp.; tom. 3 (1836, 1837; 2 parts) vi, 358, [4], 369–821 pp.; tom. 4 (1839) viii, 443 pp. Tom. 2–4 by Dezeimeris only.

A most valuable biographical dictionary with bibliographies.

PETTIGREW (THOMAS JOSEPH) 1791–1865

1102 Medical portrait gallery: biographical memoirs of the most celebrated physicians, surgeons, etc. who have contributed to the advancement of medical science. *London, Fisher, 1838.* 2 vols. Ports. 4to, 27 cms.

Vol. 1: Biographies of Aesculapius, Mark Akenside, Bernard Siegfried Albinus, Marie François Xavier Bichat, James Blundell, John Caius, Sir Anthony Carlisle, Sir Charles Mansfield Clarke, John Cooke, Sir Astley Paston Cooper, James Copland, Sir Henry Halford, Haller, Thomas Linacre, Richard Mead, Morgagni, John Radcliffe, Frederic Ruysch; Vol. 2: John Abernethy, Matthew Baillie, John Baron, Richard Bright, Sir Benjamin Collins Brodie, Henry Clutterbuck, John Hunter, William Hunter, John Huxham, Edward Jenner, James Johnson, William Lawrence, Marcellus Malpighi, Sir John Pringle, Andreas Vesalius, James Wardrop, James Wilson. Each biography separately paginated.

WINSLOW (FORBES) 1810–1874

1103 Physic and physicians: a medical sketch-book, exhibiting the public and private life of the most celebrated men of former days; with memoirs of eminent living London physicians and surgeons [*anon.*]. *London, Longman, Orme, Brown, 1839.* 2 vols. Ports. 8vo, 22 cms.

Vol. 1: xiv, 360 pp.; vol. 2: [i], ii, 393 pp. MS *index* at end.

Contains amusing and sometimes important biographical details (note Wardrop especially). Among others covered are Baillie, Bright, Cheyne, Freind, Haller, Harvey, Hope, Hunter, Jenner, Sydenham, Thomas Willis, and Thomas Young.

SKETCHES

1104 Sketches of eminent medical men. *London, Religious Tract Society, [1847].* 192 pp. 12mo, 15 cms.

Includes biographical sketches of William Harvey, Thomas Sydenham, Hermann Boerhaave, William Hey, Thomas Bateman, Edward Jenner, John Mason Good, Robert Gooch, Sir William Knighton, and James Hope.

Knighton was physician to George IV, and with Sir Henry Halford attended him in his final illness, when they quarrelled with Wardrop who diagnosed gouty heart.

BETTANY (GEORGE THOMAS) 1850–1891

1105 Eminent doctors: their lives and work. *London, John Hogg [1885].* 2 vols. 8vo, 20 cms.

Vol. 1: ix, 311 pp.; vol. 2: vi, 318 pp.

Bettany was lecturer in botany at Guy's. This useful biographical work includes Harvey, Addison, Bright, C. J. B. Williams, Stokes and Corrigan, among many others.

WILKS (Sir SAMUEL) 1824–1911 and BETTANY (GEORGE THOMAS) 1850–1891

1106 A Biographical history of Guy's Hospital. *London, Ward, Lock, Bowden & Co., 1892.* viii, 500 pp. Ports (6 plates), map. 8vo, 23 cms.

Autograph: John O. Garland, Guy's Hospital, London, S.E. (John Owneworth Garland, *d.* 1966?, L.S.A.).

Biographies include among others those of Bright, Gull, Mahomed and Moxon.

BASHFORD (Sir HENRY HOWARTH) 1880–1961

1107 The Harley Street calendar. *London, Constable, 1929.* [ix], 272 pp. Bibliog. 8vo, 20 cms.

Contains biographical essays on Gilbert the Englishman (*c.* 1165–*c.* 1230), John of Gaddesden (*c.* 1280–*c.* 1360), Thomas Linacre (1460–1524), William Harvey (1578–1657), Thomas Sydenham (1624–1689), Hans Sloane (1660–1753), John Hunter (1728–1793), Edward Jenner (1749–1823), James Young Simpson (1811–1870), Joseph Lister (1827–1912), and William Osler (1849–1919).

SIGERIST (HENRY ERNEST) 1891–1957

1108 The Great doctors: a biographical history of medicine; trans. by Eden & Cedar Paul. *London, George Allen & Unwin, [1933].* 436 pp. 8vo, 22 cms.

Translation of *Grosse Aerzte: eine Geschichte der Heilkunde in Lebensbildern.* 2. Aufl. (München, Lehmann, 1932).

Covers Hippocrates, Galen, Vesalius, Paré, Harvey, Malpighi, Santorio, Sydenham, Boerhaave, Haller, Morgagni, Auenbrugger, Jenner, Corvisart, Laennec, Rokitansky, Skoda, Lister, Pettenkofer, and Osler among others.

MOYNIHAN (BERKELEY GEORGE ANDREW MOYNIHAN) baron, 1865–1936

1109 The Truants; the story of some who deserted medicine, yet triumphed. (Linacre Lecture, 1936). *Cambridge, University Press, 1936.* [iii], 109 pp. 12mo, 19 cms.

Deals with Linacre, Lower, Mayow, Wollaston, Woodward, Guillotin, Clemenceau, Rabelais, Samuel Garth, Mark Akenside, Smollett, Goldsmith, Paget, Conan Doyle and others.

POWER (Sir D'ARCY) 1855–1941

1110 British masters of medicine; ed. by Sir D'Arcy Power. *London, Medical Press & Circular, 1936.* xv, 242 pp. Ports. 8vo, 22 cms.

Includes biographies of William Harvey, Thomas Sydenham, John Floyer, William Cheselden, Percival Pott, John Hunter, John Coakley Lettsom, Edward Jenner, Robert Willan, Richard Bright, Thomas Addison, William Stokes, William Fergusson, Robert Bentley Todd, James Young Simpson, James Paget, Joseph Lister, William Turner, Hugh Owen Thomas, Robert Jones, Patrick Manson, William Osler, James Mackenzie, and Ernest H. Starling.

BAILEY (HAMILTON) 1894–1961 and BISHOP (WILLIAM JOHN) 1903–1961

1111 Notable names in medicine and surgery. *London, H. K. Lewis, 1944.* viii, 202 pp. Illus, ports. 8vo, 19 cms.

Garrison and Morton 6737. Cardiovascular eponymous terms include the veins of Galen, the circle of Willis, the Malpighian bodies, Bright's disease, Graves' disease and Trendelenburg's operation (pulmonary embolectomy).

OSLER (Sir WILLIAM) 1849–1919

1112 Selected writings of Sir William Osler, 12 July 1849 to 29 December 1919; with an introduction by G. L. Keynes. *London, Oxford University Press, 1951.* xx, 278 pp. Illus, ports. 8vo, 23 cms.

The biographical introduction by G. L. Keynes is valuable. Contents include biographical essays on Sir Thomas Browne (pp. 40–61), Gui Patin (pp. 62–4), Robert Burton (pp. 65–99), Michael Servetus (pp. 100–25), William Beaumont (pp. 126–51), and the young Laennec (pp. 152–5), together with Osler's Harveian Oration, 1906 (pp. 205–36). Inserted is Sir Geoffrey Keynes' Oslerian Oration, 1968, from *British medical Journal*, 1968, **4**, 599–604.

NAME INDEX

Names of persons and institutions, including titles of a few periodicals and anonymous works, indexed by serial number; numbers preceded by (*biog.*) relate to biographical and critical material – monographs, articles in periodicals, and chapters in books.

SUBJECT INDEX

The list of contents indicates broadly where subjects are to be found and blocks of numbers, followed by a semi-colon serve the same purpose in this subject index, numbers following the semi-colon indicate books on the subject elsewhere in the catalogue. This index is intended to act as a guide to cardiological information in the annotations, and to those chapters in books to which special attention is drawn.

INDEX OF ASSOCIATIONS

Donors, autographs, bookplates, previous owners, etc. An asterisk against a number indicates that an autograph letter is included.